Cybernics

Yoshiyuki Sankai • Kenji Suzuki
Yasuhisa Hasegawa
Editors

Cybernics

Fusion of human, machine and information systems

Springer

Editors
Yoshiyuki Sankai
Center for Cybernics
Research/Faculty of Engineering
Information and Systems
University of Tsukuba
Tsukuba, Japan

Kenji Suzuki
Center for Cybernics
Research/Faculty of Engineering
Information and Systems
University of Tsukuba
Tsukuba, Japan

Yasuhisa Hasegawa
Center for Cybernics
Research/Faculty of Engineering
Information and Systems
University of Tsukuba
Tsukuba, Japan

ISBN 978-4-431-54158-5 ISBN 978-4-431-54159-2 (eBook)
DOI 10.1007/978-4-431-54159-2
Springer Tokyo Heidelberg New York Dordrecht London

Library of Congress Control Number: 2013955609

Printed on acid-free paper

Springer is part of Springer Science+Business Media (www.springer.com)

Preface

"Cybernics: Fusion of Human, Machine, and Information Systems," selected as the Global Center of Excellence program in Japan from 2007 to 2011, is a new domain of science that centers on cybernetics, mechatronics, and informatics; it integrates humans and robots functionally, organically, and socially with information technology. It is a fused and complex interdisciplinary area in which robotics, brain science and neuroscience, information technology, ergonomics, human society, Kansei engineering, physiology, sociological sciences, and even ethics are deeply intertwined.

This program aims to develop not only pioneering researchers who are able to lead the way with technological innovations, but also experts who support the field of cybernics through analysis of or teaching about the sociological issues associated with the introduction of cybernics-related technologies into society. This program therefore offers unique disciplines, such as Cybernics Tutorial Studies, Cybernics Project Research and Cybernics Internship Program as well as standard course subjects. This volume is edited based on the course materials of the cybernics educational program. We have digested the lectures in this book for self-learning of the interdisciplinary knowledge.

Cybernics Tutorial Studies are implemented with the emphasis on nurturing the ability of students to develop the ability to think from multiple perspectives. The learning format utilizes instructors from many different fields, which is a critical part in developing this field that is marked by alliances among medicine, engineering, and the humanities. The course is taught in a practical tutorial format that is designed to discuss specific issues in small groups and reach a conclusion within the space of 1 h. The format is designed as an engineering-type tutorial. It is based on a combination of tutorial formats widely used in medical fields and is the fruit of interviews with British researchers who are pioneers in this methodology. The focus in these tutorials is on developing the ability of students to adopt a multifaceted approach to solving practical issues in the composite field of human–machine–information systems. Unlike courses that consist mainly of lectures by instructors, students here actively examine case studies. Instructors from various disciplines in medicine, engineering, and the humanities teach these small classes, and they discuss with the students special topics related to unresolved and unexplored fields. The results of these discussions are announced as a research presentation.

In addition, project-type research programs—called Cybernics Project Research—are undertaken by students as research leaders. Together with other graduate and undergraduate students, a student research leader proposes and executes a project that drives the research. This involves a series of processes, including proposals for research plans, interviews, conducting research, interim evaluations, compiling reports on results, and post-completion evaluations. During this process, student research leaders proceed with their project research and receive both internal and external evaluations, which help cultivate their leadership and management capabilities.

Through the Cybernics Internship Program, students gain valuable experience in research and development with companies that have academic alliances. As well, they garner experience in such areas as running clinical trials and dealing with medical organizations, both in Japan and overseas. As a result, students acquire the ability to understand the importance of safety-risk assessment as they recognize and implement the high research standards that can be used for clinical trial standards, and they discover how to solve problems within real-life situations.

Cybernics Standard Course subjects were established to provide basic knowledge and techniques in advanced interdisciplinary academic fields through various innovative lectures. The knowledge acquired becomes a basis for discussions in the Cybernics Tutorial Studies and helps the students advance their own research efforts. This academic field covers a broad range of disciplines and is categorized into three groups: cybernoid research, next-generation interface management, and technologies for next-generation systems. Students make their own course notes in this area in a target-oriented fashion by compiling information from a variety of different lectures in different fields.

The interdisciplinary knowledge acquired in this way will help promote human resources with abilities in diverse academic fields: individuals will be able to approach problems from multifaceted perspectives, thereby contributing to innovative research through a synthesis of leading areas of interdisciplinary research. With robotics as their standard, students thus educated will be able to rise to the challenge facing future generations through this novel synergy of science and the humanities.

With the growing profusion of next-generation robotics systems, robotics scholars have become aware of the ethical, philosophical, social, and cultural implications in adopting robot technology into social fields. Thus, we have published a book entitled *Cybernics Technical Reports: Special Issue on Roboethics* (University of Tsukuba, 2011), based on the results of two international workshops on roboethics organized as part of the cybernics program. For further information on the fascinating topic of roboethics, readers are advised to consult that book.

Owing to its extremely low birthrate and the rapid aging of its population, Japan is facing a difficult future. We hope that the cybernics program will continue to contribute a great deal to the education of researchers who will aim to solve the problems of the future by advancing interdisciplinary research based on the fusion of human, machine, and information systems.

Finally, on behalf of the editors of these lecture notes, we gratefully acknowledge the assistance of Ms. Ayumi Shiibayashi in managing this publication.

Tuskuba, Japan Yoshiyuki Sankai
Tuskuba, Japan Kenji Suzuki
Tuskuba, Japan Yasuhisa Hasegawa

Contents

Part I
Overview of Cybernics

Chapter 1
Cybernics: Fusion of Human, Machine and Information Systems

Yoshiyuki Sankai

Abstract Cybernics is a frontier science centered on cybernetics, mechatronics, and informatics, and it aims toward an integration of humans with robotics by means of information technology A pioneering development in Cybernics is the exoskeletal robot suit HAL (Hybrid Assistive Limbs), which is able to enhance and reinforce human limb motions by detecting weak bioelectrical signals. The development of HAL is particularly important in light of the rapidly aging population in both Japan and other advanced countries. In promoting HAL as a new piece of medical equipment, the manufacturer faced considerable obstacles from administrative bodies. Japan clearly needs a world-class permit-approval process for nascent technology that can serve as an international certification standard. Education also needs to be addressed, and for this reason the Cybernics Program was established. The program aims to create and establish technology for the functional, organic, and sociological integration of human, machine, and information systems.

Keywords Cybernics • HAL • International standardization • Human resource development • Cybernetics • Mechatronics • Informatics

1.1 Introduction

Japan's extremely low birth rate and the rapid aging of its population will present the country with considerable societal problems in the future. These social challenges will have to be addressed through sophisticated interdisciplinary advances in the fusion of human, machine and information systems, and this fusion will in turn

Y. Sankai (✉)
Center for Cybernics Research/Faculty of Engineering,
Information and Systems, University of Tsukuba, Tsukuba, Japan
e-mail: sankai@kz.tsukuba.ac.jp

Y. Sankai et al. (eds.), *Cybernics: Fusion of human, machine and information systems*,
DOI 10.1007/978-4-431-54159-2_1, © Springer Japan 2014

forge a new level of coexistence and interdependence between technology and humankind. However, as innovative areas of science and technology are developed that can better meet the future needs of individuals and society, having to deal with real-life subjects and handle complex interdisciplinary problems will inevitably demand a new approach to multidisciplinary issues. In this regard, the conventional vertical divides of academia act as a hindrance.

It is against this background that we at the University of Tsukuba have developed the new research field of Cybernics. This novel domain of frontier science centers on cybernetics, mechatronics, and informatics, and it aims toward an integration of humans with robotics technology in a functional, organic, and social manner by means of information technology (IT). Cybernics constitutes a complex interdisciplinary area, in which robotics, brain science and neuroscience, IT, ergonomics, Kansei engineering, physiology, social sciences, and ethics are deeply intertwined. And in this revolutionary field, the exoskeletal robot suit HAL (Hybrid Assistive Limbs) is a pioneering achievement. HAL is able to enhance and reinforce the limb motions of the human body by detecting weak bioelectrical signals traveling through the body from the brain, which generates the nervous impulses that control the musculoskeletal system (Figs. 1.1 and 1.2).

This chapter will begin with an overview of Cybernics. Several perspectives relating to the development of innovative technology will then be presented, with the focus being on HAL. Based on these considerations, a proposal will be made that a center of excellence be established in research and education that will amount to an alliance of people and society, cutting-edge technologies, legal systems, ethics, and management systems to explore the future challenges facing humankind. The details of organizing a program toward this end will be presented before the conclusions to this chapter are given.

1.2 Cybernics

Cybernics is a new domain of science and technology, uniting people, machines, and information systems to create research and development (R&D) environments that extend from basic concepts to practical applications within a social context. It aims to explore technologies that sustain people and society. The core disciplines of Cybernics are cybernetics, mechatronics, and informatics; however, it also embraces such various fields of science and technology as those listed below in addition to nonscientific areas, for example, social science, law, and business administration:

- Cranial nerve science
- Behavioral sicience
- Robotics
- IT

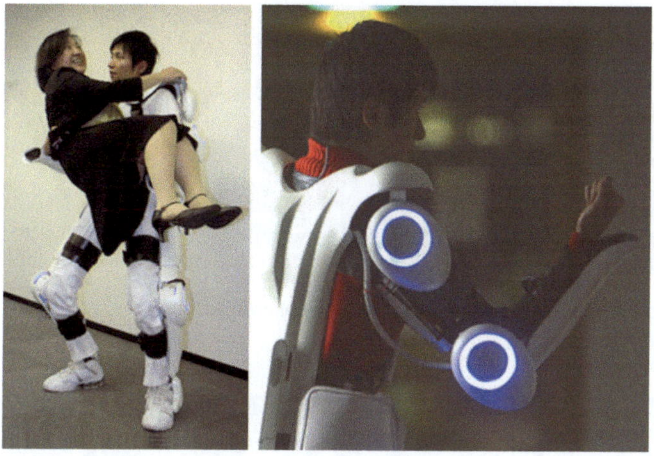

Fig. 1.1 Robot-Suit, HAL-5 is the world's first cyborg-type robot

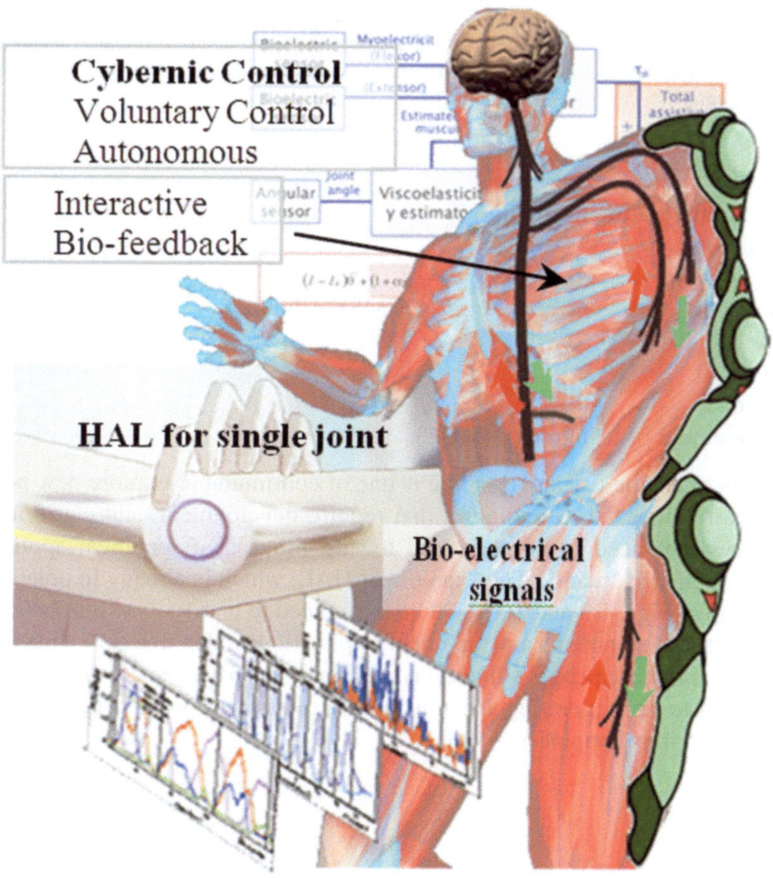

Fig. 1.2 Theory of operation for HAL

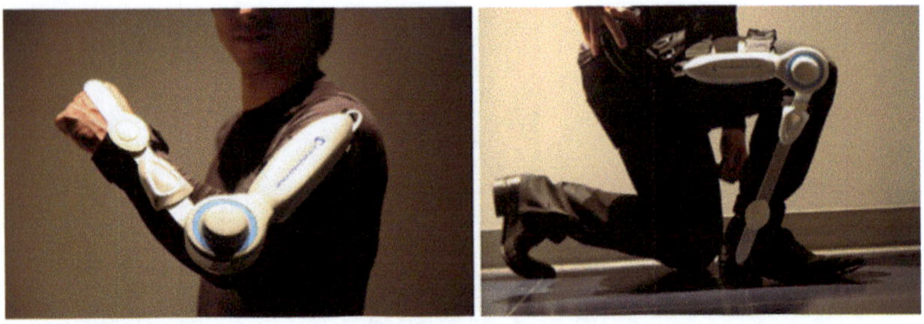

Fig. 1.3 Robot Suit HAL™for single joint of the upper/lower limb

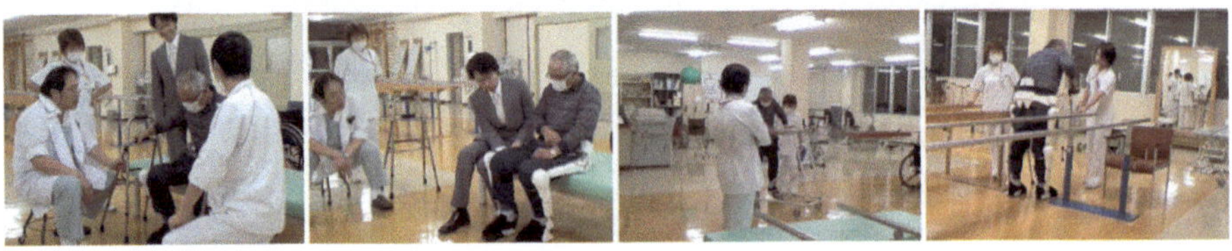

Fig. 1.4 HAL trials at the hospital. A patient succeeded in standing up, sitting down, and moving (bend and extend) his feet according to his intention by using HAL. He could also walk with walker and cane

- System integration technology
- Physiology
- Psychology
- Microelectromechanical systems (MEMS) technology
- Law
- Ethics
- Kansei
- Management of technology (MOT)

In Cybernics, the researcher's role is one of continuing to explore new possibilities, investigating the technologies that require development, and clarifying specific issues that need to be addressed toward the goal of practical applications serving people and society. The example of HAL, which is already in practical use (For example, Figs. 1.3 and 1.4), will be introduced to clarify its evolution in terms of research, development, and practical application under my own direction. In addition to enriching people's lives, it is the aim of the HAL project to make a direct contribution to reinvigorating Japan as a scientific superpower in pursuit of technology that brings happiness to others.

1.3 The Robot Suit HAL

HAL, which was developed at the University of Tsukuba, augments, extends, and supports the physical functions of the user. The equipment is designed to support the user's movements according to their particular needs by means of sensors that detect weak or potentially weak biological signals issued by the upper/lower limbs hands and other bodily movements. When wearing HAL, those unable to walk or move as they wish owing to degenerative conditions or physical problems receive locomotive or other muscular support. HAL has received worldwide attention, and there are high expectations that it will become the world's first cyborg-type robot.

1.3.1 Innovative Technology and Industry

Technology will play an increasingly important role in Japan's future aging society. Toward the goal of enabling people to live energetic lives and helping to counteract the inevitable decline that comes with age, I have focused my research efforts on the practical application of HAL since I first created it as a prototype model at university. In 2004, a university-based venture company called Cyberdyne was established to promote research efforts toward such a practical application and basic researches based on the important information fed back from the practical application for the human and society. I call this cycle between basic researches and practical applications for promoting the innovative challenges "Innovation Spiral". According to this structure of the upward Innovation Spiral, R&D and cultivation/ education of human resources will be enhanced. University-based venture company would function like a University Hospital where professors and students and medical staffs work together in order to develop difficult diseases. As part of its R&D work, the company is exploring methods of safety technology, high quality and reliable production so as to make HAL an actually useful and economically viable product for users such as the patients, medical doctors, physical therapists, elderly persons, care-givers in nursing center, workers in factory and so on.

So that HALs could be used by as many people as possible, Cyberdyne began full-scale rental of the robot suits in 2010. Thus far, HALs have been introduced to 130 facilities such as hospitals and nursing care centers around Japan, and about 270 units are in service.

To realize the company's objective of researching, developing and producing innovative technological products, particularly those targeted at assisting the human body, it has been necessary to cross many hurdles. In the case of existing product types, developing new forms of the products can progress with relative ease because various channels for R&D, obtaining government permit approval, production, and sales have already been established. However, putting entirely new technology into practical application faces major obstacles.

Japan has continuously striven to become a scientific and technological powerhouse. However, this target cannot be achieved simply by focusing on the development of innovative technology. In addition to promoting R&D, it is essential that a suitable environment be created in which fledgling technologies are able to develop. To cultivate new innovative technology, measures have to be taken in terms of systems, human resource development collaborating with universities and companies, and the establishment of an international hub of collaborative research with companies and universities. In the course of developing HAL and putting it into practical use, various problem areas in Japan, which are detailed in the sections below, became evident.

1.3.2 Medical Product Approval

HALs are currently sold as human assistive robots funded by welfare/medicare programs. When HAL is used as rehabilitation equipment for therapy in a hospital, it has to be approved as medical equipment. However, obtaining approval for innovative medical equipment is a long and arduous task. Medical equipment manufacturers are obliged to observe manufacturing and control procedures in accordance with the international standard ISO 13485(ISO for medical equipment). Severe constraints are imposed on the manufacturers, such as having to hire experts in medical equipment control to monitor and assess the new devices. HAL started to distribute as "robot suit HAL for wellbeing" to hospitals and nursing care centers according to ISO13485 procedure. However, the robot suit's development team devoted itself to promoting HAL and it began to be put into operation after various procedures had been established regarding securing human resources and developing rules and documentation relating to the suit's operation.

As the development team went through the step-by-step application process so that HAL could be utilized as medical equipment, it came as a surprise how differences between the new product and existing ones as well as HAL's distinct advantages had to be clearly emphasized for approval to be granted. The approval process of new medical equipment operates within a different framework from that of other types of equipment. Authorization of new medical equipment requires permit approval not only from the Pharmaceuticals and Medical Devices Agency but also that of the Ministry of Health, Labour and Welfare. It is clear that major reforms are needed to speed up the approval procedure with such equipment, and this in turn will have an impact on the international strategy of equipment manufacturers.

1.3.3 Social Factors

An example here will illustrate the point cited in the previous section. Though some countries have achieved global preeminence in electronic technology, there are no domestic manufacturers of pacemakers. From a technological standpoint, it would not be at all difficult for Japan to manufacture pacemakers. However, to spread the domestic use of such products, which very directly affect human life, involves social factors: a promotion system would have to be instigated that sought the cooperation of the public and private sectors. The prerequisite here would be that the potential benefits of such devices outweighed the possible risks. Many new products are available in Japan, but with devices that deal with human life or health, the approval hurdle is suddenly much higher. Naturally, this tends to dampen the entrepreneurial spirit of pioneering companies and individuals. A technology product used by society has to go through a development phase as well as a practical application process in its early days so that the technology can be refined and improved. The major obstacles imposed in this application process effectively prevent any enterprise whose product involves the social dimension, mentioned above, from succeeding in its business. With the development of certain kinds of medical equipment, there is a need to examine ways of moving away from the profit-oriented business model.

1.3.4 International Standardization

It is often the case that there is a lag of several years between the approval of certain technologies in advanced countries and approval being granted in Japan. This naturally raises the question of how new technologies can be introduced so quickly in such other countries.

In most cases in Japan, an administrative body is responsible for permit approval. As a consequence, the administrative body tends to avoid approval because the responsibility this carries can lead to scrutiny and criticism by the media. Even though Japan faces increasingly fierce international competition in areas of technology, its government bodies are not sufficiently organized to fast-track the approval of innovative technology.

Because a strategic approach has been adopted by many European countries, hundreds of private certification bodies there are in competition with one another, so much so that certification has already entered the arena of branding. European consumers now pay attention to which certification body has given a permit approval. These private certification bodies cooperate flexibly and dynamically with new business developments. Proven market results testify to the fact that conducting certification with greater international competitiveness and speed helps to promote international business. International standards or certifications are directly connected to industrial development the world over.

A world-class permit-approval process with respect to nascent technology has to be developed in Japan at the state level as an international certification standard that enjoys brand power. Once Japan is universally recognized as an international base for promoting dynamic new business development, its role in the world will be substantially enhanced.

1.3.5 International Collaboration and Globalization

It was with high societal expectations that Cyberdyne was founded as a pioneering company responding to the challenges of the future. Since its establishment, it is finally able to proceed with acquiring domestic and overseas permit approval. The company, a university-based company, will function like university hospitals where professors, students and staffs in medicine work together to research and cure difficult diseases together for patients. It will strongly promote the international collaboration and globalization through human resource development, R&D including basic research and actual treatment in hospital, and international social activities such as international approval collaboration.

Progress in Europe has been surprisingly fast. For example, Sweden's Karolinska Institute, where the Nobel selection committee is located, offered full support for clinical tests and permit-approval acquisition in Europe. Bergmannsheil hospital (BG group) in German also offered full support for clinical tests like Karolinska Institute. They can be great teams to promote the international collaboration and globalization. Recently, the president of Europe's top notified body, TÜV in Germany, visited us, and TÜV is now actively involved in the certification of HAL. Europe has been quick to launch into certification because being involved in pioneering new fields improves the brand power of a notified body or a certification body in Karolinska Institute, and attracts positive publicity.

If a Japanese manufacturer of medical equipment placed the emphasis on overseas certification, it would receive faster approval there than in Japan. However, Cyberdyne initially focused its efforts on Japan, EU and USA because it was hoped that it would thereby promote human resource development in these countries and engender international appreciation of Japanese achievements in this field. It is the aim that companies and researchers with technologies that could lead to next-generation industries would wish to develop them.

1.3.6 Intellectual Property Strategy

If some countries aim to be an intellectual property powerhouse, it must promote intellectual property strategies boldly in the international arena. This will require cooperation between the public and private sectors with respect to strong patents that will be used on a global scale rather than concentrating efforts on intellectual property applications that are limited to domestic patents. As an example of such strategy, HAL's international patents were evaluated by the World Intellectual Property Organization in 2005 and the Japan Institute of Invention and Innovation (Twenty-first Century Invention Award) in 2009.

1.3.7 Business and Branding Strategy

As noted above, various obstacles have to be overcome before state-of-the-art medical equipment integrated with robot technology is accepted by society. However, we are taking on this difficult challenge because we predict an energetic world in the future. Success in achieving international certification requires branding. At the heart of successful branding are human resources as well as a system of cooperation between the public and private sectors. The quality of nation and its products amounts to the quality of its human resources.

Although expertise in various disciplines is of course important, a balanced education is essential when developing human resources when there is a strong emphasis on high ethical standards. This has become all the more important now that the number of young people in Japan, who represent a vital asset to the country, is on the decline. A balanced education is necessary in developing individuals with firm spirit and character. However, few junior or high schools incorporate broad educational aspects within their regular curriculum. Japan now has the opportunity to undertake reform in this area. To become the envy of the world with respect to practical applications of high-quality innovative technology, Japan has to recognize the reality of its current situation, take appropriate steps to rectify it, and thereby set itself as an example of an engine of growth on the global scale.

1.4 Developing Human Resources

The Japanese government and various administrative bodies appear to be struggling with regard to making the kind of social reforms mentioned in the previous section. And it is clear that the vertical divisions of administrative systems hamper reform efforts. However, we hope that the government will boldly tackle the reform efforts. I believe that Japan is able to cultivate and develop new world-leading technologies. This will involve creating an environment in which innovative technology can be delivered, budding innovation be promoted, and emerging innovative technology be properly developed. Such an environment will attract innovative technologies from around the world, and it will help develop essential human resources. Both people and technology need to be nurtured. And it was for this reason that Cyberdyne was established.

1.4.1 Fostering Pioneer-Type Leaders

Engineering colleges in Japan play a prominent role in human resource development for various manufacturing fields, including system development. However, it is necessary to expand the types of professors and lecturers that teach such subjects as product design, development, and quality control at a practical level. Such changes in college teaching staff can be addressed by both industry and academia.

In the field of medicine, all professors at a medical college are capable of carrying out clinical treatment of patients. However, the equivalent situation does not apply in the case of an engineering college: lecturers at such colleges generally have few chances of becoming involved in high-quality manufacturing. I am uncomfortable with the notion of lecturers in engineering colleges who teach aspects of manufacturing to their students yet they themselves lack a practical background in this area. The ability to nurture top-level professionals that can be next-generation leaders will be limited unless at least 20–30 % of university lecturers in the engineering field can provide advanced practical education based on personal experience.

It is vital that Japan rapidly develops its human resources so as to support its industry and create the technologies of the future. It is likewise essential to build an environment that allows enthusiastic young entrepreneurs to devote themselves to intensive research efforts and encourages the flourishing of lively, innovative minds.

1.4.2 Developing a Positive Environment

Because the R&D of HAL required more than engineering knowledge, a new scientific system called Cybernics was established, which, as noted above, combines such diverse fields as behavioral science, cranial nerve science, physiology, psychology, social science, ethics, and law. The philosophy behind Cyberdyne is that if something is not available, then it should be created.

Most medical colleges have teaching hospitals, where college professors, medical personnel, and graduate students devote their energies to conducting research on the cause and treatment of various diseases, including incurable and rare conditions. In the process, they develop world standard treatments. A teaching hospital serves as a pioneering field for state-of-the-art medical care, and it acts as a bridge between basic research, practical application, and human resource development.

However, engineering colleges lack an environment similar to that of teaching hospitals. One of the reasons for establishing Cyberdyne was that engineering disciplines need an environment in which state-of-the-art R&D is promoted alongside human resource development while at the same time making a real contribution to society—as is the case with the teaching hospitals in medical colleges. If facilities exist for developing necessary technologies, it is highly probable that meaningful research themes and the human resources required will likewise be advanced.

1.5 A Center of Excellence: Cybernics

As Japan's era of an aging population and declining birth rate progresses, there is an urgent need to develop technologies to counter the associated problems, including the demand for new-generation medical welfare and technology to extend and generate physiological functions. However, current approaches based on IT, robotics, or a combination of the two—information and robot technology (IRT)—are inadequate to meet the demand.

Japan has led the world in robotics research in recent years. However, the gap with other countries is diminishing rapidly. IT itself has also reached a peak of development in Japan, and it will soon reach a point of saturation, which will mean that the field will have to rise to a new stage of development. Under these circumstances, simply expanding conventional research strategies, where there is a strong bias toward technological development, is not the solution for future scientific progress in this country. It is necessary to pursue a course in which scientific research directly contributes to people and society (Fig. 1.5). This is vital if Japan is to become a world leader in R&D.

The Cybernics Program has the advancement of Cybernics as its central purpose, and it has the potential to serve both the international community and Japanese society in the future. Breakthrough technology in the field of Cybernics will not result from the combination of human, machine, and information technology alone. The interrelationships among medicine, engineering, and humanity will also play an important role, and from an early stage the Cybernics Program incorporates consultation with specialists in ethics, legislation, and security as well as representatives from various communities. We believe that such an integration of technology with the humanities is essential for the future development of Cybernics as well as for ensuring the usefulness of Cybernics in society.

The program therefore aims to create and establish technology for the functional, organic, and sociological integration of human, machine and information systems. With cybernetics, mechatronics, and informatics at its core, we aim to develop the new scientific field of Cybernics. Through the generation of this new area of science, we aim to achieve the following:

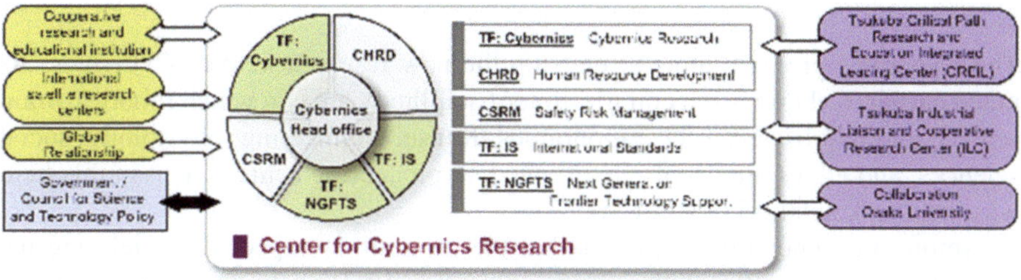

Fig. 1.5 Strategic initiative of Cybernics

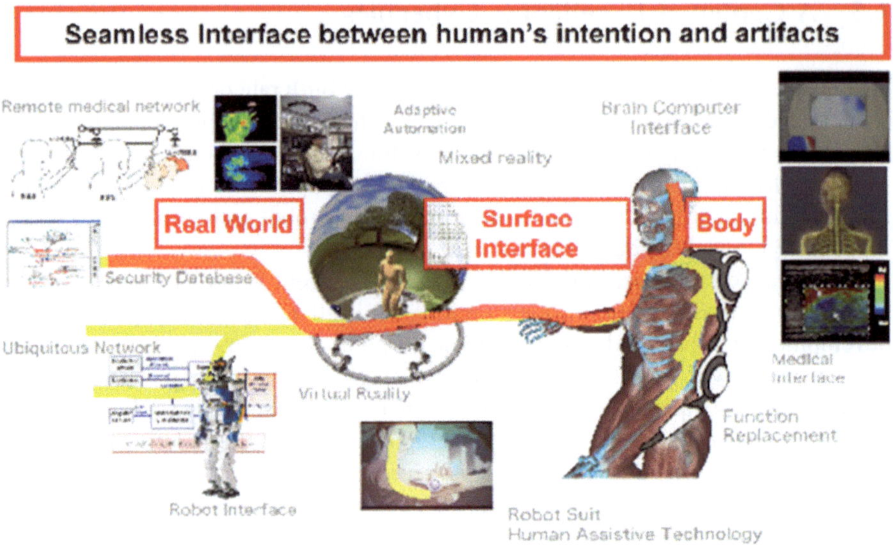

Fig. 1.6 Research target of Cybernics

(a) Create a new industry and new academic discipline;
(b) Dynamically and comprehensively reform the academic system (Fig. 1.6);
(c) Establish a management framework that integrates the creation of frontier multidisciplinary research with education and human resource development;
(d) Achieve sustainable operation of the program through the development of industries and human resources via pioneering research.

The multidisciplinary integration approach of the Cybernics Program is expected to yield a large number of innovations. The primary emphasis of our research is the social application of leading technology to support society in the future.

1.5.1 Objectives

The Cybernics program aims to develop the new research field of Cybernics. As noted earlier, Cybernics is a complex interdisciplinary area, in which robotics, brain science and neuroscience, IT, ergonomics, Kansei engineering, physiology, social sciences, and ethics are deeply intertwined. A pioneering achievement in this field was the exoskeletal robot suit HAL.

Among the innovative creations that the program is expected to yield are the following: a new academic discipline; a new industry for commercializing innovations in Cybernics, such as HAL; a dynamic and comprehensive reform of the academic system; and integration of advanced interdisciplinary research,

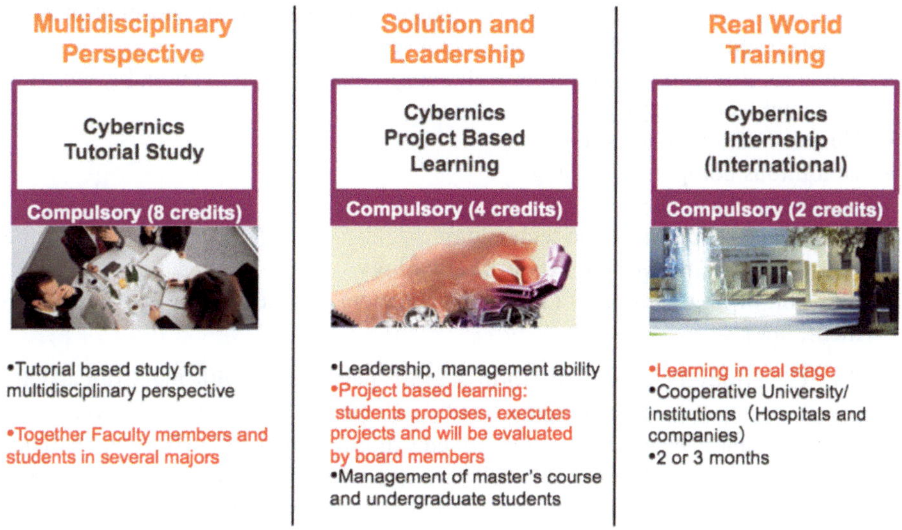

Fig. 1.7 Cybernics educational program (20 credits for Ph.D. students)

development of human resources, and education (Fig. 1.7). In this way, the program will facilitate a system in which industrial development, through the creation of new fields and consequent generation of job opportunities, engenders a self-sustaining management.

From an educational viewpoint, the program aims to cultivate pioneering researchers who lead the way with technological innovations. It also endeavors to nurture experts who support the field of Cybernics through analysis and teaching on the social issues associated with the introduction of Cybernics-related technologies into society.

1.5.2 Project Outline

In addition to the disciplines mentioned in the previous section, research in Cybernics will also cover the following fields, which will interact with those domains of science (Fig. 1.6):

- Cyborg studies
- Implantable devices (micro- and nanotechnology)
- Tissue engineering/function replacement
- Neuroscience/brain interfacing
- Kansei engineering/ergonomics
- Medical welfare engineering

- Life-support technology for elderly people (remote, in-home, hospital, institutional, community medical welfare, vital sensing)
- Robotics (life support, assistive technology, human support, middleware, fundamental technology)
- Human-machine interfacing
- Ubiquitous computing/sensing
- Secure database IT
- Vital database construction technology
- Frontier medicine welfare network technology
- Creation of new industries (MOT, management, intellectual property management, law)

The Cybernics Program will form a close partnership with the Critical Path Research and Education Integrated Leading Center (CREIL) at the University of Tsukuba to establish an infrastructure for education on medical welfare and patient-based clinical testing. We are also collaborating with two universities to systematically evaluate the medical applications of Cybernics technology developed by the program. Young researchers from the two universities will undertake research in medical engineering, and at the same time they will acquire first-hand knowledge and experience in regenerative medicine in medical wards.

1.6 Conclusion

With respect to technological innovation, it is appropriate now for Japan to change its role from that of being just a birth parent to one of being a foster parent: not only must new technology be created, it must also be nurtured. With Japan's aging society, fewer people means that there is less potential for creating new technology. Japan will develop significantly if it can acquire the potential of fledgling technology developed abroad and promote it just as well as it promotes its own domestically created technology. This will allow outstanding new technologies to be consistently acquired from abroad and then developed along with domestic technologies while rapidly expanding peripheral technology.

In this way, Japan will be transformed into an international hub for promoting technological development. A number of European countries are eager to collaborate with Japan through bases in their own countries, which will oblige Japan to establish overseas affiliated firms instead of working through domestically based organizations. In setting up affiliated firms in other countries and introducing Japan-derived technology there, those countries will be able to accumulate the know-how related to peripheral technology even if they possess no innovative technology of their own. By the time the term of the intellectual property expires, sufficient knowledge will have been acquired in those countries such that they will be able to launch new business development in that technical field.

Public officials from such countries as Denmark, Sweden, Germany, and France visit Japan in an official capacity as do other officials engaged in administration, technology, medical care, finance, and insurance. They enthusiastically explain the advantages of the tax system in their respective countries compared with Japan and try to persuade Japanese industrialists and researchers how it is more efficient to establish affiliated firms in Europe than to engage in R&D in Japan. We have much to learn from the power and operation of European countries in this area and, through the cooperation of the public and private sectors in Japan, we need to do likewise.

Having a dream or passion for one's work is important in research, but it is not enough in engineering, where it is necessary also to cultivate a concern for others. In engineering, it is essential to conduct research and develop technology that will be appreciated by others. Researchers who lack a deep concern for their fellow human beings will be unable to conceive of research themes that will have a positive impact on other people's lives. In their work, such researchers would be more likely just to follow lines of investigation based on information derived from the government, administrative bodies, or the media.

It is difficult to conduct pioneering R&D with such a "passive" approach. In the past, good research in engineering started with a general theory; within this, the researcher would concentrate on only one particular aspect and a new hypothesis would be developed, which could then be presented to the world at large. However, in reality, a combination of problems is involved in research, and it is impossible to deal in terms of a single theory alone.

In engineering, which deals with devices and systems that have a direct impact on people's lives, focusing on particular problems can lead to generalization. In other words, developing technology that is originally applicable to a single user can result in the development of a generalized technology that is applicable to many. This is certainly the case with HAL. For the developers of the robot suit, the pleasure in seeing mobility-impaired people stand, walk, or move their legs for the first time in their lives by wearing HAL was an unforgettable experience. The growth in the use of HAL thus far has been gradual: the number of users of HAL has increased in ones and twos. Though some people may regard HAL as a completely exotic piece of technology, it is able to bring great happiness to an individual. And it is certain that HAL will develop into a general-purpose technology for people with physical needs.

Under the proper control and management by physicians and physiotherapists currently active in medicine and welfare, HAL has developed steadily in social and academic terms. And the fact that the development of HAL has called for the cooperation of industrial, governmental, and academic sectors marks it out as a very rare piece of technology. In addition, the users of the technology are invited to be involved right from the basic research phase as well as in the ongoing development and improvement of the robot suit.

When various individuals with physical problems were involved in the R&D of HAL, they were treated with the utmost sympathy. What this amounted to for the development team was a people-centered way of thinking, a complete sense of responsibility, and the will for mutual cooperation in that the research they were conducting was going beyond mere technology and knowledge. Based on this experience, we realized that it is of the greatest importance to create a structure in which various fields are involved and develop in a well-balanced manner as technologies useful for society. But it is vital too to create a structure of human resource development, in which well-balanced personnel resources are promoted within a comprehensive educational system for the purpose of establishing an energetic and healthy society in the future.

A Cybernics ethics board has been established, and it has obtained approval from the ethics boards of every organization that Cyberdyne deals with in the course of promoting the company's R&D. It is a concern to us that very few people in Japan are educated to respect their communities at a regional or national level. It is through concern for others, their families, their local communities, and their countries that the importance of interregional and international tolerance and cooperation can be appreciated. And it is of course highly important that people be encouraged to consider others based on the premise that everyone lives in an organization in one form or another.

In Japan, however, discussion tends to leap from the concern for individuals to the importance of world peace. This is because patriotic education in this country has long been ignored owing to the deep remorse over the national education during the Second World War. As a result, the importance in Japan of thinking about one's local society tends to be overlooked. This point is particularly important when helping the next generation of young researchers to develop a concern for others. Such a spirit of concern is certain to lead to an increase in the number of significant research themes.

In conducting state-of-the-art research, what sorts of fields should researchers in Japan engage themselves in? Japan is a rare country that is committed to peace. Consequently, Japan should find a way for new opportunities not in military research but in medical care and welfare.

To a greater or lesser degree, all advanced countries are heading along the path of low birth rate and longevity. The era of mass production based on the premise of population growth and social prosperity has ended. As a result, it is only by developing technologies that help users with varied symptoms and disabilities achieve a happy life that Japan will advance as a true scientific and technological powerhouse. Toward this end, human resource development and establishing an international hub of technology in Japan are essential if the potential for innovative technologies is to be achieved in the future.

Part II
Cybernoid

Chapter 2
Wearable Robot Technology

Hiroaki Kawamoto

Abstract Exoskeletal robots, i.e., robots integrated with the human body, have been developed since the 1960s, but these were initially not effective. Recently, these robots have been actively developed as wearable robots, with a wide range of practical applications expected for them in the near future. In this chapter, as an important feature of wearable robots, we explain the force interaction conditions between the wearer and the wearable robot for each application. As an example, we introduce the HAL (Hybrid Assistive Limb) robot suit and present, in particular, the interaction technologies and several clinical case studies related to it.

Keywords Wearable robot • Exoskeleton • Power assist • Robot suits • HAL

2.1 Introduction

Robots integrated with humans to enhance human strength have been developed since the 1960s as exoskeletal robots, which were initially teleoperation robots [1]. However, these developments declined due to a lack of actual applications. Moreover, exoskeletal robots in the early days were faced with a deficiency in control techniques and sensing technologies, which became a safety issue in transporting hundreds of kilograms of heavy load.

Recently, robots integrated with humans have been actively developed as wearable robots owing to the progress in miniaturization and the high performance of elemental technologies for robots. The purpose of these new wearable robots is not to enhance, impractically, the lifting strength far above human capability by wearing a bulky robot, but to support human capability within its range by wearing lightweight and compact robots. Wearable robots with a wide range of applications

H. Kawamoto (✉)
Center for Cybernics Research, University of Tsukuba, Tsukuba, Japan
e-mail: kawamoto@golem.kz.tsukuba.ac.jp

Y. Sankai et al. (eds.), *Cybernics: Fusion of human, machine and information systems*,
DOI 10.1007/978-4-431-54159-2_2, © Springer Japan 2014

as human friendly robots and capable of being integrated into a living environment, are needed in society. Therefore, practical applications of wearable robots are expected in the near future.

The most popular practical use of wearable robots is to support the body motion of people with motor disorders, in particular to support the walking function. The application to body motion is important because the elderly population is increasing, and solutions are required to help them stay fit. The application of wearable robots to rehabilitation is similarly expected to help recover or maintain the motor functions of people with disabilities. The robots can improve rehabilitation thanks to longer periods of motion training that can be conducted.

Application of heavy work support such as carrying heavy loads at construction sites and in logistical services, or lifting and transfer assistance of patients by nursing personnel wearing assistive robots are also expected to see an increase in demand. If, additionally, wearable robots were to enable elderly people to do heavy work, it would be possible to ensure a stable workforce in countries with low birthrates like Japan.

Other than strength support and enhancement, there are applications that have not yet been considered. In the fields of entertainment or sports, for example, wearable robots could be used as a force display device for the wearers' extremities in order to provide force feedback.

In this chapter, the force interaction conditions between the human and the wearable robot are explained for each application. Thereafter, as an example of a wearable robot, the HAL robot suit is introduced. In particular, interaction technologies and clinical case studies related to the HAL are presented.

2.2 Force Interaction Between Wearer and Machine for Wearable Robots

Man-Amplifier and Hardyman were full body type exoskeletal robots developed in America in the 1960s [1, 2]. These robots consisted of a master–slave system, composed of an exoskeletal internal master mechanism to detect human motion and an exoskeletal external slave mechanism containing large output actuators. As its motion mechanism, the external slave follows the human motion that is detected by the internal master. As such, these exoskeletons are systems that operate by providing the slave with position commands. The purpose of these developments was to assist soldiers in walking while carrying a large payload.

Later, an arm type exoskeletal installation, called Extender, was proposed by Kaserooni in the 1990s [3–5]. This installation was a kind of manipulator that consisted of a motorized arm that could lift a heavy load directly, without direct manipulation by the wearer. The arm enhanced the force that the wearer exerted

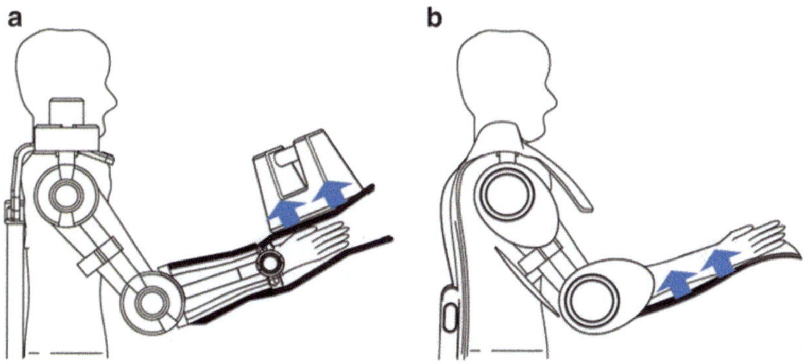

Fig. 2.1 Direction of force generated by a wearable robot: (**a**) while lifting a heavy load, (**b**) when assisting the wearer's limbs

with his arm in order to provide sufficient force to hold heavy loads. This exoskeleton thus provided a system that operated by sending force commands to the exoskeleton arm. Through application of this method, an assist system has been developed to reduce the physical burden of lifting people receiving care in health care facilities.

In power assist systems as described above, an object (heavy load) exists apart from the wearer and the exoskeletal robot. The force generated by the robot acts directly on the heavy load as shown in Fig. 2.1a. The task of the robot is thus, to decrease the force that the wearer needs to exert to move the heavy load. The operating information is the position or force that the wearer generates toward the robot. So, the wearer operates the robot by direct action from the human body to the robot.

There is also another type of power assist system that supports the forces that are needed to move the limbs by using the force generated by the exoskeletal robot. This form of assistance is applied, for example, to walking support for people with gait impairments. The force that the robot generates acts directly on the wearer's limbs as shown in Fig. 2.1b. In this case, the position or force information is not available as operating information.

The two methods for power assistance are organized as shown in Fig. 2.2. In the power assist method for lifting heavy loads (Fig. 2.2a), the wearer controls the position or force to operate the robot, and then the robot manipulates the heavy load based on the detected position or force. The force generated by the robot acts directly on the load, outside of the exoskeleton. On the other hand, in the power assist method for physical assistance (Fig. 2.2b), the wearer's intentions for the desired movement are transmitted to the robot via sensors on his/her skin that can detect bioelectrical signals of the muscles. The robot then manipulates the wearer's limbs based on this intended information. The force generated by the robot acts directly on the wearer's body.

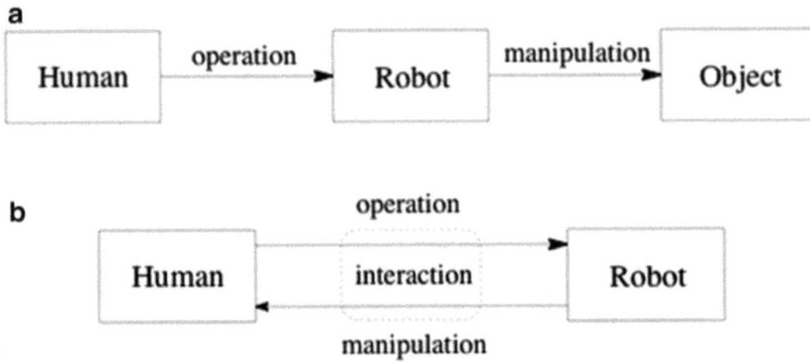

Fig. 2.2 Power assist method for a wearable robot: (**a**) when lifting a heavy load, (**b**) when assisting the wearer's limbs

2.3 The HAL Robot Suit

The HAL (Hybrid Assistive Limb) robot suit is a human-integrated, wearable robot developed by Cybernics. This is a new field of technology that inherits mainly from Cybernetics, Mechatronics and Computer Engineering, but also integrates other disciplines such as Neuroscience, Robotics, Systems Engineering, Information Technology, "Kansei" Engineering, Ergonomics, Physiology, Social Science, Law, Ethics, Management, and so on. The HAL, which enhances or supports the human physical function, is expected to be applied in various fields. The concept of the HAL basically comes from a fusion of the strengths of both humans and machines. The human assumes the role of advanced intelligence, such as judgment, recognition or intention, while the machine implements the heavy physical work or precise work. While co-dependency between the wearer and the machine is moderately established, the human physical abilities are enhanced, supported or extended. The HAL can be applied to a wide range of application fields, including medical and the machine is moderately established, the human physical abilities are enhanced, supported or extended. The HAL can be applied to a wide range of application fields, including medical and welfare, heavy work, and rescue.

The HAL has been developed over the past dozen years or so, with continuous progress still being made in increasing performance, reducing size and weight, and extensions to fit various parts of the human body such as lower limb, upper limb, whole body, single joint, and so on. Marketing of the HAL in the welfare field is being carried out by CYBERDYNE Inc., which was established as a university venture to mass-produce the robot suit. In this section, we explain the mechanism, function, and control of the HAL.

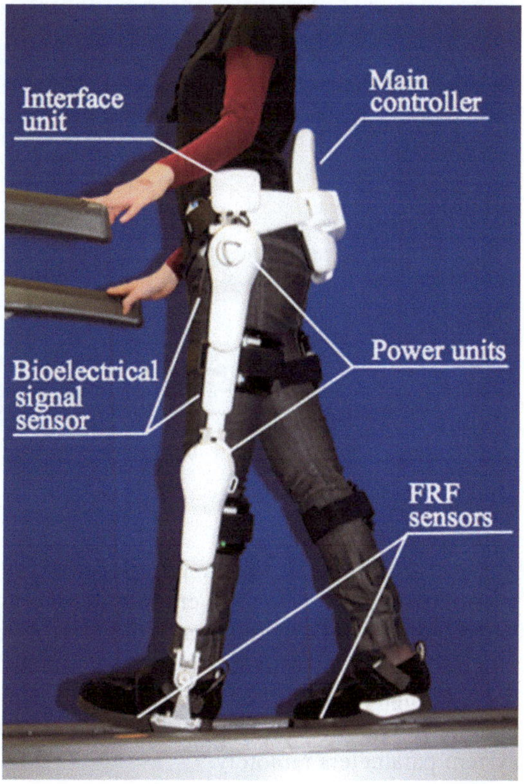

Fig. 2.3 HAL robot suit for welfare

2.3.1 The HAL System

The system configuration for the welfare version of the HAL is shown in Fig. 2.3. The HAL is basically composed of an exoskeleton, several power units, a main controller, interface units (to allow the user to adjust the HAL's behavior) and a sensing system. The exoskeleton of the HAL system is an articulated structure designed to support the mechanical functions of the human lower body. It consists of a frame and active joints, and is attached to the user's hips and legs with belts. The joints of the exoskeleton (hip, knee, and ankle) each have one DOF in the sagittal plane. The torques required by the system's dynamics are generated by the power units. Each unit integrates an actuator, a motor driver, a microprocessor, and a communication interface into one sub-system. The motion support is achieved by transmitting the torques of the power units to the user's legs through the exoskeleton's frames. Depending on which of the wearer's limbs needs support or enhancement, a single power unit or a combination of power units can be used with different configurations, including a version with two legs, a single leg version, a single joint HAL, a full body HAL, and an upper limb HAL, as shown in Fig. 2.4.

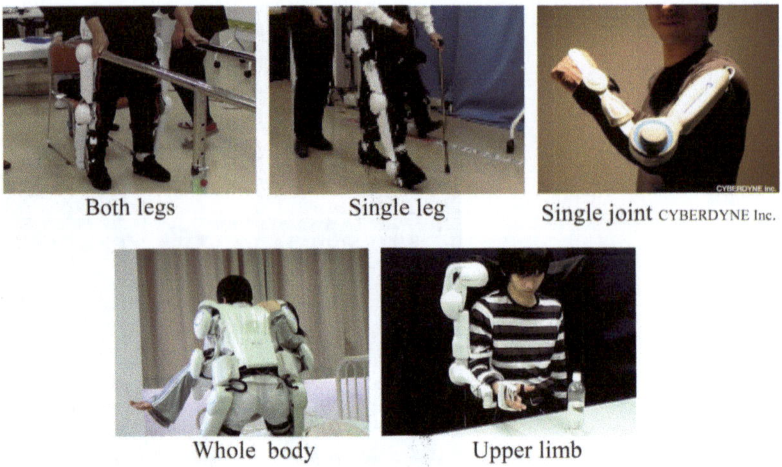

Fig. 2.4 HAL robot suit series

Control of the HAL system is performed by the main controller. Its purpose is to control and supervise the power units, monitor the batteries, and communicate with the system operator. It modulates the assist torque of each power unit to perform motion support for walking, standing up, and sitting down. Furthermore, it sends the information of the sensors and the system condition to a remote monitoring system, providing visual feedback to the operator and allowing him to adjust the system parameters remotely.

The interface units contain an interface to adjust the parameters of the HAL and the batteries. The interface includes the HAL's power switch and the digital potentiometers to tune the assistive gain. This interface allows the wearer to turn the HAL on and off easily and adjust the assist torque depending on his/her physical condition or desired level of comfort.

The HAL is equipped with a sensing system containing several types of sensors to detect the HAL's state as well as the wearer's bioelectrical signals. Potentiometers are mounted on each HAL joint and used as angular sensors to measure the joint angles. The bioelectrical sensors are attached on the skin surface of the extensor and flexor muscles of the wearer's knee and hip joints to detect muscle activity. Additionally, the insole of each of the wearer's shoes contains two floor reaction force (FRF) sensors to measure the FRFs generated at the front and the rear of the foot (heel and ball areas).

2.3.2 Motion Controller for the HAL

The HAL robot suit has been applied to physical assistance through power assist. To implement the power assist method for physical assistance, the HAL has a Cybernic Control System, which is a hybrid control algorithm consisting of

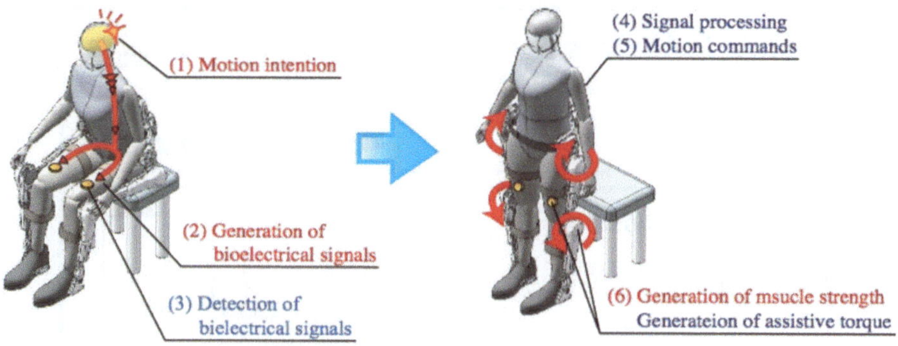

Fig. 2.5 Cybernics voluntary control

a Cybernic Voluntary Control (Bio-Cybernic Control) and aCybernic Autonomous Control (Cybernic Robot Control). This subsection introduces these controllers.

Cybernic Voluntary Control. This provides physical support according to the wearer's voluntary muscle activity (Fig. 2.5) [6]. The power units of the HAL generate assistive torques, thereby amplifying the wearer's own joint torques. The joint torques are estimated from the wearer's bioelectrical signals, which are detected at the surface of the muscles. These signals are then used as input commands to control the HAL according to the wearer's intentions to move. By using this property of the human body, the controller can predict the start and the generation of the muscles' forces, and use these as the motion commands.

In fact, the relationship between the joint torque and the processed bioelectrical signal during isometric contractions has been reported to be approximately linear, and the joint torque can thus be directly estimated from the bioelectrical signal. The required assist torque of the power units can then be calculated from the estimated joint torque, and is thus indirectly based on the bioelectrical signal.

Cybernic Autonomous Control. When the measured motion control signals include strong components of involuntary signals, Cybernic Voluntary Control may not be suitable, as, for example, in the case of patients suffering from stroke related paralysis. In these cases, Cybernic Autonomous Control would be more suitable to provide efficient physical support. Cybernic Autonomous Control provides a predefined functional motion based on recorded motion patterns from able-bodied persons [7]. Using this control method, possible involuntary signals have no influence on the physical support, as Cybernic Autonomous Control does not use the wearer's bioelectrical signals to generate assistive torque.

Cybernic Autonomous Control uses the phase sequence method with human motion characteristics to enable HAL to generate human-like motion in an autonomous way. The phase sequencing was constructed according to the three stages shown in Fig. 2.6. First, the functional motion of an able-bodied person is recorded, and analyzed based on motion variables and the wearer's physiological data. Then, the reference motion patterns are divided into motion sequences or motion

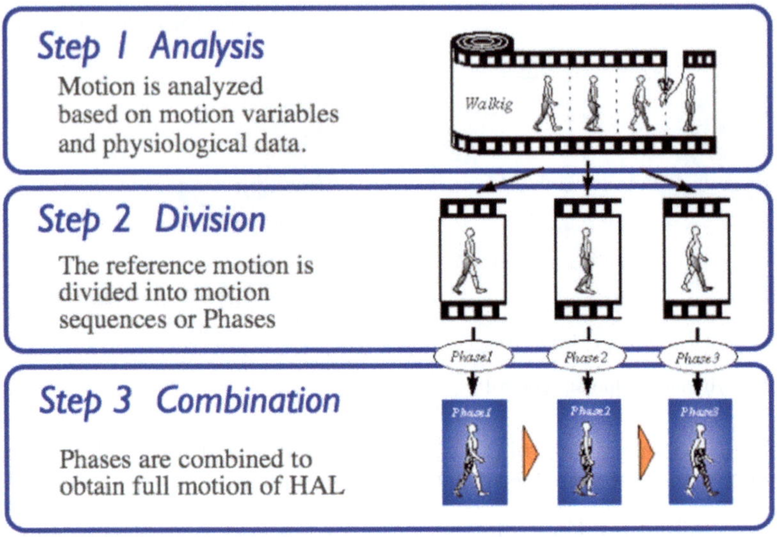

Fig. 2.6 Phase sequence

phases. This division is made according to specific intended motions such as "swinging the leg" or "lifting the body". The motions of the resulting phases are then stored in the HAL. Each phase is further adjusted in terms of duration and amplitude depending on the wearer's characteristics such as his/her body parameters or medical condition. Finally, the phases are combined to obtain the whole motion to be executed by the HAL. As a result, the HAL allows the wearer to perform functional motions such as walking, sitting, and so on, in an autonomous way.

2.4 Clinical Applications of the HAL Robot Suit

This section introduces clinical applications of the HAL to a spinal cord injury (SCI) patient and a stroke patient, and a case study of rehabilitation using the HAL. For more details, the reader is referred to the references.

2.4.1 Walking Support for a Spinal Cord Injury Patient Based on Wearer's Intention

In this section, we introduce an algorithm to estimate human intentions related to walking based on Autonomous Control in order to comfortably and safely support the walking motion of paraplegic patients [8]. Estimation of the patient's intentions contributes to providing not only comfortable support but also safe support, because

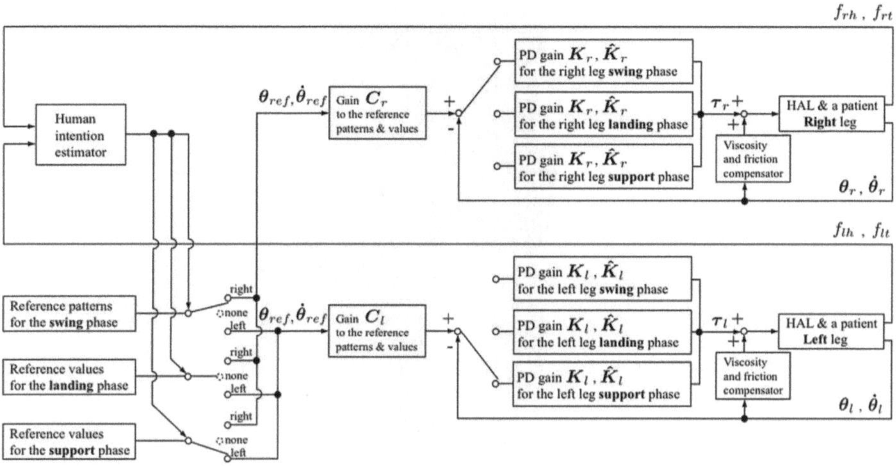

Fig. 2.7 Block diagram for tracking control and phase synchronization [8]

any nonconformity between the motion of the robot suit and that of the patient may result in his/her stumbling or falling. The proposed algorithm estimates a patient's intentions from the FRF, reflecting the patient's weight shift during walking and standing. The effectiveness of this algorithm was investigated through experiments on a paraplegic patient with sensory paralysis in both legs, but more extreme in the left leg. We show that the HAL adequately supports the patient's walk.

Methods. Bipedal locomotion using a patient's legs is achieved by tracking control and phase synchronization of motion support with the patient's intention. This control consists of PD (proportional-derivative) control using reference walking patterns based on a healthy person's walk in the swing phase and constant-value control in the landing and support phase.

Figure 2.7 shows a block diagram of this tracking control and phase synchronization. The human intention estimator (HIE) located in the upper left of Fig. 2.7 takes the FRF as input for the estimation algorithms. The three blocks directly below the HIE represent a library of reference patterns in the swing phase, and the reference values in the landing and support phases. The HIE allocates these references to the two legs during walking. There are six ordinary PD control blocks on the right side of the HIE and the library. The upper three blocks are controllers for the right leg, while the lower ones are for the left leg. For more details, refer to the reference [8].

The subject in this case is a 57-year-old male SCI patient with incomplete sensory and motor paralysis in the left leg, especially the left lower thigh. He was diagnosed with incomplete SCI; the sixth and seventh thoracic vertebra (T6 and T7) are damaged. While he has good voluntary control of the upper body and limited voluntary control of both legs, he has little voluntary control of the muscles below the left knee joint. His deep sensitivity, including angle sensitivity, remains

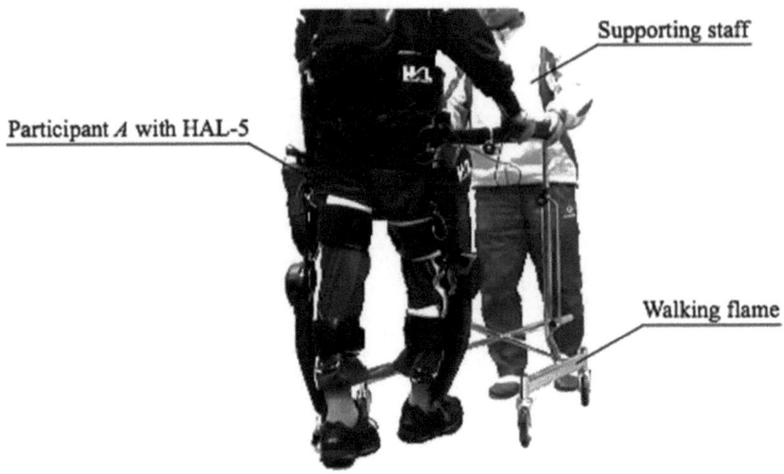

Fig. 2.8 Experimental setting

partially intact in his lower thigh; however, tactile, pain, and temperature sensitivities have been lost. He has trouble lifting his own leg against gravity, and thus experiences significant difficulty climbing up stairs. In addition, he has stiffening in his left knee joint and sometimes spasticity of his left lower thigh muscles. The subject gave his informed consent before participating in this study.

The aim of the HAL support is to help his leg swing forward without a limp and sustain his weight (65 kg), since he can stand on his own using two canes. This support contributes to stabilizing his walk by pushing the swing leg forward, avoiding collisions of the swing leg with the floor, and preventing sudden knee bends. This walking support was conducted 16 times with the subject, and he was required to start walking from a standing posture and stop walking in his own time. In each trial, the subject walked 5–7 m using 12–18 steps. Moreover, since he was experiencing walking support embedded with the proposed intention estimation algorithm for the first time, the subject was supposed to maintain his own stability by holding onto a walking frame with his arms while a staff member supported the walking frame for the sake of the subject's safety as shown in Fig. 2.8.

Results. Figure 2.9 shows the joint and reference angles, and the torque of the power units during walking support. Torque data was estimated based on the amount of current provided to each power unit. In Fig. 2.9a, the left hip and knee joints follow the reference angles based on a healthy person's walk for most of one cycle of the supported walk. In Fig. 2.9b, the right hip and knee joints follow the reference angles based on a healthy person's walk for most of one cycle of the supported walk. Compared to the right leg support shown in Fig. 2.9b, the left hip and knee joints, which have more severe sensory and motor paralysis, require larger torque than the right joints.

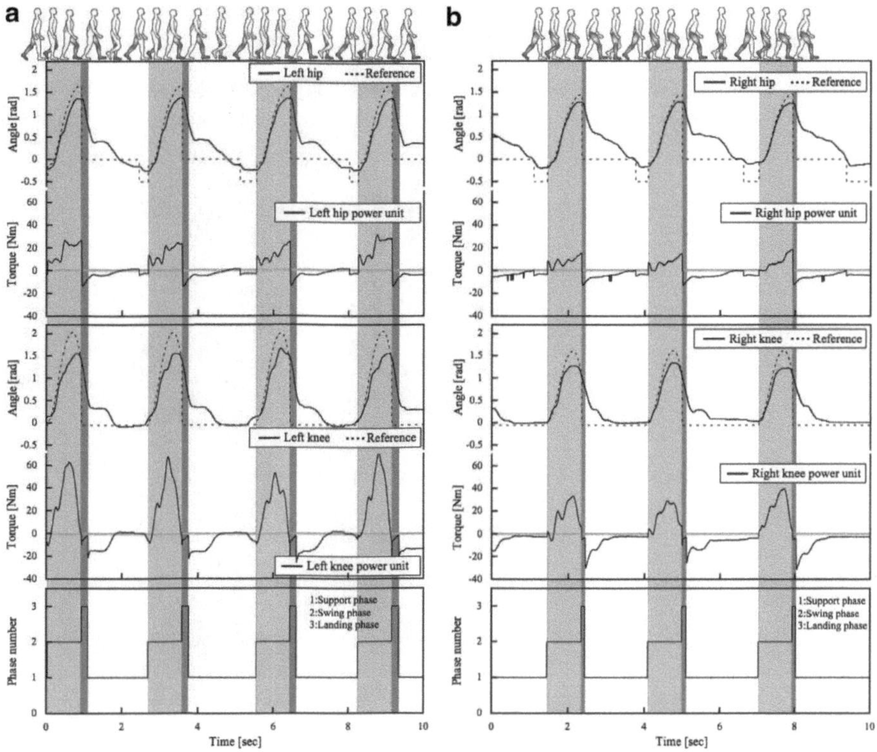

Fig. 2.9 Joint angles together with reference angles and power unit torques for three steps during walking support: (**a**) *left* side, (**b**) *right* side

Discussion. From the results of the joint angles in these figures, the subject's hip and knee joints follow the reference angles most of the time during one cycle of the supported walk. This means that the HAL supports his walk based on a healthy person's walk and the subject performs a more natural walk with greater step length than his own normal walk. The HAL also successfully reduces the risk of his stumbling and falling by assisting his hip and knee flexor muscles during swinging of the leg, by lifting up his drop foot, and by assisting his supporting leg to sustain his weight and prevent sudden knee bends.

2.4.2 Walking Support for a Stroke Patient Using a One Leg Version of the HAL

The case study presented in this section involves the development of the HAL for use as an assistive device providing walking motion support to patients with hemiplegia [9]. This includes the realization of a single leg version of the HAL

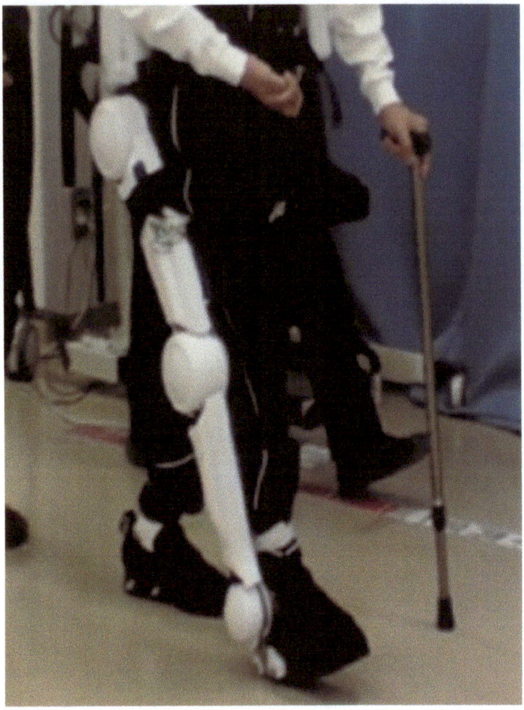

Fig. 2.10 Single leg version of the HAL fitted to a subject

and redesign of the original HAL's Autonomous Controller to execute human-like walking motion in an autonomous way. Clinical trials were conducted to assess the effectiveness of the developed system. The first stage of the trials described in this section involved the participation of one hemiplegic patient who has difficulty in flexing his right knee.

Methods. A single leg version of the HAL was developed to support leg motion on the affected side. Actually, the single leg version consists of two power units and an exoskeletal frame on one side. No device was attached to the unaffected side. Figure 2.10 shows the single leg version of the HAL fitted to a subject.

The subject in this case is a 59 year old male with right hemiplegia, resulting from a stroke (Brunnstrom recovery stage IV). In his daily life, he wears an ankle orthosis, and walks with the support of a cane. His walking is characterized by a circumduction gait, due to difficulty in flexing the right knee joint without flexing the right hip joint. The subject gave his informed consent before participating.

As the subject can move his hip joint by himself, the actuator of the hip joint was replaced by a free joint. Usually in Cybernic Autonomous Control, an assistive torque is generated for flexion and extension during the swing phases. However, as the patient can voluntarily extend the knee of his right leg, the action of the Cybernic Autonomous Control was limited to flexion.

The trials were organized in 1 h sessions, which were performed once a week, for 4 weeks. In each session, the subject was asked to walk a required distance (about 5 m in the first two sessions and then gradually extending the distance up to 10 m). Once the subject has covered the required distance, the HAL's parameters are adjusted to improve the walking. The parameters involved are the amplitude of the assistive torque, the timing of the phase switching, and the motion velocity.

An evaluation of the walking support was carried out by comparing the data measured with and without the HAL support. The comparison is based on the time to cover the required distance, the length of the stride, the knee joint angle, the hip joint angle, and the right foot FRF.

Results. Figure 2.11 illustrates the data recorded during one walking cycle. The following conventions apply to the measured data. The reference used for the joints angle is the value measured for the standing posture. The angles are considered positive during flexion and negative during extension. The assistive torque is positive during flexion and negative during extension. It appears that the HAL generates assistive torque in the flexion direction and knee flexion of the subject is performed during the right leg swing phase.

Figure 2.12 shows the knee joint angle and the hip joint angle with and without assistive support during one walking cycle (starting when the right foot touches the ground). It is clear that the right knee angle and the hip joint angle measured during the swing motion are greater when using the HAL.

Figure 2.13 presents the FRF measured at the front and back of the right foot with and without the HAL during one cycle of walking, starting with contact of the right foot. When the subject is walking without the HAL, it appears from the FRF that the right foot makes contact with the floor over the whole surface of the foot simultaneously. Then, the FRF remains almost constant while the weight shifts forward. This means that the weight is not shifted smoothly from the rear to the front of the right foot.

On the other hand, in the case of walking with the HAL, the FRF shows clearly that the foot makes contact with the ground from the rear of the foot first, and then the weight is shifted smoothly to the front. This phenomenon can be explained by the support of the active knee flexion, which makes it faster and smoother to transfer the weight forward.

Table 2.1 shows the left and right stride lengths and the walking times to cover 10 m with and without using the HAL. When the subject is wearing the HAL, the length of the right stride is longer and the walking speed is higher than without the HAL.

Discussion. The single leg version of the HAL was used to assess the support provided to a person with hemiplegia for the bending motion of the knee. The stride of the right leg increased significantly, due to a wider motion of the knee joint and the hip joint during the swing phase. Furthermore, the use of the HAL resulted in a decrease in the walking time, because the HAL allows a shift forward. This confirms that the single leg version of the HAL could effectively improve the walking of a patient with hemiplegia.

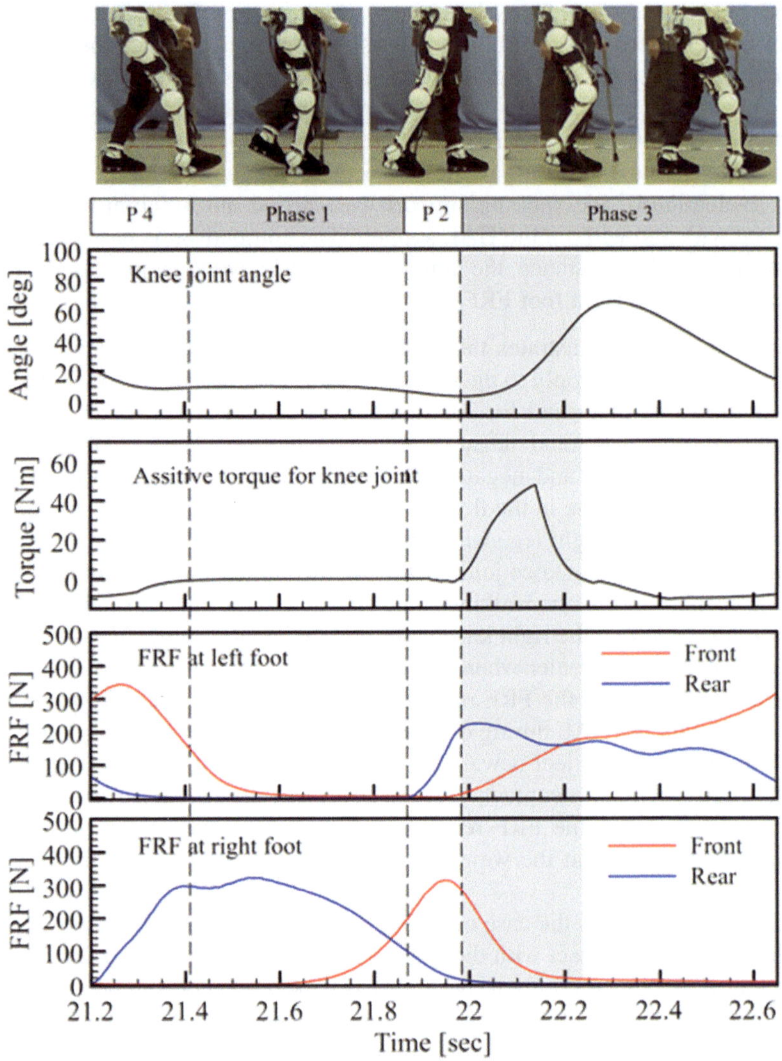

Fig. 2.11 Metrics for one cycle of walking support with the HAL

2.4.3 Locomotion Improvement for a Spinal Canal Stenosis Patient Using the HAL

The case study presented in this section concerns locomotion improvement through continued use of the HAL [10]. Locomotor training is conducted by applying the HAL for 8 weeks to a spinal canal stenosis patient who has difficulty in walking (Fig. 2.14).

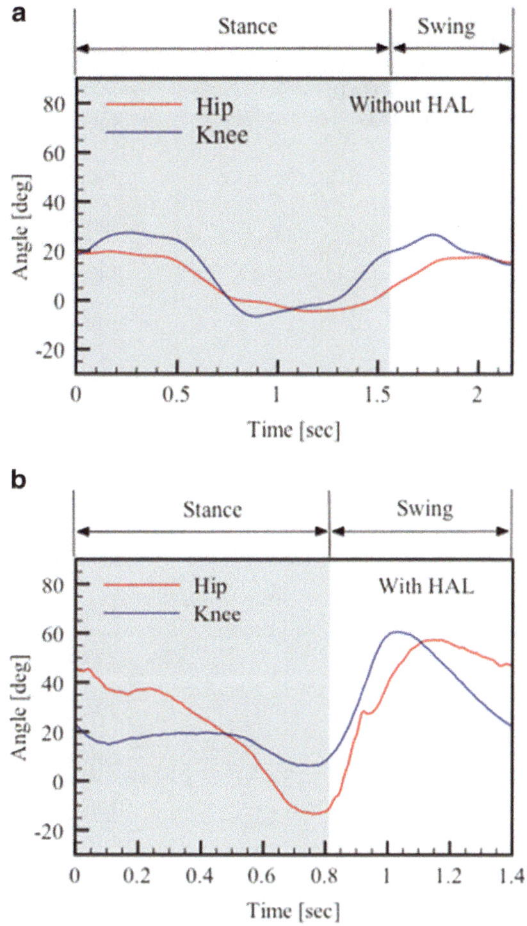

Fig. 2.12 Angles of the knee and hip joints on the right side while walking: (**a**) without the HAL, (**b**) with HAL

Methods. The subject is a 67-year-old man who suffers from paralysis due to spinal canal stenosis: he had a posterior cervical spinal fusion 1 year previously. At the time of training, his right leg muscle strength was Grade 2 or less according to the manual muscle test (MMT), while his left leg muscle was Grade 3–4. He had neither dysesthesia nor pain. The subject's main impairment was muscle weakness of the lower limbs. He was able to walk with a pick-up walker and an ankle-foot orthosis (AFO). He provided his informed consent for participation in this study. All the procedures employed were approved by the ethics committees of the relevant facilities.

The trials were organized in 1-hour sessions, which were performed twice a week for 8 weeks. In each trial, the subject walked on a treadmill for around 5 sets of 3 min each. The assistive torque for each joint was adjusted to provide motion support that was comfortable for the subject.

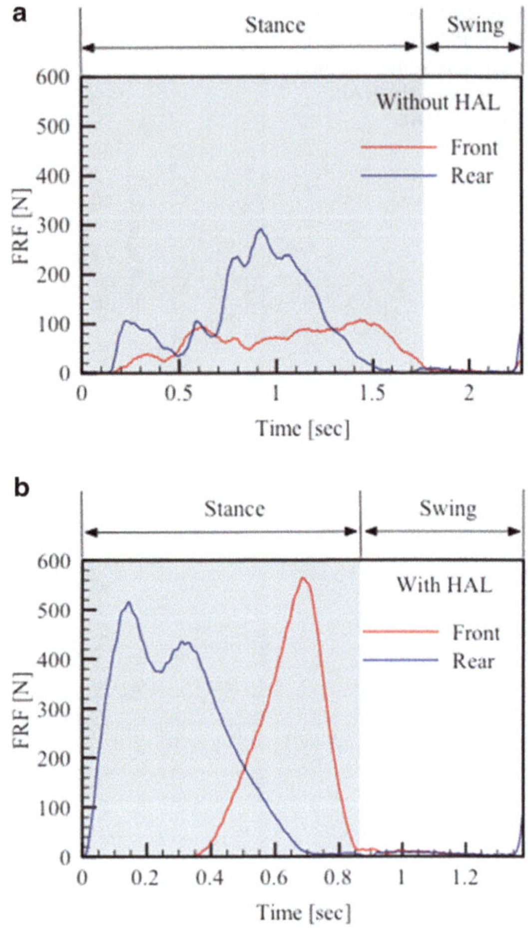

Fig. 2.13 FRF on the front and the rear parts of the right foot while walking: (**a**) without the HAL, (**b**) with the HAL

Table 2.1 Left and right stride lengths and walking times with and without the HAL

	Without the HAL	With the HAL
Left stride length [cm]	115	157
Right stride length [cm]	118	171
Walking time (10 m) [sec]	33.2	13.4

The changes in walking ability were evaluated during the 8-week training period. The walkingability was assessed by a 10 m walking test (10MWT) and a 3 m timed up and go test (TUG). We also evaluated the balance ability according to the Berg Balance Scale (BBS), the range of motion (ROM), the MMT for each leg joint, and the activity of daily living (ADL) according to the Barthel Index (BI).

Results. Figures 2.15a–d show, respectively, the walking speed and walking rate during the 10MWT, the time for the TUG, and the total BBS score, before

Fig. 2.14 Gait rehabilitation with the HAL for spinal canal stenosis

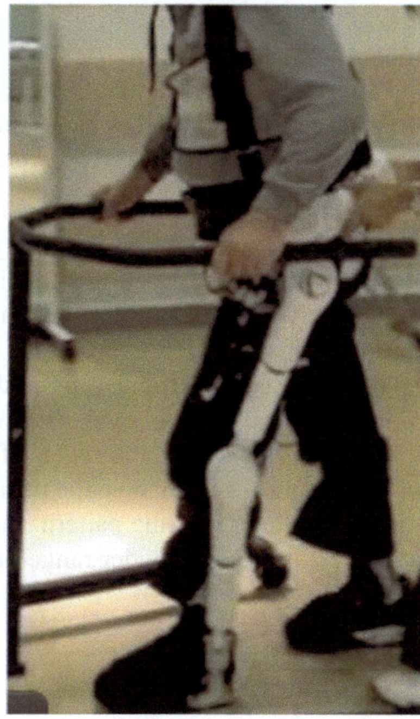

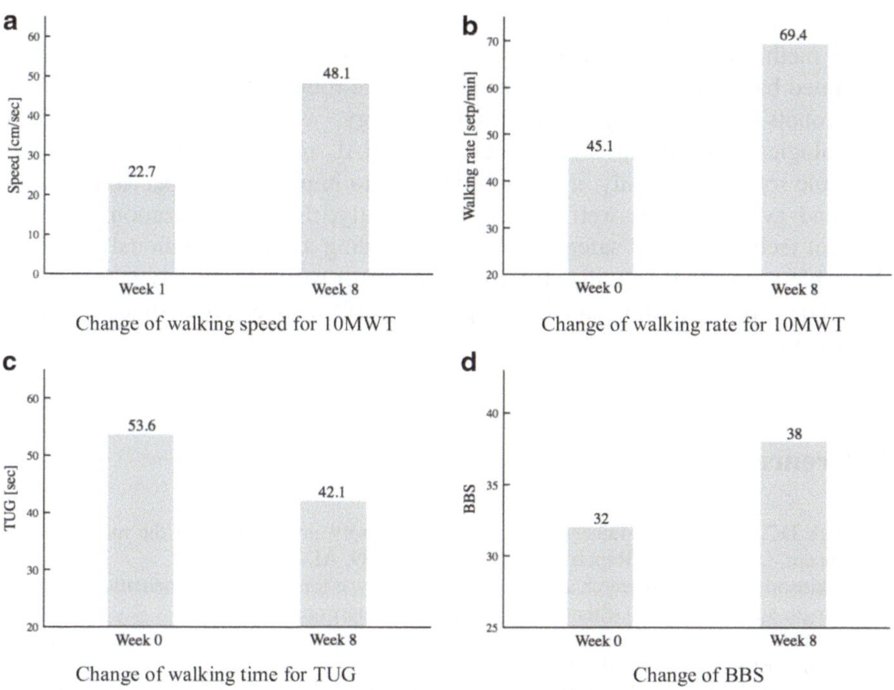

Fig. 2.15 Experimental results for walking speed and walking rate for the 10MWT, walking time for the TUG, and BBS before and after the 8-week training period (**a**) Change of walking speed for 10MWT (**b**) Change of walking rate for 10MWT (**c**) Change of walking time for TUG (**d**) Change of BBS

and after the 8-week training period. All these measurements showed improvement after 8 weeks. On the other hand, there were no obvious changes in the MMT and the ADL based on the BI. However, the patient reported that he was able to walk around the room using two T-canes and an AFO instead of the pick-up walker.

Discussion. The results of this study show that the walking ability of the subject improved after the 8-week gait training with the HAL. This suggests the feasibility and effectiveness of training for patients with spinal canal stenosis. The HAL's motion support, which is based on a voluntarily controlled bilaterally symmetric gait as well as a left-right weight shift, strengthened the patient's own ability to control his walking, as evidenced by the improved walking rate and balancing ability once the HAL was taken off. This gait training also increased voluntary walking control and enabled the patient to increase his walking balance and acquire a more rhythmic walking pattern. In the near future, we will report the results of a study performed on a wider range of patients.

2.5 Conclusion

In this chapter, we introduced wearable robots which enhance and support human physical functions by integrating human and machine. First, two types of power assist methods (lifting a heavy load and assisting the wearer's limbs) were explained based on force interaction for wearable robots. As an example of wearable robots developed by Cybernics technology, we introduced assist control technologies and clinical case studies of the HAL robot suit. In order to apply wearable robots practically, it is also important to improve performance technologies and availability as well as safety. Currently, the standardization of safety element technology and safeguarding is proceeding as an International Standard. Wearable robots will be utilized in living spaces or worksites as a type of friendly robot coexisting with humans, by integrating performance technologies, availability and safety.

References

1. Clark DC, Deleys NJ, Matheis CW (1962) Exploratory investigation of the man amplifier concept, U.S. Air Force Report No. AMRLTDR-62-89, AD-290070
2. Makinson BJ (1971) Research and development prtotype for machine augmentation of human strength and endurance, General electric company report no. S-71-1056
3. Kazerooni H (1990) Human-robot interaction via the transfer of power and information signals. IEEE Trans Syst Man Cybern 20(20):450–463
4. Kazerooni H, Mahoney SL (1991) Dynamics and control of robotic systems worn by humans. J Dyn Syst Meas Control Trans ASME 113:379–387
5. Kazerooni H (1993) Jenhwa Guo: human extenders. J Dyn Syst Meas Control Trans ASME 115:281–290

6. Kawamoto H, Sankai Y (2002) Power assist system HAL-3 for Gait disorder person. Lect Notes Comput Sci 2398:198–203
7. Kawamoto H, Sankai Y (2005) Power assist method based on phase sequence and muscle force condition for HAL. Adv Robot 19(7):717–734
8. Suzuki K et al (2007) Intention-based walking support for paraplegia patients with robot Suit HAL. Adv Robot 21(12):1441–1469
9. Kawamoto H, Hayashi T, Sakurai T, Eguchi K, Sankai Y (2009) Development of Single Leg Version of HAL for Hemiplegia. In: Proceedings of the 31st Annual International Conference of the IEEE Engineering in Medicine and Biology Society, pp 5038–5043
10. Yamawaki K, Kawamoto H, Eguchi K, Nakata Y, Sankai Y, Ochiai N (2011) Gait training for a spinal canal stenosis patient using robot suit HAL. A case report. In: Proceedings of the 5th world congress of the international society of physical and rehabilitation medicine, pp 66–68

Chapter 3
Robot Motion Control for Physical Assistance

Yasuhisa Hasegawa

Abstract This chapter introduces some motion control algorithms for a mechanical system that has a redundant degree of freedom. Human motions are intelligently and dexterously controlled by sensory and motor nerve systems based on sophisticated sensory organs, intelligent environment recognition, task planning, and redundant and soft mechanical structures. An assistive robot, such as an exoskeleton robot, should be capable of achieving the same level of motions as humans when it compensates for some of the impaired motions of the patient using the device. Human sensorial and motional properties, including a musculoskeletal system, will be introduced in Chap. 4. This chapter focuses on motion control of the redundant mechanical structure, such as an arm system, and the whole body of the exoskeleton. Some basic and advanced control algorithms for a redundant mechanical structure of a robot are introduced to make the physically assistive robot useful and comfortable.

Keywords Redundant degree of freedom • Control algorithm • Assistive robot

3.1 Introduction

Robot dynamics has several characteristics, among which is that it involves multiple inputs and outputs. A robot has multiple sensors to discern both its environment and itself, and it has multiple degrees of freedom in its operations. It sometimes has redundant degrees of freedom, and the redundancy in its motion can contribute to its dexterity or efficiency. Humans also have redundancy in the upper limbs. For example, when we put our hand on the table, the hand is supported by the table. In this case, six degrees of freedom of the hand are constrained by the

Y. Hasegawa (✉)
Faculty of Engineering, Information and Systems, University of Tsukuba, Tsukuba, Japan
e-mail: hase@iit.tsukuba.ac.jp

Y. Sankai et al. (eds.), *Cybernics: Fusion of human, machine and information systems*,
DOI 10.1007/978-4-431-54159-2_3, © Springer Japan 2014

table; however, we may change the position of the elbow, so that only one degree of freedom remains. We can say that the human upper arm has seven degrees of freedom and is a redundant system.

Robot dynamics is generally nonlinear, because serial links rotate around its joints. The gravitational force that affects the link is a function of sine or cosine. The point of contact between a robot and its environment can change in the course of its operations. An equation of motion for the robot changes when its point of contact with the environment changes. For example, the structure of a biped robot changes with each step as it walks: a single-support phase alternates with a dual-support phase. In addition, the conditions of contact with the environment vary. It is difficult to identify or calibrate a model that is able to accommodate changes in friction, elasticity, and viscosity. These characteristics make robot control a highly complex matter.

3.2 Equation of Motion

An equation of motion for a robot that has multiple inputs and outputs is generally derived by Lagrange's equation of motion, which is a very powerful tool for the purpose. Let us consider this two-link manipulator with two joints as an example, as illustrated in Fig. 3.1.

At first, we consider the system kinetic energy:

$$K = \frac{1}{2}J_1\dot{q}_1^2 + \frac{1}{2}J_2(\dot{q}_1 + \dot{q}_2)^2 + \frac{1}{2}m_1 l_1^2\dot{q}_1^2 + m_2 l_2 a_2 \dot{q}_1(\dot{q}_1 + \dot{q}_2)\cos q_2 \tag{3.1}$$

where $J = (J_1, J_2)$ is link inertia and $Q = (q_1, q_2)$ is the joint angle. The first and second terms are rotational energy. The third and fourth terms are translational energy.

The potential energy is

$$P = m_1 a_1 g \sin q_1 + m_2 g(l_1 \sin q_1 + a_2 \sin(q_1 + q_2)) \tag{3.2}$$

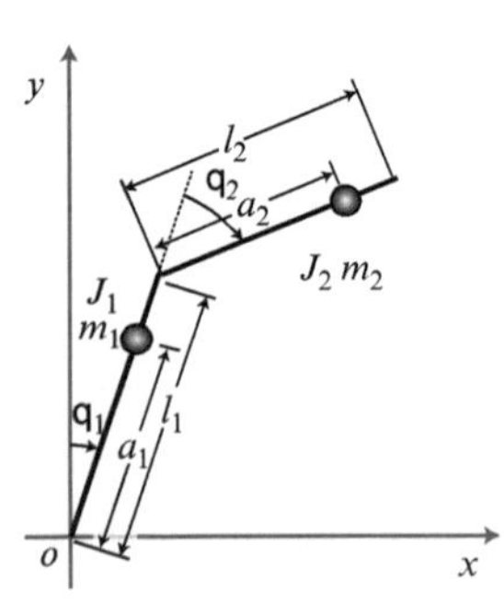

Fig. 3.1 Model of two-link manipulator

The first term is the potential energy of the first link; the second term is that of the second link. Lagrangian L is kinetic energy, K, minus potential energy, P:

$$L = K - P \tag{3.3}$$

Using Lagrange's equation of motion below, we derive an equation of motion for the two-link manipulator. In the first term, the Lagrangian is partially differentiated with respect to the angular velocity of joint angle q and then differentiated with respect to time. In the second term, the Lagrangian is differentiated with respect to the joint angle.

$$\frac{d}{dt}\left(\frac{\partial L}{\partial \dot{q}_i}\right) - \frac{\partial L}{\partial q_i} = \boldsymbol{\tau} \tag{3.4}$$

where τ is the external joint torque vector. The equation of motion is generally a second-order differential equation. The equation of motion of the two-link manipulator is composed of two equations, because it has two degrees of freedom.

$$\begin{aligned}&(J_1 + J_2 + m_1 l_1^2 + 2m_2 l_2 a_2 \cos q_2)\ddot{q}_1 + (J_2 + m_2 l_2 a_2 \cos q_2)\ddot{q}_2 \\ &-2m_2 l_2 a_2 \sin q_2 \dot{q}_1 \dot{q}_2 + m_1 a_1 g \cos q_1 + m_2 g\big(l_1 \cos q_1 + a_2 \sin(q_1 + q_2)\big) = \tau_1\end{aligned} \tag{3.5}$$

$$(J_2 + m_2 l_2 a_2 \cos q_2)\ddot{q}_1 + J_2 \ddot{q}_1 - m_2 l_2 a_2 \sin q_2 \dot{q}_1 \dot{q}_2 + m_2 a_2 g \cos(q_1 + q_2) = \tau_2 \tag{3.6}$$

These equations are rewritten in state-space representation as follows:

$$\begin{aligned}&\begin{bmatrix} J_1 + J_2 + m_1 l_1^2 + 2m_2 l_2 a_2 \cos q_2 & J_2 + m_2 l_2 a_2 \cos q_2 \\ J_2 + m_2 l_2 a_2 \cos q_2 & J_2 \end{bmatrix}\begin{pmatrix} \ddot{q}_1 \\ \ddot{q}_2 \end{pmatrix} \\ &-\begin{pmatrix} m_2 l_2 a_2 \dot{q}_2 \sin q_2 & m_2 l_2 a_2 \dot{q}_1 \sin q_2 \\ m_2 l_2 a_2 (\dot{q}_1 + \dot{q}_2) \sin q_2 & m_2 l_2 a_2 \dot{q}_1 \sin q_2 \end{pmatrix}\begin{pmatrix} \dot{q}_1 \\ \dot{q}_2 \end{pmatrix} \\ &+\begin{pmatrix} m_1 a_1 g \cos q_1 + m_2 g\big(l_1 \cos q_1 + a_2 \sin(q_1 + q_2)\big) \\ m_2 g a_2 \sin(q_1 + q_2) \end{pmatrix} = \begin{pmatrix} \tau_1 \\ \tau_2 \end{pmatrix}\end{aligned} \tag{3.7}$$

Generally, robot dynamics is expressed by the following form:

$$\frac{d}{dt}(\mathbf{M}(\boldsymbol{\Theta})\dot{\boldsymbol{\Theta}}) - \frac{1}{2}\frac{\partial}{\partial \boldsymbol{\Theta}}\left(\dot{\boldsymbol{\Theta}}^T \mathbf{M}(\boldsymbol{\Theta})\dot{\boldsymbol{\Theta}}\right) - \mathbf{G}(\boldsymbol{\Theta}) = \boldsymbol{\tau} \tag{3.8}$$

The first term is an inertia matrix and angular acceleration. The second term is the Coriolis torque or centrifugal torque. The third term is gravity. The right side of the equation is a joint torque.

3.3 Trajectory of the Human Hand and Its Control Laws

There are very interesting phenomena in the trajectory of human hand movement. Morasso [1] found that the hand path is straight in the action of reaching. The human upper limb is modeled as serial links. Thus, the trajectory of the hand tends to be arc-shaped. If the hand moves in a straight line, the shoulder and elbow synchronize the movement very precisely. Abend, Bizzi, and Morasso [2] found that the velocity of the trajectory of the hand has a bell-shaped profile. Hogan [3] showed that motion can be achieved if the jerk associated with the hand is minimized. Velocity is the first-order differential of the position with respect to time. Acceleration is the second-order differential of the position. The jerk is the third-order differential of the position. For the third phenomenon, Flash and Hogan [4] found that the velocity profile remains invariant when normalized with respect to the movement time and amplitude. We consider here a control algorithm that can achieve these phenomena.

First, we consider that the velocity of the trajectory has a bell-shaped profile. To achieve the bell-shaped profile, Flash and Hogan found the evaluation function like this:

$$C_j = \frac{1}{2}\int_0^T \|\widetilde{x}(\tau)\|^2 \, d\tau \tag{3.9}$$

This evaluation function is just the integration of the jerk of the trajectory of x. The trajectory that minimizes the evaluation function is expressed by this fifth-order polynomial:

$$x(t) = x_0 + (x_f - x_0)\left\{-15\left(\frac{t}{T}\right)^4 + 6\left(\frac{t}{T}\right)^5 + 10\left(\frac{t}{T}\right)^3\right\} \tag{3.10}$$

where x_0 is the initial position, x_f the final position, and T the final time. What we have to do is determine the initial position, final position, and final time. This algorithm is very simple, but such robot dynamics as inertia and mass are not considered.

Uno et al. [5] proposed a minimum torque-change model to design a trajectory that takes into account the physical parameters of the manipulator:

$$C_j = \frac{1}{2}\int_0^T \|\dot{u}(\tau)\|^2 \, d\tau \tag{3.11}$$

This evaluation function has a differential of torque. The trajectory of joint angle x that minimizes the evaluation function can be derived by solving these differential equations:

$$\frac{dX}{dt} = f(X, \dot{u}) \tag{3.12}$$

$$\frac{d\varphi}{dt} = -\left(\frac{\partial f}{\partial X}\right)^T \varphi \tag{3.13}$$

$$\dot{u} = \varphi_u \tag{3.14}$$

where $x = \left(q^{\mathrm{T}}, \dot{q}^T, u^T\right)$, φ is Lanrangian vector.

These design algorithms—the minimum jerk model and the minimum torque-change model—can be applied to normal industrial manipulators that have the necessary degrees of freedom for a particular task. If a manipulator has redundant degrees of freedom, these algorithms are not sufficient.

3.4 Control Law of a Redundant System

Redundant degrees of freedom of a manipulator allow multiple arm configurations such that the end effector can achieve a unique position and orientation. For example, if a manipulator with three degrees of freedom works in two-dimensional space, there are multiple configurations for reaching the target position. The redundancy in the manipulator's motion could contribute to its dexterity or efficiency because the manipulator can either avoid or use the singular configuration. Another advantage of the redundancy is "bracing." We use the environment to fix our bodily position or decrease joint torque. For example, if we pick up a small object from a table, the wrist is fixed by the table to increase precision with regard to position. Even if the wrist is fixed, the hand has sufficient degrees of freedom (DOF) to handle the object. When we relax, we may place our elbow on the table to decrease the torque of the shoulder. However, we have to determine one configuration to utilize the redundancy of the manipulator.

Joint torques, u, of each joint of a normal manipulator are generally calculated by

$$u(t) = H(q_d(t))\ddot{q}_d(t) + \left\{\frac{1}{2}\dot{H}(q_d) + S(q_d, \dot{q}_d)\right\}\dot{q}_d - k_p(q - q_d) \\ - k_v(\dot{q} - \dot{q}_d) \tag{3.15}$$

The first term compensates for link inertia. The second term compensates for the Coriolis and centrifugal torque. The third term is position feedback. The fourth term is velocity feedback. A redundant manipulator, however, has null space in the Jacobian matrix. The Jacobian matrix is the first derivative of the position vector of the end effector. We therefore add additional constraints or criteria to fix the motions of all joints. Manipulability [6], kinetic energy [7], and the sum of squared torque [8] are proposed as the criteria to degenerate the redundancy.

Minimum angular velocity control is the simplest of these criteria. Using a pseudo-inverse matrix of the Jacobian matrix, the reference angular velocity is determined by

$$\dot{q}_d(t) = J^+(q_d)\dot{x}_d \tag{3.16}$$

where $J^+ = J^T(JJ^T)^{-1}$

As another criterion, the angular velocity of all joints is designed by maximizing the manipulability of the hand. Manipulability is the ability of the manipulator to move uniformly in all directions. The angular velocity is determined by

$$\dot{q}_d(t) = J^+(q_d)\dot{x}_d + (I - J^+(q_d)J(q_d))\eta \tag{3.17}$$

where $\eta = k\left(\frac{\partial c_m}{\partial q}\right) = k\left(\frac{\partial}{\partial q}\sqrt{\det J(q)J^T(q)}\right)$

This algorithm is very useful to avoid a singular point of the manipulator.

Arimoto [9] proposed another algorithm to control a redundant system. This algorithm can achieve similar properties to the human reaching trajectory explained in the previous section. This algorithm uses a virtual spring that conducts the hand to a target position. We consider here the virtual spring connecting the hand to the target position. Δx is the position error and $f(=-\ k\Delta x(t))$ is the spring force. Using a transfer of the Jacobian matrix, the conducting torque, u, of each joint is calculated by

$$\begin{aligned} u &= -C\dot{q} - J^T(q)k\Delta x(t) \\ &= -C\dot{q} - J^T(q)f \end{aligned} \tag{3.18}$$

where C is the damping coefficient in the joint space. An advantage of this algorithm is that it can realize the bell-shaped velocity profile of the hand trajectory. In addition, this algorithm does not require the pseudo-inverse matrix, the calculation of which demands great effort. The trajectory to the target position is, however, not straight. The trajectory becomes almost straight when a damping factor in the operating space is employed, as follows:

$$u = -C\dot{q} - J^T(q)\{\alpha\dot{x} + k\Delta x(t)\} \tag{3.19}$$

where α is a positive damping coefficient.

Two phenomena of the human reaching motion—the bell-shaped profile and the straight trajectory—are achieved with this control algorithm. The third one is not achieved, and for this further studies are required.

3.5 Passive Dynamic Autonomous Control

Passive dynamic autonomous control (PDAC) is one of the control methods for the redundant mechanical system based on point contact and a virtual holonomic constraint. The point contact denotes that the robot contacts the ground at a certain point (i.e., the first joint is passive) and makes it possible to achieve adaptability to ground irregularity and energy efficiency. The concept of the virtual holonomic constraint was proposed as the virtual constraint by Grizzle et al. [10] and Westervelt et al. [11]. It is defined as a set of holonomic constraints on the robot's actuated DOF parameterized by the robot's unactuated DOF. The virtual holonomic constraint enables a robot to satisfy the desired path of postural motion.

3.5.1 *Dynamics of PDAC*

Assuming that PDAC is applied to the serial n-link rigid robot shown in Fig. 3.2, the point contact is achieved by zero torque applied to the ground around the contact point. The point contact is therefore expressed by

$$\tau_1 = 0 \tag{3.20}$$

The virtual holonomic constraint is written by

$$\Theta = [\theta_1, \quad \theta_2, \quad \cdots, \quad \theta_n]^T = [f_1(\theta), \quad f_2(\theta), \quad \cdots, \quad f_n(\theta)]^T := f(\theta) \tag{3.21}$$

where θ is the angle around the contact point in the absolute coordinate system. The angle is

$$\theta = \theta_1 + \zeta \tag{3.22}$$

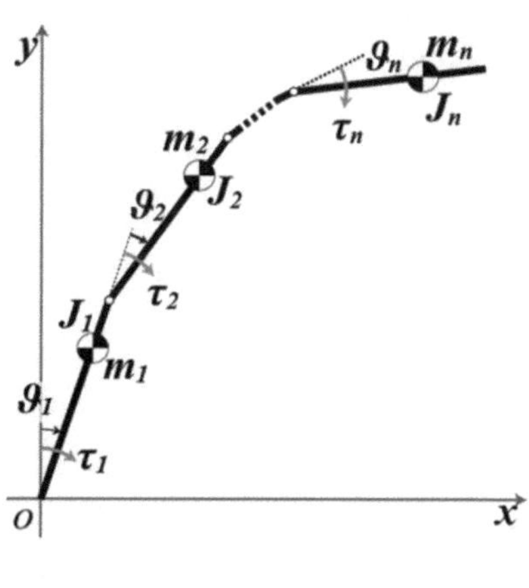

Fig. 3.2 Mechanical model of the serial n-link rigid robot. θ_i and τ_i are the angle and the torque of i-th joint, respectively. m_i and J_i are the mass and the moment of inertia of i-th link, respectively

where ζ is the angle of the ground slope (ascent is positive, and descent is negative). On flat, level ground,

$$\theta = f_1(\theta) = \theta_1 \tag{3.23}$$

The virtual holonomic constraint interlocking robot joints $f_1(\theta)$, $f_2(\theta)$, $\cdots$, $f_n(\theta)$ are adequately designed in accordance with the target motion.

The dynamic equations of this model are also given by Eq. 3.8. The first term is inertia and the centrifugal terms are written as

$$\mathbf{M}(\boldsymbol{\Theta}) = \begin{bmatrix} m_{11}(\Theta) & m_{12}(\Theta) & \dots & m_{1n}(\Theta) \\ m_{21}(\Theta) & m_{22}(\Theta) & \dots & m_{2n}(\Theta) \\ \vdots & \vdots & \ddots & \vdots \\ m_{n1}(\Theta) & m_{n2}(\Theta) & \dots & m_{nn}(\Theta) \end{bmatrix} := \begin{bmatrix} m_1(\Theta) \\ m_2(\Theta) \\ \vdots \\ m_n(\Theta) \end{bmatrix} \tag{3.24}$$

The second term is the Corioli force, where

$$\frac{\partial}{\partial \boldsymbol{\Theta}} = \left[\frac{\partial}{\partial \theta_1}, \quad \frac{\partial}{\partial \theta_2}, \quad \dots, \quad \frac{\partial}{\partial \theta_{n1}} \right]^T \tag{3.25}$$

$\mathbf{G}(\boldsymbol{\Theta})$ and τ denote the gravity terms and torque, respectively, which are defined below:

$$\mathbf{G}(\boldsymbol{\Theta}) = [G_1(\Theta), \quad G_2(\Theta), \quad \dots, \quad G_n(\Theta)]^T \tag{3.26}$$

$$\tau := [\tau_1, \quad \tau_2, \quad \dots, \quad \tau_n]^T \tag{3.27}$$

Since in this model, the dynamic equation around the contact point (the first equation) has no term for the Coriolis torque, it is written by

$$\frac{d}{dt}\left(m_1(\boldsymbol{\Theta})\dot{\boldsymbol{\Theta}}\right) - \mathbf{G}_1(\boldsymbol{\Theta}) = \boldsymbol{\tau}_1 \tag{3.28}$$

By differentiating Eq. 3.21 with respect to time, the following equation is acquired:

$$\dot{\boldsymbol{\Theta}} = \frac{\partial f(\theta)}{\partial \theta}\dot{\theta} = \left[\frac{\partial f_1(\theta)}{\partial \theta}, \quad \frac{\partial f_2(\theta)}{\partial \theta}, \quad \dots, \quad \frac{\partial f_n(\theta)}{\partial \theta} \right]^T \dot{\theta} \tag{3.29}$$

By substituting Eqs. 3.20, 3.21, and 3.29 into Eq. 3.22, the following dynamic equation is derived:

$$\frac{d}{dt}\left(M(\theta)\dot{\theta}\right) = G(\theta) \tag{3.30}$$

where

$$M(\theta) := m_1(f(\theta))^T \frac{df(\theta)}{d\theta} \tag{3.31}$$

$$G(\theta) := G_1(f(\theta)) \tag{3.32}$$

By multiplying both sides of Eq. 3.30 by $\mathbf{M}(\boldsymbol{\Theta})\dot{\theta}$ and then integrating with respect to time, the dynamics around the contact point is obtained as follows:

$$\int (M(\theta)\dot{\theta}) \frac{d}{dt}(M(\theta)\dot{\theta})dt = \int M(\theta)\dot{\theta}G(\theta)\dot{\theta}dt \tag{3.33}$$

$$\Leftrightarrow \frac{1}{2}(M(\theta)\dot{\theta})^2 = \int M(\theta)G(\theta)d\theta \tag{3.34}$$

Therefore, the whole robot dynamics is expressed as the following one-dimensional autonomous system:

$$\dot{\theta} = \frac{1}{M(\theta)}\sqrt{2\int M(\theta)G(\theta)d\theta} \tag{3.35}$$

$$:= \frac{1}{M(\theta)}\sqrt{2(D(\theta) + C)} \tag{3.36}$$

$$:= F(\theta) \tag{3.37}$$

Equations 3.35 and 3.36 constitute converged dynamics. By setting the desired dynamics to Eq. 3.37, a robot achieves a desired dynamic motion. However, it is quite difficult to solve the inverse problem, which involves finding the virtual holonomic constraint, Eq. 3.21, so as to satisfy the desired dynamics. Therefore, the virtual constraint is empirically designed based on the condition of the desired posture upon foot contact or perhaps a desired center of gravity (COG) trajectory.

Here, we have to consider an unsolved problem with PDAC. To obtain the converged dynamics by utilizing PDAC, Eqs. 3.33 and 3.34 should be integrable. However, the condition of virtual constraint whereby Eq. 3.33 would be made integrable has not yet been clarified. Thus, to make PDAC more practical, it is necessary to find such a condition or to propose an approximate calculation method or deriving algorithm for the converged dynamics without using integration. Making PDAC integrable is an area for future work.

3.5.2 PDAC Constant

Since converged dynamics is autonomous and independent of time, it is considered a conservative system. The integral constant on the right-hand side of Eq. 3.34, C, is a conserved quantity and is termed the PDAC constant. Its value is decided according to the initial condition (in biped walking, the state immediately after foot contact) and kept constant during a cycle of motion.

The dimension of the PDAC constant is equal to the square of angular momentum and is relevant to it. As is well known, assuming that the robot shown in Fig. 3.2 resides in the horizontal plane, the angular momentum around the contact point is conserved since there is no effect of the gravitational force on the robot dynamics. In this condition, it is clear that $M(\theta)\dot{\theta}$ (angular momentum) $= \sqrt{2C}$ from Eq. 3.36, since in Eq. 3.8 hence $D(\theta) = 0$. Note that the PDAC constant is conserved since it includes the effects of gravity, although angular momentum is not conserved when the robot dynamics is affected by gravity. In conclusion, the PDAC constant is a conserved quantity derived by embedding the gravity term into angular momentum around the contact point.

3.5.3 Interlocking Dynamics

As mentioned above, PDAC is based on two premises—passivity and virtual holonomic constraint. These premises make it possible to describe the whole robot dynamics as a one-dimensional autonomous system, and as a result a simple and valid controller based on the robot dynamics can be designed. However, there is a possibility of holonomic constraint of the joint angles causing a problem if the robot vibrates and the controller loses its stability during locomotion, especially at the moment when the impact force is applied, such as upon foot contact with a biped robot. This is because all the other active joints vibrate when the passive joint starts vibrating. Interlocking dynamics is employed as a control technique to solve this problem. In this method, all the robot joints are controlled according to the desired dynamics derived from the interlocking function Eq. 3.21 and the target dynamics Eq. 3.38 as follows:

$$\dot{\theta}_i = \frac{\partial f_i}{\partial \theta} F\left(f_i^{-1}(\theta_i)\right) \quad (i = 1, 2, 3, \cdots) \tag{3.38}$$

The joint angles derived from the desired dynamics are not always the same as the actual joint angles. The desired trajectories are adjusted slightly based on the error between the desired joint angle derived from the interlocking functions and the actual joint angles as follows:

$$\dot{\theta}_1^d = F\left(f_1^{-1}(\theta_1)\right) \tag{3.39}$$

$$\dot{\theta}_i^d = \frac{\partial f_i}{\partial \theta} F\left(f_i^{-1}(\theta_i)\right) + k_i(f_i(\theta) - \theta_i) \ \ (i = 2, 3, \cdots) \tag{3.40}$$

$$\Leftrightarrow \dot{\mathbf{\Theta}}^d := F_D(\mathbf{\Theta}) \tag{3.41}$$

where k_i is the connection strength determined empirically. This second term of Eq. 3.40 becomes zero if the robot dynamics is ideally identified and there are no physical disturbances.

3.5.4 Virtual Passive Joint

Most humanoid robots can generally be fully actuated, e.g., the ankle joints have actuators for standing on a slope. Such robots use actuators with a high reduction-ratio gear to generate sufficient joint torque with limited actuator weight. A high reduction gear has high viscosity. To apply PDAC to such robots with high reduction gears, it is necessary to diminish the joint viscosity to simulate the point-contact state.

It is generally known that viscosity is associated with angular velocity; that is, the viscous torque of joints can be expressed and compensated for as the function of the angular velocity as follows:

$$\tau_\beta = \beta\left(\dot{\theta}^d\right) = \beta \circ F(\theta) \tag{3.42}$$

Note that the viscous torque is estimated based on the desired angular velocity.

In addition, a slight departure can be made from the assumption that the point contact enhances the convergence of the robot dynamics toward the desired dynamics. For instance, the following torque is applied to the passive joint, such as the ankle of a support leg:

$$\tau_\beta = \beta\left(\dot{\theta}^d\right) + \tau_{fb} = \beta \circ F(\theta) + \tau_{fb} = \beta \circ F(\theta) + k_\beta\left(F(\theta) - \dot{\theta}\right) \tag{3.43}$$

The second term on the right-hand side of Eq. 3.43 is a feedback term. Various forms of τ_{fb} can be employed, such as PID, PI, and PD. Note that all gains in the feedback term have to be set at quite small values since the objective of this term is to attenuate the slight error that arises from the modeling error. It is believed that the controller performance can be more greatly enhanced if the controller updates the robot dynamics model adaptively according to the error of the dynamics.

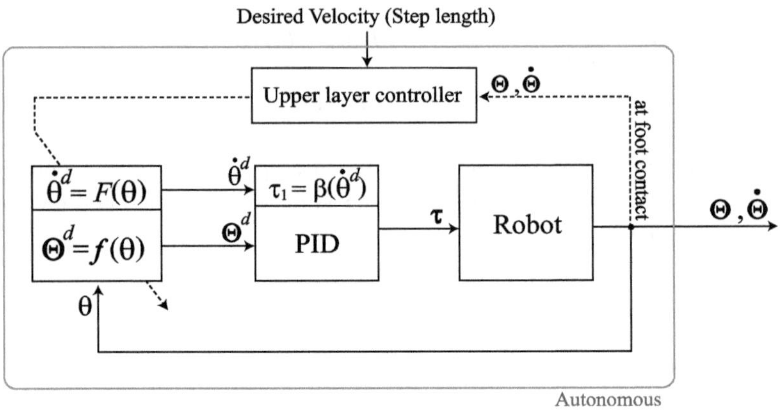

Fig. 3.3 Block diagram of PDAC in bipedal locomotion without interlocking dynamics

3.5.5 Control Architecture

Figure 3.3 is a block diagram of PDAC in bipedal locomotion without interlocking dynamics. The control loop including the robot (enclosed by the gray line) has no input from outside the controller; thus, it can be considered that the control system is autonomous. This autonomy makes it possible to achieve natural dynamic motion based on the inherent dynamics of the robot. The loop indicated by the broken line is executed only at the moment of foot contact. In this loop, the virtual holonomic constraint and the converged dynamics of the next step are updated according to both the robot status and the desired parameters, such as walking velocity. This update makes it possible to stabilize walking or vary the walking parameters, such as length of stride and walking direction.

Figure 3.4 is a block diagram of PDAC in bipedal locomotion with interlocking dynamics. The interlocking dynamics has no effect on autonomy of the controller since the interlocking dynamics affects only the left-hand block of the control loop. The angular velocity of active joints is controlled by PD control.

Additionally, the controller with a weak feedback for modeling error is shown in Fig. 3.5 The controller measures the actual angular velocity around the contact point and calculates the compensation torque to attenuate the error between the desired and the actual dynamics. Note that the feedback gain is quite small; hence this feedback has a weak effect. If there is the possibility of the robot falling over based on information from the sensors, the robot controller is switched to the falling-avoidance controller, as depicted in Fig. 3.5.

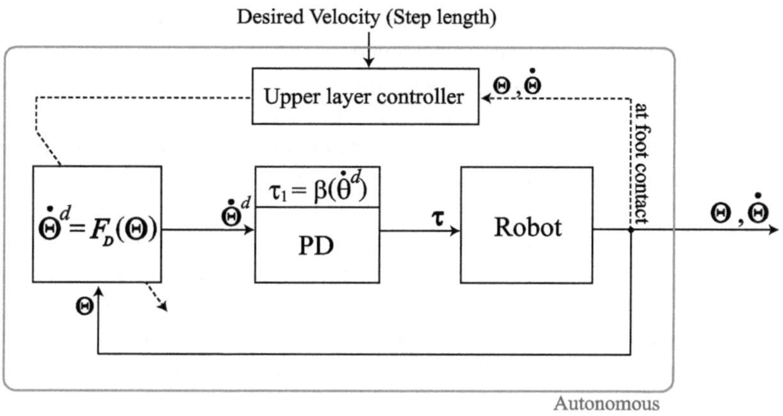

Fig. 3.4 Block diagram of PDAC in bipedal locomotion with interlocking dynamics

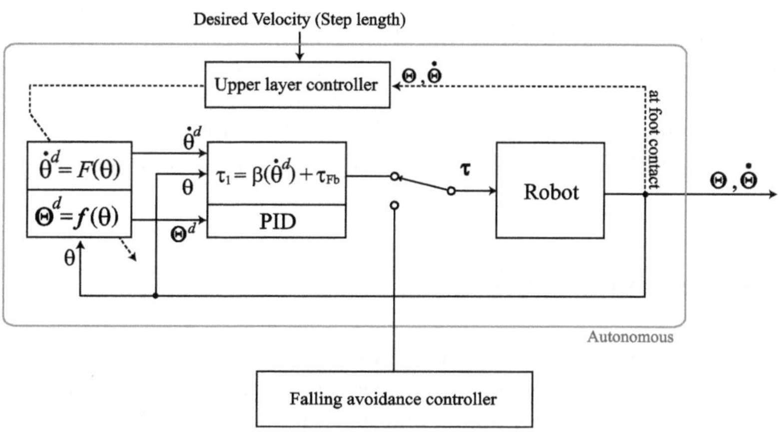

Fig. 3.5 Block diagram of PDAC in bipedal locomotion with weak feedback for modeling-error compensation

3.5.6 Advantages of PDAC

PDAC has the several advantages. The first is related to PDAC constant and converged dynamics. Although robot dynamics is a high degree-of-freedom complex system, it can be expressed as a one-dimensional autonomous system, i.e., the phase around the contact point. This one-dimensional dynamics is called converged dynamics and it facilitates robot dynamics and control over a desired motion. In addition, converged dynamics includes the conserved quantity that is theoretically maintained constant when walking even if conservation of angular momentum and energy conservation are not satisfied. This conserved quantity, termed the PDAC constant, makes it possible to stabilize motion, analyze it, and ensure the stability of the walking dynamics.

The second advantage is ease of motion design. Dynamic motion that is based on robot dynamics can be easily designed if the motion satisfies the postural constraints given by an operator or determined by environmental conditions. The PDAC method enables us to design the desired path of postural motion by adequately setting the virtual holonomic constraint. For example, a robot can avoid obstacles or maintain a certain posture at a particular inclination when performing some tasks.

The third advantage is passivity. A robot controlled by PDAC has a passive joint. The rest of the robot's joints are controlled through the passive joint. The whole motion of the robot pauses whenever rotation of the passive joint is stopped by an external force. The passive joint works as a kind of sensor to detect a robot's conflict with the environment. To achieve the same function in active walking, a robot is equipped with extensive touch sensors all over its body.

The fourth is to compensate for the disadvantages of active walking and passive walking, when it is applied to a biped walking design. It is basically difficult for active walking to utilize the natural dynamics of the robot since all the joints are controlled by a high-gain feedback. Hence, active walking has the following disadvantages compared with passive walking: (1) unnatural walking motion; (2) vulnerability to ground irregularities; (3) low energy efficiency. Passive walking has the following disadvantages: (1) highly limited capability to walk; (2) low tolerance of disturbances; (3) inability to perform another task while walking.

3.6 Application of PDAC

PDAC is applied to various kinds of motions of a mobile robot. Doi et al. [12] utilized PDAC to design three-dimensional biped walking based on two two-dimensional dynamics in the lateral and sagittal planes. Doi et al. [13, 14] enhanced the two-dimensional dynamics to three-dimensional dynamics and then applied proof stability to the dynamics. Doi et al. [15] also designed a brachiation controller. Brachiation is arboreal locomotion using the arms to swing like a monkey from branch to branch through the trees. Asano et al. [16] developed a controller for quadruped walking using the PDAC concept. An example of the controller design using PDAC is introduced in this section.

3.6.1 Biped Walking Design

We designed the lateral motion by means of PDAC, as depicted in Fig. 3.6. In phase A, a robot starts to turn over toward its swing-leg side and is accelerated by gravitation from the tilting position at a standstill on the stance-leg side to foot contact. In phase B, after foot contact, the robot achieves the tilting position at standstill by the energy obtained in phase A. Since the mechanical energy is lost at

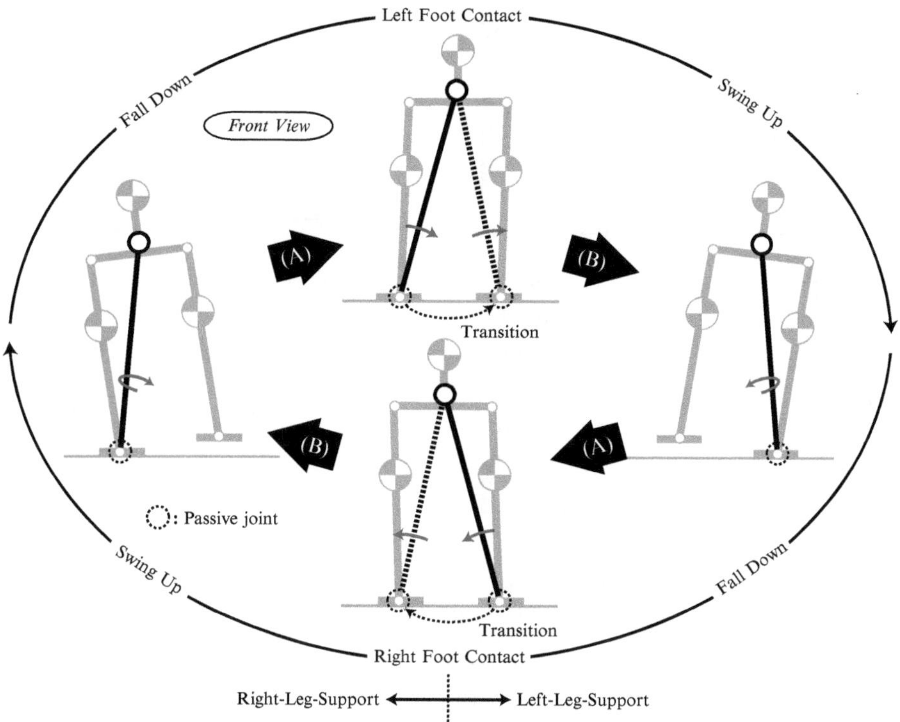

Fig. 3.6 Lateral motion of lateral-based walk (*front view*). The inverted pendulum falls in phase A and swings up in phase B

foot contact, the robot compensates for the lost energy by lifting its pelvis in both phases to continue the side-to-side rocking motion. It is possible to consider the lifts of the pelvis approximately as the change in pendulum length. The model shown in Fig. 3.7 is used as a model of the lateral motion: two inverted pendulums, which are opposite each other, continue to rock, iterating the collision between them. The right-hand figure in Fig. 3.7 shows the trajectory of COG and two coordinate systems, $\sum^R$ and $\sum^L$, which correspond to the right- and left-leg-support period, respectively.

3.6.2 Phase Portrait Coalescence

Lateral motion is considered in terms of dynamics. Figure 3.8a shows the phase portrait of an inverted pendulum in the coordinate system $\sum^R$ and $\sum^L$.

Lateral motion continues by switching these coordinate systems at foot contact. Coalescence of the phase portrait in $\sum^R$ and $\sum^L$ yields that of lateral motion, as shown in Fig. 3.8b. As can be seen in this figure, in the gray tetragon surrounded by

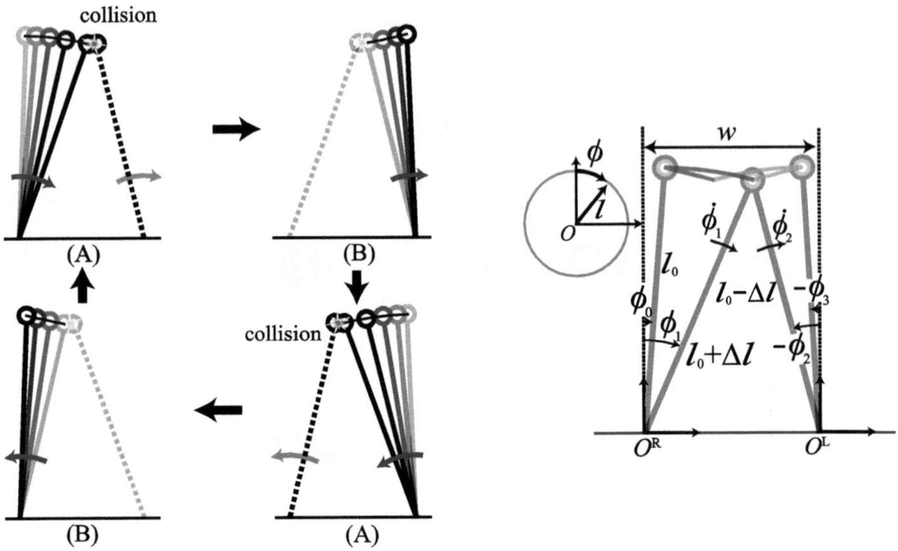

Fig. 3.7 (*Left figure*) Motion of CIPM. The impact between the foot and the ground is regarded as that between two pendulums. *A* and *B* correspond to *A* and *B* in Fig. 3.6. *Figure on the right*: trajectory of COG and polar coordinate systems. l and ϕ denote the length and the angle of an inverted pendulum. (l_0,ϕ_0) and $\left(l_0 + \Delta l, \dot{\phi}_1\right)$ are the coordinates in $\sum^R$ at the beginning and ending of phase A, ($l_0 + \Delta l$, ϕ_2),and (l_0,ϕ_3) is that of $\sum^L$ of phase B, respectively. ϕ_1 and $\dot{\phi}_2$ denote the angular velocity at the end of phase A and the beginning of phase B, respectively

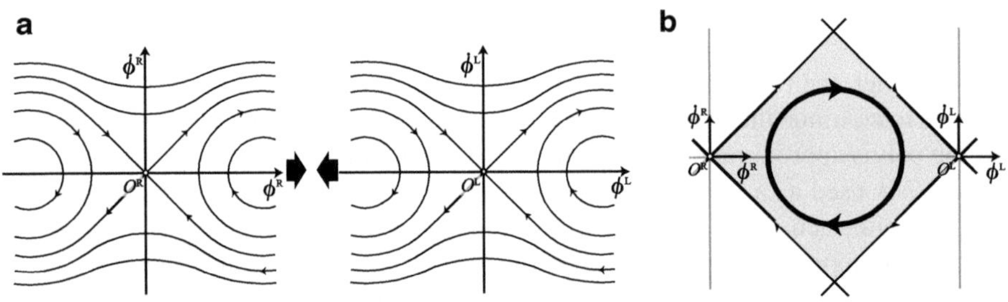

Fig. 3.8 (**a**) Phase portraits of ϕ^R and ϕ^L (**b**) Coalescence of the phase portrait in $\sum^R$ and $\sum^L$

the pair of separatrices, the dynamics has the property to rotate, which implies lateral sway motion. Stable lateral motion is achieved only in this zone. That is, if the actual dynamics is outside it, an inverted pendulum—i.e., a robot—falls over, and stable motion cannot be continued unless some compensation takes place.

The effect of the pelvis lift on lateral dynamics is explained by use of the virtual COG trajectory shown in Fig. 3.9a. In this trajectory, the pendulum length is switched virtually from l_0 to $l_0 + \Delta l$ instantaneously at the shift from phase B to A, which, however, cannot be actually achieved in practice. The pendulum length is kept at $l_0 + \Delta l$ in phase A and l_0 in phase B. If $l = l_0 - \Delta l$, the absolute

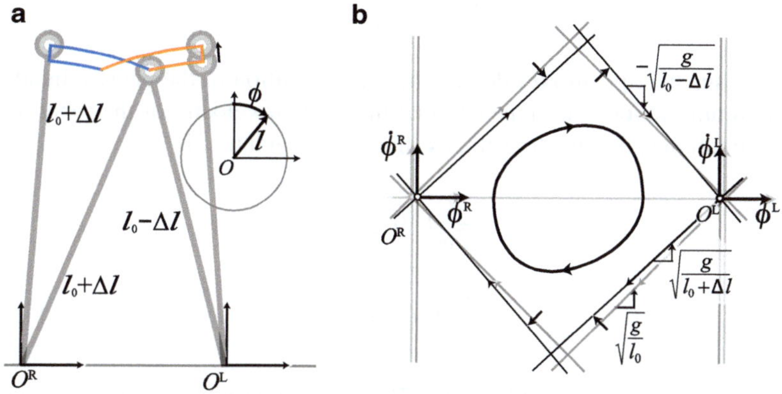

Fig. 3.9 (**a**) Virtual trajectory designed as follows: $l = l_0 + \Delta l$ in phase A and $l = l_0 - \Delta l$ in phase B, and the pendulum lengthens instantly and discontinuously $l_0 - \Delta l \rightarrow l_0 + \Delta l$ at the shift from phase B to A (**b**) CIPM map of this trajectory. Pendulum separatrices are approximately linear near the saddle points, and their gradients are $\pm\sqrt{g/l}$

value of the separatrices' gradient near the origin is lower than that of $l = l_0$, and if $l = l_0 + \Delta l$, the gradient is higher (see Fig. 3.9b). This deformation of the solution trajectory makes it possible to achieve the continuous side-to-side rocking motion.

3.6.3 *Virtual Holonomic Constraint of Lateral Joints*

A virtual constraint that is pendulum length l is described as the function of φ. It is clear that the right side of Eq. 3.44 can be integrated if $f(\varphi)$ is a polynomial equation. Thus in this section, $f(\varphi)$ is decided as follows:

$$l = f(\varphi) \tag{3.44}$$

$$= a\varphi^2 + b\varphi + c \tag{3.45}$$

where a, b, and c are determined so as to satisfy the conditions described below.

At first, the conditions of the pendulum length at the beginning and ending of phase A and phase B introduce the following four equations:

$$f^A(\varphi_0) = l_0 \tag{3.46}$$

$$f^A(\varphi_1) = l_0 + \Delta l \tag{3.47}$$

$$f^B(-\varphi_2) = l_0 - \Delta l \tag{3.48}$$

$$f^B(-\varphi_3) = l_0 \tag{3.49}$$

where the superscript suffixes denote the differentiation of the phases. In addition, the pendulum motion is designed so that the angular velocity of the robot joints is not discontinuous, that is, the velocity along the pendulum is zero:

$$\frac{\partial}{\partial \varphi} f^A(\varphi_1) = 0 \tag{3.50}$$

$$\frac{\partial}{\partial \varphi} f^B(-\varphi_2) = 0 \tag{3.51}$$

Using Eqs. 3.46, 3.47, 3.48, 3.49, 3.50, and 3.51, the coefficients a, b, and c in each phase are calculated.

3.6.4 Converged Dynamics

The dynamic equation of a general inverted pendulum is described as follows:

$$\frac{d}{dt}\left((ml^2 + J)\dot{\varphi}\right) = mgl \sin\varphi \tag{3.52}$$

Multiplying both sides of this equation by $(ml^2 + J)\dot{\varphi}$ and integrating with respect to time yields the following equations:

$$(ml^2 + J)\dot{\varphi}\frac{d}{dt}\left((ml^2 + J)\dot{\varphi}\right) = mgl(ml^2 + J)\dot{\varphi} \sin\varphi \tag{3.53}$$

$$\Leftrightarrow \frac{1}{2}\left((ml^2 + J)\dot{\varphi}\right)^2 = \int mgl(ml^2 + J)\dot{\varphi} \sin\varphi dt \tag{3.54}$$

$$\Leftrightarrow \dot{\varphi} = \frac{1}{ml^2 + J}\sqrt{2\int mgl(ml^2 + J)\dot{\varphi} \sin\varphi dt} \tag{3.55}$$

The phase around the contact point (phase of passive joint) is obtained from Eqs. 3.44 and 3.55 as follows:

$$\dot{\varphi} = \frac{1}{mf(\varphi)^2 + J}\sqrt{2\int mgf(\varphi)\left(mf(\varphi)^2 + J\right)\dot{\varphi} \sin\varphi dt} \tag{3.56}$$

$$:= \frac{1}{M_l(\varphi)}\sqrt{2(D_l(\varphi) + C_l)} \tag{3.57}$$

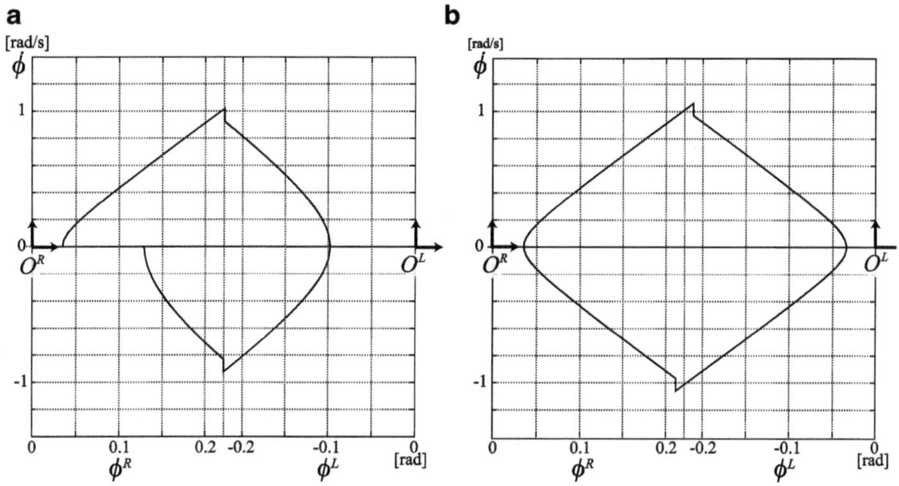

Fig. 3.10 Phase portrait of the lateral motion (simulation, $l_0 = 0.46$[m], $\phi_0 = \phi_3 = 0.28$[rad], $w = 0.2$[m]) (**a**) with no lift, (**b**) with lift

$$:= F(\varphi) \tag{3.58}$$

Finally, the value to lift the pelvis, Δl is determined. Δl has to be determined so that Eq. 3.58 satisfies the initial condition of phase A and the end condition of phase B, that is:

$$F_l^A(\varphi_0) = F_l^B(-\varphi_3) = 0 \tag{3.59}$$

$$\Leftrightarrow \frac{\sqrt{2\left(D_l^A(\varphi_1) - D_l^A(\varphi_0)\right)}}{M_l^A(\varphi_1)} \cos(\varphi_1 + \varphi_2) = \frac{\sqrt{2\left(D_l^B(-\varphi_2) - D_l^B(-\varphi_3)\right)}}{M_l^B(-\varphi_2)} \tag{3.60}$$

where the superscript suffixes denote the differentiation of phases. Δl is so small that it is possible to find the appropriate value that satisfies Eq. 3.60 by the use of quadratic approximation.

3.6.5 Simulation

Figure 3.10 shows the simulation results of the above-mentioned motion design under the condition $\varphi_0 = \varphi_3$. Although the motion is attenuated without lengthening the pendulum, as shown in Fig. 3.10a, the periodic motion is generated with lift, as shown in Fig. 3.10b.

3.6.6 Control of the Lateral Period

We designed the period controller of the lateral motion described in the previous subsection. The period of lateral motion is determined by the amplitude of the pendulum motion, i.e., if the period is long, the amplitude is large; if it is short, the amplitude is small. The period is adjusted by controlling the lateral amplitude.

Assuming that the pendulum angle at the transition from phase B to phase A is φ_3, the motion period T can be calculated using the following equation:

$$\int_{-\varphi_3}^{-\varphi_2} \frac{1}{F_B(\varphi)} d\varphi + \int_{\varphi_3}^{\varphi_1} \frac{1}{F_A(\varphi)} d\varphi = T \tag{3.61}$$

However, it is not easy to solve this equation for φ_3. The pendulum extension is so small that the desired amplitude is determined approximately by use of the model of the inverted pendulum, the length of which is not variable, as follows:

$$\varphi_3 = \frac{\varphi_C}{\cosh\left(\sqrt{\frac{g}{l_0}}\frac{T}{2}\right)} \tag{3.62}$$

where φ_C is the pendulum angle in the standing posture, i.e., the pendulum angle at foot contact under the condition of $\Delta l = 0$.

3.6.7 Stabilization by Landing Position Control

Various methods to stabilize the lateral motion were proposed by Hemami and Wyman [17], Miura and Shimoyama [18], Sano and Furusho [19], and Kuo [20]. This subsection introduces another stabilizing method to adjust the pendulum length and angle at foot contact according to the error between the phase around the contact point derived by PDAC and actual motion. With regard to the robot motion shown in Fig. 3.11, the state at foot contact is varied by opening or closing the swing leg in phase A. This motion has the following two effects:

- Change of the pendulum angle of the swing leg at foot contact, φ_2.
- Variation of the pendulum length on the side of swing leg at foot contact, $l_0 - \Delta l$.

Strictly speaking, the pendulum angle on the side of the stance leg at foot contact, φ_1, is also changed by this motion; however, its effect is so small that we do not consider it. Hence, in this section, it is assumed that φ_1 does not vary.

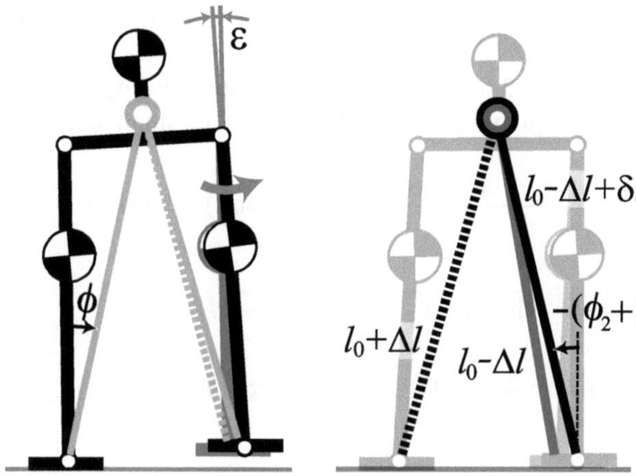

Fig. 3.11 Stabilization of lateral motion

We can describe the condition of the pendulum angle at the end of phase B as φ_3 below:

$$\frac{2\left(D_l^A(\varphi_1)+C_l\right)}{\left(M_l^A(\varphi_1)\right)^2}=\Phi(\varphi_2,l_0-\Delta l) \tag{3.63}$$

From Eq. 3.60, the right-hand side of Eq. 3.63 is described as

$$\Phi(\varphi_2,l_0-\Delta l)=\frac{2\left(D_l^B(-\varphi_2)-D_l^B(-\varphi_3)\right)}{(l_0-\Delta l)^2\cos^2(\varphi_1-\varphi_2)} \tag{3.64}$$

Here, we assume that the actual C_l has the error between the desired value and actual one, δC_l, and determine the landing position of a swing leg.

To stabilize the motion, it is necessary for the robot to satisfy the desired state at the end of phase (B), that is, $F_l^B(\varphi_3)=0$. Assuming that the robot opens its swing leg by ε and consequently φ_2 and $l_0-\Delta l$ are changed to $\varphi_2+\delta\varphi_2$ and $l_0-\Delta l+\delta l$, respectively. Equation 3.63 can be rewritten as follows:

$$\frac{2\left(D_l^A(\varphi_1)+C_l+\delta C_l\right)}{\left(M_l^A(\varphi_1)\right)^2}=\Phi(\varphi_2+\delta\varphi_2,l_0-\Delta l+\delta l) \tag{3.65}$$

In addition, from the geometric condition, the following two equations are obtained:

$$(l_0-\Delta l)\cos\varphi_2=(l_0-\Delta l+\delta l)\cos(\varphi_2+\delta\varphi_2) \tag{3.66}$$

$$(l_0 - \Delta l + \delta l)\cos(\varphi_2 + \delta\varphi_2) - (l_0 - \Delta l)\sin\varphi_2 = L_\varepsilon \tag{3.67}$$

ε is calculated by Eqs. 3.63, 3.64, 3.65, 3.66, and 3.67 by assuming that it is possible to neglect the squared term of Δ because of its small size.

$$\varepsilon = \frac{(l_0 - \Delta l)\cos\varphi}{L}(\tan(\varphi_2 + \delta\varphi_2) - \tan\varphi_2) \tag{3.68}$$

$$\delta\varphi_2 = \frac{\cos\varphi_2}{\Phi_{\varphi_2}\cos\varphi_2 + \Phi_{l_0-\Delta l}(l_0 - \Delta l)\sin\varphi_2}\delta C \tag{3.69}$$

where $\Phi_{\varphi_2} = \frac{\partial\Phi}{\partial\varphi_2}(\varphi_2, l_0 - \Delta l)$ and $\Phi_{l_0-\Delta l} = \frac{\partial\Phi}{\partial(l_0-\Delta l)}(\varphi_2, l_0 - \Delta l)$.

3.6.8 Simulation

The simulation result of this feedback control is shown in Fig. 3.12, where $\varphi_0 = \varphi_3$. In this simulation, we assign a certain error to the robot and confirm the convergence by the control method described above. As shown in Fig. 3.12a, c, if the actual angular velocity is higher than the desired one, the lateral dynamics diverges; if the actual angular velocity is lower than the desired one, it is attenuated.

However, as shown in Fig. 3.12b, d, the controller with the feedback makes the stated error and converges on the desired state after foot contact.

3.7 Concluding Remarks

This chapter introduced some motion control algorithms of a mechanical system with a redundant degree of freedom, especially PDAC. PDAC is also a control method for a redundant mechanical system based on point contact and virtual holonomic constraint. These control algorithms will be useful in helping a powered orthotic system, prosthesis, and exoskeleton with a redundant degree of freedom to support human motion in a dexterous, synchronized fashion. In addition, the converged dynamics of the two-dimensional inverted pendulum model has been introduced as an example of PDAC applications; its stabilization has been discussed using the results of numerical simulations. Though this chapter has been limited to a two-dimensional model, a converged dynamics of the three-dimensional inverted pendulum model has been proposed by Doi et al. [21]. The stability of this converged dynamics has been confirmed by Doi et al. [14]. Aoyama et al. [22] has been able to control walking direction by means of two PDAC constants. For further details on these studies, consult the papers listed in the References section.

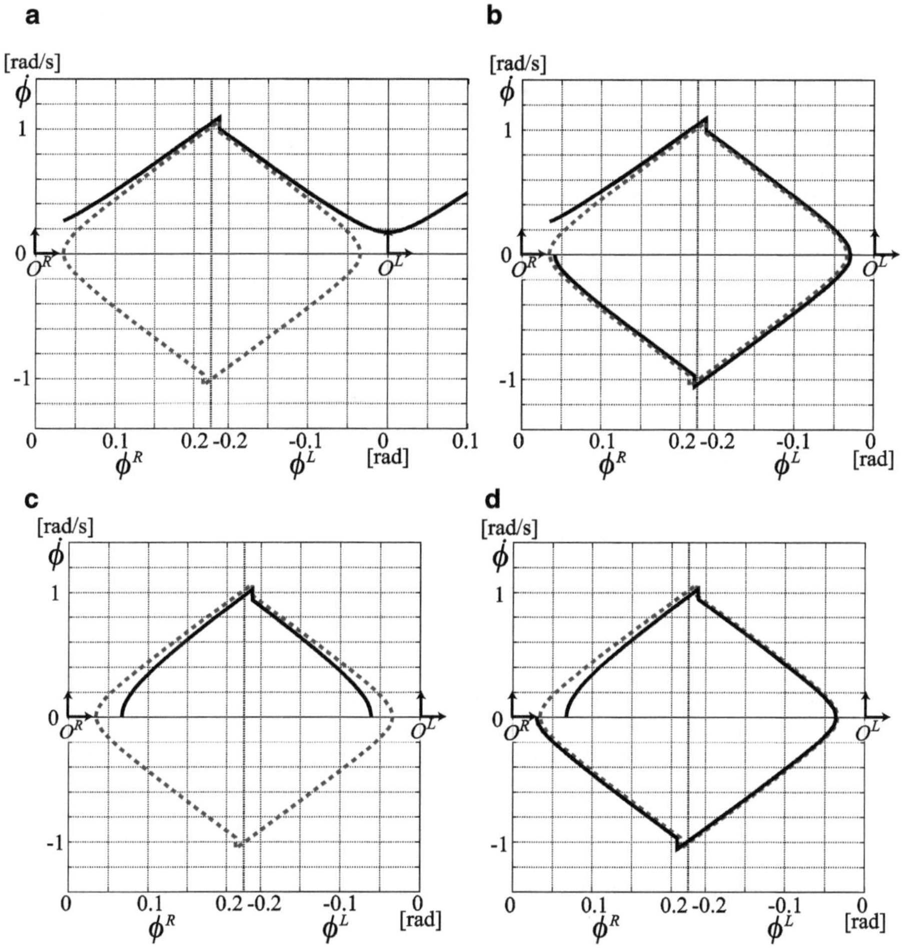

Fig. 3.12 Simulation results of the feedback of lateral motion (**a**) $\delta\dot{\phi} > 0$ without the feedback, (**b**) $\delta\dot{\phi} < 0$ with the feedback, (**c**) $\delta\dot{\phi} > 0$ without the feedback, (**d**) $\delta\dot{\phi} < 0$ with the feedback

References

1. Morasso P (1981) Spatial control of arm movements. Exp Brain Res 42:223–227
2. Abend W, Bizzi E, Morasso P (1982) Human arm trajectory formation. Brain 105:331–348
3. Hogan N (1984) An organizing principle for a class of voluntary movements. J Neurosci 4 (11):2745–2754
4. Flash T, Hogan N (1985) The coordination of arm movement: an experimentally confirmed mathematical model. J Neurosci 5(7):1688–1703
5. Uno Y, Kawato M, Suzuki R (1989) Formation and control of optimal trajectory in human multijoint arm movement. Minimum torque-change model. Biol Cybern 61(2):89–101
6. Yoshikawa T (1985) Manipulability of robotic mechanisms. J Robot Res 4(2):3–9

7. Khatib O (1987) A unified approach for motion and force control of robot manipulators: the operational space formulation. IEEE J Robot Autom RA-3(1):43–53
8. Hollerback JM, Suh KC (1987) Redundancy resolution of manipulators through torque optimization. IEEE J Robot Autom RA-3(4):308–316
9. Arimoto S, Hashiguchi H, Sekimoto M, Ozawa R (2005) Generation of natural motions for redundant multi-joint systems: a differential-geometric approach based upon the principle of least actions. J Field Robot 22(11):583–605
10. Grizzle JW, Abba G, Plestan F (2001) Asymptotically stable walking for biped robots: analysis via systems with impulse effects. IEEE Trans Automat Contr 46(1):51–64
11. Westervelt ER, Buche G, Grizzle J (2004) Experimental validation of a framework for the design of controllers that induce stable walking in planar bipeds. Int J Robot Res 23 (6):559–582
12. Doi M, Hasegawa Y, Fukuda T (2004) Passive dynamic control of bipedal walking. In: Proceedings of IEEE-RAS/RSJ international conference on humanoid robots. Los Angeles, CA, USA, pp 3049–3054
13. Doi M, Matsuno T, Hasegawa Y, Fukuda T (2006) Proposal of smooth biped walking control by means of heel-off motion. In: Proceedings of the 2006 I.E. international conference on robotics and automation (ICRA2006). Orlando, Florida, USA, pp 1591–1596
14. Doi M, Hasegawa Y, Matsuno T, Fukuda T (2007) Stability proof of biped walking control based on point-contact. Proceedings of the 2007 I.E. international conference on robotics and automation. Roma, Italy, pp 3204–3209
15. Doi M, Kojima S, Matsuno T, Fukuda T, Hasegawa Y (2006) Analytical design method of Brachiation controller on the irregular ladder. In: Proceedings of the first IEEE/RAS-EMBS international conference on biomedical robotics and biomechatronics, (BIOROB 2006). Pisa, Tuscany, Italy
16. Asano Y, Doi M, Hasegawa Y, Matsuno T, Fukuda T (2007) Quadruped walking by joint-interlocking control based on the assumption of point-contact: comparison between pace gait and crawl gait based on the energy consumption. Trans JSME C73(725):230–236 (in Japanese)
17. Hemami H, Wyman BF (1979) Modeling and control of constrained dynamic systems with application to biped locomotion in the frontal plane. IEEE Trans Automat Contr AC-24 (4):526–535
18. Miura H, Shimoyama I (1984) Dynamic walking of a biped. Int J Robot Res 3(2):60–74
19. Sano A, Furusho J (1991) Realization of dynamic quadruped locomotion in pace gait by controlling walking cycle. International symposium on experimental robotics. Toulouse, France, pp 491–502
20. Kuo AD (1999) Stabilization of lateral motion in passive dynamic walking. Int J Robot Res 18 (9):917–930
21. Doi M, Hasegawa Y, Fukuda T (2005) 3D dynamic walking based on the inverted pendulum model with two degree of underactuation. In: Proceedings of 2005 IEEE/RSJ international conference on intelligent robots and systems. Edmonton, Alberta, Canada, pp 2788–2793
22. Aoyama T, Hasegawa Y, Sekiyama K, Fukuda T (2009) Stabilizing and direction control of efficient 3-D biped walking based on PDAC. IEEE/ASME Trans Mechatron 14(6):712–718

Chapter 4
Motor Control and Learning

Kiyotaka Kamibayashi

Abstract Human movements are controlled by the interaction between the central program and peripheral feedback. In this chapter, to understand the human motor control mechanism, the physiological basis of the sensory-motor systems for the movement is explained. In particular, a detailed explanation of the neural mechanism for locomotion is provided. Next, the mechanism of motor learning is described. Finally, our experimental results from using a robotic gait orthois, on how somatosensory inputs influence the excitability of neural circuits during human locomotion, are shown.

Keywords Human movement • Motor system • Walking • Brain • Spinal cord • Corticospinal tract • Spinal reflex

4.1 Introduction

From waking in the morning to going to sleep at night, we perform many kinds of movements. Even though these actions involve many muscles and joints, they are made smoothly without much attention. Executing action towards a goal requires a process of correctly recognizing the surroundings, selecting the corresponding movement for them, and making a plan. Because external environments change moment by moment during movement, we need to update our movements to correspond to sensory information. Furthermore, even for a novel movement, by repeatedly practicing, the necessary motions are learned, and it becomes possible to control the movement more effectively. In this section, the physiological basis of the sensory-motor systems for the generation of movement will be explained. In particular, a detailed explanation of the neural mechanism for walking, a locomotor

K. Kamibayashi (✉)
Faculty of Health and Sports Sciences, Doshisha University, Kyoto, Japan
e-mail: kkamibay@mail.doshisha.ac.jp

Y. Sankai et al. (eds.), *Cybernics: Fusion of human, machine and information systems*,
DOI 10.1007/978-4-431-54159-2_4, © Springer Japan 2014

behavior specific to humans, will be provided. Next, the mechanism of motor learning will be described. Finally our research results regarding human bipedal locomotion, on how somatosensory inputs influence the excitability of neural circuits, will be shown.

4.2 Motor Systems

4.2.1 Motor Unit

The skeletal muscle which generates movement is formed of muscle fibers, and the muscle fibers are subdivided into bundles of myofibrils (Fig. 4.1). The myofibril contains contractile proteins, thick filaments called myosin and thin filaments called actin. In a contracting muscle, thick and thin filaments slide past each other, and form cross-bridges between the myosin and actin which generate a contractile force. This contractile machinery is called the "sliding filament hypothesis" [1]. Skeletal muscle fibers are classified into slow-twitch fibers (type I) and fast-twitch fibers (type II) depending on its contractile characteristics. The slow muscle fibers produce a relatively small force for a long time without fatigue. The fast muscle fibers can contract quickly and exert a large force. The fast muscle fibers are further categorized into two subtypes (IIA and IIB) depending on differences in oxidative enzyme activity. The fast fatigue-resistant (type IIA) fibers have relatively fast twitch dynamics and fatigue-resistance for several minutes. The fast fatigable (type IIB) fibers have the highest contractile velocity but low resistance to fatigue.

The command to the muscle fibers to contact is transmitted from the motor neurons (MNs) in the spinal cord. One MN is connected to multiple muscle fibers (Fig. 4.1). Therefore, when one MN excites, all of the multiple muscle fibers which are connected to it receive a command to contract. A functional unit which consists of one MN and the muscle fibers that it innervates is called a motor unit. A muscle consists of a number of motor units. Motor units are also classified into fast twitch

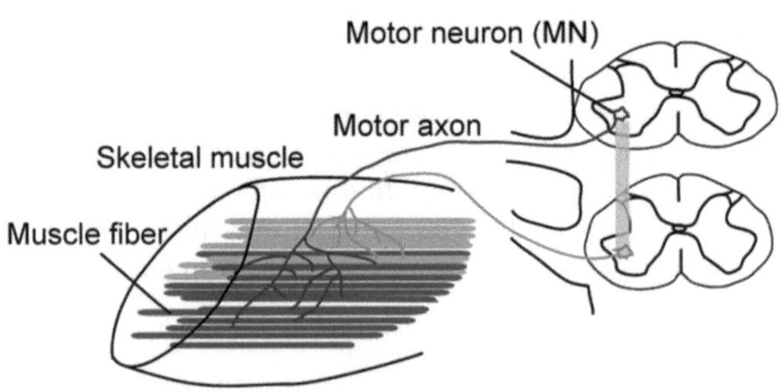

Fig. 4.1 Motor unit consisting of a motor neuron and muscle fibers which consist of bundles of myofibrils

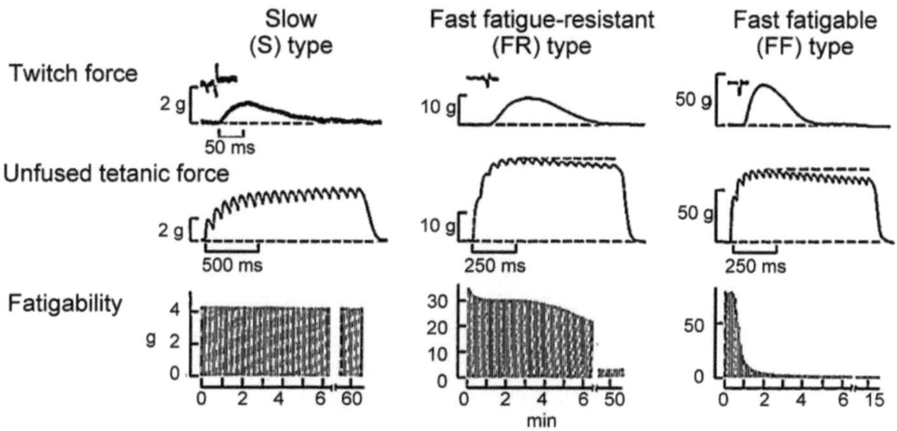

Fig. 4.2 Twitch, tetanic force, and fatigability of three motor unit types (Modified from Burke et al. [2])

(F) type, where the velocity and force of contraction are large, and slow (S) type, where the velocity and force of contraction are small [2] (Fig. 4.2). Similar to the muscle fiber types, the F type motor unit is classified into the easily-tiring fast fatigable (FF) type and the fast fatigue-resistant (FR) type.

The MNs receive descending input from supraspinal centers and peripheral input from the sensory receptors [3]. If the membrane potential of a MN is raised above the threshold potential by excitatory input to the neuron, an action potential in the neuron is produced. By firing the action potential, the signal is propagated along the axon of the MN, and the action potential releases transmitters at the nerve-muscle synapse. Because there is space between the motor axon and muscle, the signals are transmitted by the release of chemical substances. This produces electrical potentials in the muscle, which are recorded using surface electrodes on the skin as an electromyogram (EMG). The strength of muscle contraction depends on the number of recruited motor units and their individual firing rates [4]. When executing voluntary movement, type S motor units, which exert weak muscle force, are activated in weaker muscle contractions, and when the contraction level becomes stronger, type F motor units are recruited. Some of the descending systems from the supraspinal centers connect directly to the MNs to excite them, but most of descending pathways affect indirectly to the MNs via the interneurons in the spinal cord.

4.2.2 Motor Cortical Areas

The muscle contractions which generate movements are controlled by the excitation of MNs, and the inputs to the MNs are regulated by the central nervous system composed of the brain and the spinal cord. The brain is classified into the cerebral

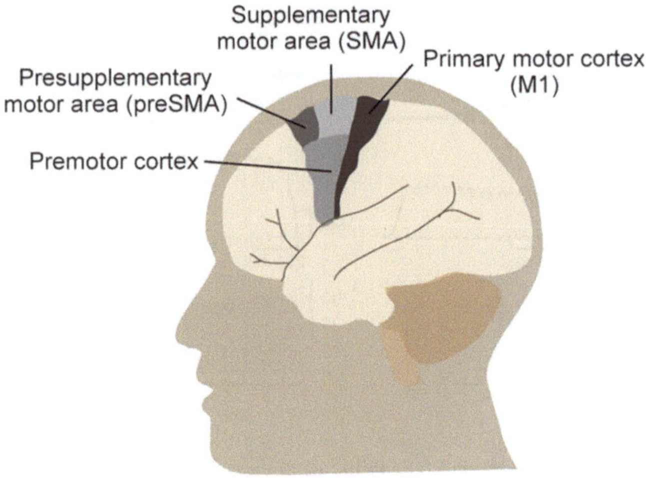

Fig. 4.3 Motor-related areas of the cerebral cortex

cortex, the diencephalon, the brainstem, and the cerebellum. The diencephalon contains two major subdivisions: the thalamus and hypothalamus. In the primates, including humans, the most recently evolved part of the brain is the cerebral cortex. Many areas of the cerebral cortex are concerned primarily with processing sensory information or transmitting motor commands. An area just rostral to the central sulcus of the cerebral cortex is called the primary motor cortex (M1), which is intimately associated with the motor systems of the spinal cord (Fig. 4.3). Penfield and Boldrey [5] electrically stimulated the motor cortical area in humans, and elucidated the relationship between the stimulated area of the brain and the evoked muscle contraction. The areas for the lower limbs, trunk, upper arms, hands, and face are arranged from the top to the bottom of the precentral gyrus. This is called somatotopic organization or somatotopic representation. The area of M1 devoted to the fingers and face are large, but the area for the trunk is small.

One of the characteristics of the M1 is that it possesses neurons which project their axons directly to the spinal cord. The output pathway of the neuron in layer V of the M1 is called the corticospinal tract. The majority of the fibers of the corticospinal tract cross at the medulla oblongata, and the signal from right side of the brain is sent to the left side of the body. Their targets of connection are the interneurons and MNs in the spinal cord. This synapse connection enables the cells of the motor cortex to send signals directly to the spinal neurons. The monosynaptic connections to MNs are well developed in humans, and they are considered to be what makes skilful movement of the hands and fingers possible. The fibers of the corticospinal tract are separated into nerve branches, so that one cell of the M1 controls multiple neurons in the spinal cord. It has actually been demonstrated that one cell of the M1 controls several hand muscles [6]. The M1 cells seem to have a variety of functions simultaneously, such as controlling interneurons to regulate the amount of somatosensory information sent to the brain at the spinal level. There are also pathways from the M1 which do not cross the medulla oblongata but descend on the same side. Regarding the question as to what firing rates of neurons in the M1 encodes, it has been hypothesized that it expresses the amount of force used in the movement [7]. There have also been reports linking cell activity to the direction of movement [8]. Regarding the direction of reaching movements, it appears that individual cells have a wide range of direction selectivity, and they act as a cell cluster of the M1 to encode the movement direction.

In addition to the M1, the premotor cortex and the supplementary motor area (SMA) are known as motor-related cortical areas (Fig. 4.3). The premotor cortex is located primarily on the lateral surface of the brain, just rostral to the M1. The SMA is located on the medial surface, also just rostral to the M1. The rostral part to the SMA is called the presupplementary motor area (preSMA). Furthermore, the cingulate motor area resides in the banks of the cingulate sulcus in the medial surface of the cerebral hemisphere. In recent years, a more detailed classification has been carried out. The premotor cortex is classified into dorsal and ventral areas, and the cingulate motor area is subdivided into rostral and caudal parts [9, 10]. The premotor cortex, the SMA, and the cingulate motor areas give information to the M1 based on sensory information and memory information.

At the start of a visual guided motor task, activity of neurons in the premotor area starts about 50 ms before activity of neurons in the M1 [11]. Thus, they are thought to be involved in the planning and preparation of a movement. The dorsal and ventral areas of the premotor cortex receive inputs from different parts of the parietal lobe. The dorsal premotor area receives inputs from the superior parietal lobule, whereas the ventral premotor area receives inputs from the inferior parietal lobule. The input from the prefrontal cortex also differs between the dorsal and ventral areas of the premotor cortex. The dorsal premotor area is crucial for motor planning to decide what to do and which action to perform. Hoshi and Tanji [10] proposed that the ventral premotor area receives information on a motor target and sends outputs to achieve an action that directly matches the information, while the dorsal premotor has a major role in indirect sensorimotor processing, retrieving multiple sets of motor information from sensory signals, and integrating components of a required action. It has also been reported that in the premotor cortex of the monkey, there are cells which activate both when the monkey performs an action and when he observes an experimenter's similar action [12]. From these research results, it is interpreted that the premotor areas have major roles in preparing and executing movements.

It is considered that the SMA has a rough somatotopic representation [9]. The neurons in the SMA receive sensory information. In the SMA, electrical stimulation is less effective than in the M1, and the induced movement is more complex. This area is involved in movements which are based on internal information like memories, such as the sequence control of finger movements [13]. In functional brain imaging studies using positron emission tomography (PET), it has been observed that the SMA is activated during sequential movements [14, 15]. It has also been reported that even when movement does not take place, merely imagining the movement causes activity in this area [14]. Thus, it is thought that the SMA plays the role of preparing a sequence of motions in response to memory and sending information to the M1. When lesion occurs to this part, actions such as the sequence control of finger movements are impaired. After a long period of practice of a simple reaction motor task, the number of cells in the SMA with movement-related activity was extremely low but after lesions of the M1, the cells in bilateral SMA were very active with a high frequency [16]. The SMA seems to involve a compensatory role for movement.

As for the preSMA, there is almost no direct projection from the preSMA to the M1 or the spinal cord, but there are some fiber connections to motor-related cortical areas other than the M1 [9]. This indicates that the SMA has a more direct access to motor effectors than the preSMA. There is no clear somatic representation, and it has been shown that it does not respond to somatosensory stimuli [9]. With increasing sequence complexity of finger movements, regional cerebral blood flow in the contralateral preSMA was increased, implicating a motor executive role [17].

The cingulate motor areas are connected to other motor-related cortical areas and the subcortical motor-related parts. The cingulate motor areas can induce limb movements in response to electrical stimuli. The PET findings indicated that the rostral cingulate motor area activated in relation to complex tasks and the caudal cingulate motor area activated during simpler tasks [9]. It is also suggested that the rostral cingulate motor area plays a part in processing the reward information for motor selection [18].

4.2.3 Subcortical Regions

In addition to the motor-related regions of the cerebral cortex, subcortical regions such as the cerebellum and basal ganglia are also deeply involved in the motor control and motor learning. The M1 for the appropriate function needs to exchange information with the cerebellum, as well as functional modification by the basal ganglia. The motor-related cortical areas output the signals to the cerebellum and basal ganglia, and receive inputs from both via the thalamus.

When performing movements, it is necessary to continuously correctly control both spatial aspects, such as the direction and size of the movement, and temporal aspects, such as speed and timing. The cerebellum is known to have a very important role in their regulation. The cerebellum is made up of three parts, the cortex, the white matter, and the cerebellar nuclei. When classified by its input–output structure, there are three main divisions. The first is the vestibulocerebellum, which receives vestibular information, and sends the results of the information processing to the vestibular nuclei. Its output is related to posture control and eye movements. The second receives somatosensory information via the spinocerebellar tract, which is called the spinocerebellum. The information processed at the spinocerebellum is sent to the reticular formation and the vestibular nuclei. Its output is related to the execution of movement. The third is the cerebrocerebellum, which receives input exclusively from the cerebral cortex. The information from the cerebral cortex passes through the pontine nuclei. The output from the cerebellum is sent to the thalamus, and via that to the premotor, motor, and prefrontal cortices. Since the cerebrum and cerebellum continuously exchange information via these pathways, it is thought that the cerebrocerebellum is part of a high-level internal feedback circuit that regulates cortical motor program.

The cerebellar cortex is composed of only five types of cells and two main types of afferent fiber. The efferent neurons which send signals from the cerebellum are all Purkinje cells, and the outputs from the Purkinje cells inhibit the deep cerebellar neurons. There are also three types of inhibitory interneurons in the cerebellar cortex, the basket cell, the Golgi cell, and the stellate cell. The activity of the Purkinje neurons is inhibited by these interneurons. On the other hand, there is only one type of excitatory cell, the granule cell, which receives signals from the mossy fibers, the major source of input to the cerebellum. The mossy fibers originate from a wide range of parts such as the vestibular organ, the spinal cord, and the pons. The fibers carry sensory information from the periphery as well as information from the cerebral cortex. The axons of the granule cells (the parallel fibers) terminate as the excitatory synapses on the four types of inhibitory neurons, including the Purkinje cells, through the fibers running parallel on the surface of the cerebellum. Another source of inputs to the cerebellum is synaptic contacts to the Purkinje cells by the climbing fibers originating in the inferior olivary nucleus in the medulla. The basket and stellate cells are excited by input from the parallel fibers, and both inhibit the Purkinje cells. In the inputs from the mossy fibers, the balance between the direct excitatory inputs to the Purkinje cells and the indirect inhibitory inputs by the inhibitory neurons determines the level of excitation in the Purkinje cells. When the cerebellum is lesioned, a variety of abnormalities in the execution of voluntary movements occur. Typical defects are delays in initiation of movement, coordination difficulty, and errors in the range of movement.

The basal ganglia consist of four nuclei: the striatum, the globus pallidus, the subthalmic nucleus, and the substantia nigra (Fig. 4.4). The striatum that consists of the caudate nucleus and the putamen receives primary inputs from the cerebral cortex. Most of outputs from the basal ganglia are sent to the brain stem and, via the thalamus, back to the cerebral cortex. The output signals inhibit their target nuclei in the brain stem and thalamus. Unlike most other components of the motor system, they do not have direct input or output connection with the spinal cord. Because the cerebral cortex is both the input and the output of the basal ganglia, this is called the cortico-basal ganglia loop. There are both a direct and an indirect pathway from the striatum to the two output nuclei. The indirect pathway passes first to the external pallidal segment and from there to the subthalamic nucleus and finally to the output nuclei. When the direct pathway from the striatum to the internal pallidal segment is activated, the thalamus is disinhibited, thereby increasing thalamocortcial activity. In contrast, activation of the indirect pathway increases inhibition of the thalamocortical neurons. Further, the two pathways are affected differently by the dopaminergic projection from the substantia nigra pars compacta to the

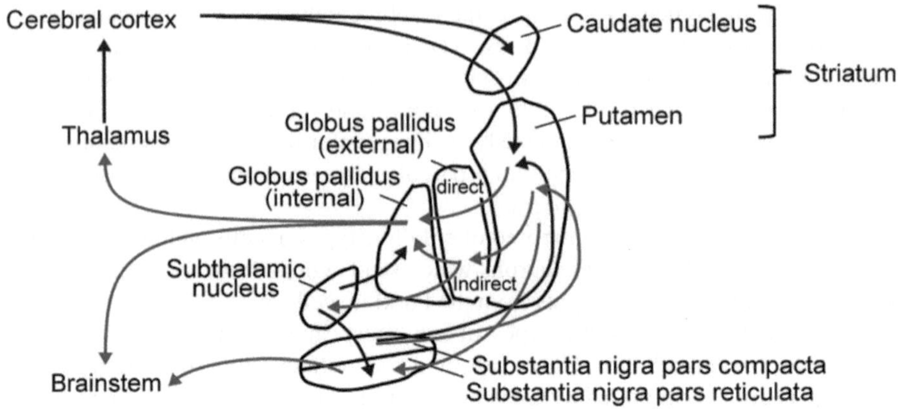

Fig. 4.4 Anatomic connections of the basal ganglia

striatum. With this arrangement, the inputs from the indirect pathway might assist in braking the movement, while those in the direct pathway facilitate the movement. It is considered that this reciprocal regulation would be related with the role in modulating voluntary movements by both reinforcing the selected movement pattern and suppressing potentially conflicting patterns. Clinical observations suggest that disorders of the basal ganglia may result in either diminished movement (as in Parkinson disease) or excessive movement (as in Huntington disease). In addition to the cortico-basal ganglia loop for the voluntary movement, the basal ganglia also contribute to the occulomotor, cognitive, and emotional functions by a variety of circuits.

4.2.4 Somatosensory Information

To make the action for some goal, the parts of the brain which control movement need information about muscles and joints and about the objects which are touching the skin. A variety of somatosensory information such as pressure, vibration, and the proprioceptive sensations from muscles and joints are transmitted from receptors to the spinal cord, through the ascending pathways to the cerebral cortex. The area behind the central sulcus is called the postcentral gyrus, also known as the somatosensory cortex. The somatosensory cortex contains a somatotopic representation like the one in the motor cortex. In Brodmann's classification, the primary somatosensory cortex corresponds to areas 1, 2, and 3. Basic processing of tactile information takes place in area 3, while more complex or higher-order processing occurs in area 1. In area 2 information on both the tactile and limb position are combined to mediate the tactile recognition of objects. In area 2, there are projects to the motor cortex. The somatosensory information is used to guide directed movement.

Proprioception is the sense of position and movement of one's limbs and body. Three types of mechanoreceptors in muscle and joints signal proprioceptive information. One of the representative receptors is the muscle spindle. The muscle spindle is located within the fleshy part of the skeletal muscles, a sensor which detects change in the muscle length and rate of change of length. The information from muscle spindles is used by the central nervous system to sense relative positions of body segments. There are two kinds of intrafusal fibers in the muscle spindle, called the nuclear chain fiber and the nuclear bag fiber. Nuclear bag fibers are divided into two types, dynamic and static, depending on their functional and morphological properties. The intrafusal fibers are terminated to two kinds of sensory fiber endings, called the primary ending (Ia fiber) and secondary ending (II fiber). When a muscle is stretched, the muscle spindles are also stretched, and the activity in the sensory endings is increased. When a muscle is held in an extended state, the primary and secondary endings increase their activity. Since the frequency of discharge is almost proportional to the length of the muscle, this is thought to transmit information about the length of the muscle. In addition, the primary endings are highly sensitive to the velocity of the muscle stretch. Thus, the primary endings are related to dynamic responses of the muscle stretch, and they provide information about the speed of movements. In contrast, secondary endings show very little dynamic response.

When the intrafusal fibers are contracted by the action of gamma MNs, the sensory receptor's responsiveness increases, and the sensitivity of the muscle spindles to muscle stretch increases. There are two types of gamma MN (dynamic and static neurons) that innervate different intrafusal fibers. When dynamic gamma MNs are active, only dynamic nuclear bag fibers are contracted. When static gamma MNs are active, static nuclear bag fibers and nuclear chain fibers are contracted. During movement in the cat, it has been observed that dynamic gamma MNs are activated during rapid movements, while static gamma MNs are active during activities in which muscle length changes slowly [19].

The second type of the mechanoreceptors in muscle and joints is the Golgi tendon organ at the junction between muscle fibers and tendon. The tendon organs are sensors which monitor the changes in the tension produced by the muscles. Each tendon organ is innervated by the group Ib fiber. The signals from the tendon organs are transmitted to the spinal interneurons (the Ib inhibitory interneurons) that inhibit the MN. The Golgi tendon organs are generally thought to have a protective function, preventing muscle damage. The third type is the joint receptors which exist in joint capsules. They are thought to detect extreme flexion or extension of the joint.

The sense of the touch is detected by the mechanoreceptors in the skin. There are four types of cutaneous and subcutaneous mechanoreceptors: Meissner's corpuscle, Merkel disk receptor, Pacinian corpuscle, and Ruffini endings. The Meissner's corpuscle and the Merkel disk receptor are principal mechanoreceptors in the superficial layers of the skin, while the Pacinian corpuscle and the Ruffini ending are situated in the deep subcutaneous tissue. These mechanoreceptors have different size and structure of their receptive fields. Mechanical information sensed by these receptors contributes to perception of stroking, pressure, texture, vibration, and skin stretch.

4.2.5 Spinal Cord

The spinal cord is the most caudal part of the central nervous system, and it is divided into the cervical, thoracic, lumbar, and sacral regions. The spinal cord receives sensory inputs from the skin, muscles and joints, and descending commands from the brain. The output pathways from the spinal cord are motor nerves that are the axons of the MN, and the ascending tracts to the brain. Sensory inputs from various receptors are sent to the interneurons and the MNs in the spinal cord and via the ascending tracts to the supraspinal centers. The spinal cord consists of white matter and gray matter. The ascending tract, which sends sensory information to the brain, and the descending tract, which mediates motor commands from the brain, pass through specific locations in the white matter. In contrast, the gray matter, in which various types of neurons exist, is divided cytoarchitecturally into layers I to X. The layers I to IV of the dorsal horn are sensory areas, and the MNs exist in the layer IX of the ventral horn. The interneurons are located in layers V to VIII. Sensory information from the receptors is transmitted to the spinal cord through the dorsal root, while the motor nerves come out through the ventral root (Fig. 4.1). Because the motor commands from supraspinal centers finally act through the MNs of the spinal cord, the MNs are called the "final common pathway".

4.2.6 Spinal Reflexes

Some movements are automatic, and do not require any attention to be paid. The most pronounced examples are movements which can be induced by reflexes. In particular, reflexes which are produced by neuronal circuits in the spinal cord are called spinal reflexes. Sensory information from the various receptors on the muscles, joints, and skin induce excitatory or inhibitory reflex inputs to the MN through neuronal circuits in the spinal cord [3].

Of the spinal reflexes, the patella tendon reflex (knee jerk) is a typical stretch reflex deriving from the muscle spindles. Due to the muscle stretching by a tendon tap to the quadriceps muscles, the activity in the sensory endings of muscle spindles is increased and the action potentials which propagate along the axon to the terminal are generated. The sensory neurons make excitatory synaptic connections to the MNs and the stretched muscle is contracted by the firing of the MNs. The Ia afferents from the primary spindle endings have direct synaptic connections to the MNs, and because it is mediated by only one synapse, it is called a monosynaptic reflex. However, sensory information evoked by the muscle stretch is also transmitted to the interneurons in the spinal cord. The spinal interneurons inhibit the MNs in the muscle (hamstring muscles) which is antagonistic to the stretched muscles (quadriceps muscles) by the knee jerk. So because the antagonistic muscle is inhibited, it does not prevent the contraction of the quadriceps muscles. This phenomenon that inhibits the antagonistic muscle via one inhibitory interneuron (Ia inhibitory interneuron) is called reciprocal Ia inhibition.

The excitatory responses of the stretch reflex are often observed at longer latency compared to that of monosynaptic reflex, and oligosynaptic inputs from the group Ia afferents and synaptic inputs from the group II are speculated [3]. Further, at the long-latency components of the stretch reflex, it is considered that the reflex response is at least partly mediated by a transcortical reflex pathway [20].

Monosynaptic stretch reflex which is induced by mechanical muscle stretch can be induced by transcutaneous electrical stimulation to the sensory fibers. The responses induced by the electrical stimulation are called the Hoffman reflex (H-reflex) [21]. The excitability of the reflex pathway can be assessed by the evoked EMG response. For this reason, the H-reflex technique is used not just in clinical tests, but also in research to investigate the spinal reflex excitability during human movements, and has led to insights into the mechanism of motor control [22, 23]. For example, the H-reflex amplitudes in the soleus muscle become smaller from supine to sitting, and then from sitting to standing posture [24, 25]. Thus, it has been shown that the spinal reflex excitability is modulated by changes in posture.

Cutaneous stimuli to the skin can evoke responses in the muscles. If a stumble occurs during walking, cutaneous reflex responses to a lot of muscles are evoked by the sensory information due to the stumble, correcting the posture. In humans, non-noxious electrical stimulation to cutaneous afferents is used to investigate the cutaneous reflex responses in the muscles [26–28]. The cutaneous reflex pathway is a polysynaptic pathway that contains a number of spinal interneurons interposed between the first order afferent terminals and the MNs. It has been observed that excitatory or inhibitory response is evoked to various muscles by the stimulation, and that reflex response varies from excitation to inhibition depending on the state of movement [27].

4.3 Locomotion

Locomotion is the rhythmical alternate movements of the left and right limbs, and it is a complex movement involving many muscles. During walking, posture is stabilized without conscious effort, and the walking pattern is altered temporally and spatially to deal with changes in the path such as uneven surface. The basis of locomotion is timely excitation and inhibition in the flexor and extensor muscles. Regarding the neural mechanism of locomotion, in decerebrate cats in which the brain stem is completely transected at the level of midbrain, and in spinalized cats in which the spinal cord is transected at the lower thoracic level, interneurons in the spinal cord rhythmically burst, and locomotor-like muscle activities occur during passive stepping movement on a treadmill [29, 30]. From these results, it is indicated that the spinal cord has a neuronal network which generates the basic locomotor pattern. This neuronal circuitry in the spinal cord is called the central pattern generator (CPG) [31, 32]. Since the CPG is under the supraspinal control, start and cessation of the locomotion as well as the characteristics of its pattern are decided by the supraspinal centers. However, after locomotion has begun, it can continue activation of the CPG even without input from supraspinal centers. In experiments with cats which have their spinal cord completely transected, the locomotor EMG activities driven by CPG were observed with only the sensory input elicited by passive stepping on a treadmill [33]. The CPG appears to be a simple system, but most of the alternating bursts which are necessary for locomotion can be explained by it.

In experiments with decerebrate cats, it has been reported that it is possible to induce locomotion by electrical stimuli to specific locations of the midbrain, subthalamic region, and the cerebellum, which suggests existence of the locomotor regions in the brain [30, 34]. In the experiments with decerebrate cat preparations, the connection between the diencephalon and midbrain was completely cut. In this condition, standing on four limbs was impossible. However, if the cat with body weight support was placed on a treadmill, locomotion was generated by electrical stimulation to the brainstem. It is considered that the signals from the midbrain locomotor region descend the reticulospinal tract to the spinal cord, and activate the CPG, making locomotion possible. The reticulospinal tract has many branches, which terminate at layers VII and VIII in the spinal cord. In the layer VII, there are many interneurons. These interneurons receive descending inputs and inputs from sensory receptors, and the integrated result is sent to MNs as an output signal.

In the cerebral cortex, it is shown that the neurons of the M1 in the cat fire rhythmically during locomotion [35]. In particular, in a situation such as walking to avoid an obstacle, the discharge frequency of the neurons in the M1 particularly increases, so it is supposed that regulation by the motor cortex plays an important role in conditions where visuomotor integration is needed. Regarding the influence of peripheral input, it is reported that the rhythm of locomotion is reset by stimulation to the cutaneous and group Ib afferents during locomotion [27, 36]. Therefore, it is considered that these sensory inputs enter the neuronal networks which form the rhythm. However, even without input from the periphery, a locomotor rhythm is generated, so sensory input seems not to be indispensable for rhythm generation. It is considered that sensory information is involved in modification of locomotor pattern.

As discussed above, from results of electrophysiological experiments on quadrupedal locomotion, understanding of the mechanism for locomotion is advanced in the spinal and supraspinal levels. Humans, on the other hand, have evolved a specific locomotor pattern of upright and bipedal movement. Since it is not possible to perform invasive experiments in humans, many points remain unclear about the neural mechanisms of locomotion. Regarding the CPG, its presence is indirectly suggested on the basis of experimental results from patients with complete spinal cord injury [37–39]. However, compared to results from animals with complete spinal cord injury which can step on a treadmill with their body weight unloaded, humans with complete spinal cord injury cannot walk independently. Therefore, it seems that compared to quadrupedal locomotion, for humans the descending input from the supraspinal system is strongly involved in locomotion [40].

The importance of sensory input during walking has also been reported in human subjects [36, 41]. It has been shown that in the stance phase of walking, feedback from the load-related receptors is involved in generating muscular activity in the plantar flexor muscle [42]. The main receptors involved in detecting load-related information are the Golgi tendon organs and the cutaneous receptors of the foot sole. The muscle spindles and joint receptors also play a supplementary role [41, 43]. Generally, the group Ib fibers which connect to the Golgi tendon organs inhibit excitability in the homonymous muscle and facilitate the excitability in the antagonistic muscle. However, it has been reported in the experimental data from cats and humans that during locomotion the effect of Ib input to the MN in the homonymous muscle changes from inhibition to facilitation according to the step phase of locomotion [31, 44]. The effect of Ib fibers from extensor muscles is excitatory in the extensors in the stance phase of locomotion. It is considered that this serves to modulate the muscle activity in the extensors in accordance with the amount of loading. It is also observed in patients with complete spinal cord injury that muscle activities cannot be induced by passive stepping movement of the lower limbs without loading of the body weight, therefore rhythmic load inputs to the lower limbs are necessary for muscle activity [45].

4.4 Motor Learning

In typing on a keyboard, both hands need to execute complex continuous movements. Even if you first find the typing hard, by repetition, it becomes possible to type accurately and quickly without paying particular attention. In recent years, a great deal of knowledge about the neural mechanisms of motor learning has been obtained from electrophysiological experiments in animals and brain imaging experiments using functional magnetic resonance imaging (fMRI) or PET in humans. In this section, the neural basis of motor learning will be discussed.

Of the parts of the cerebral cortex involved in movement, the most important is the M1 which sends motor commands to the spinal cord. In a human experiment using fMRI that subjects practiced finger-to–thumb opposition movements with complex sequence over several weeks, Karni et al. [46] found that activation areas in the M1 changed corresponding to the amount of training. It has also been reported that besides the M1, a lot of the motor-related cortical areas change their activity in response to training. In exploratory motor learning for pushing buttons in a correct sequence while getting true-false feedback, activities in multiple areas such as the prefrontal cortex, premotor cortex and cerebellum increased, while for button pushing in an already-learned sequence, the SMA was activated [47]. Compared to the later stage of learning, the premotor cortex showed a stronger level of activity in the early learning stage. It appears that in the early learning stage, sensory information is important role for learning the motor behavior. Then, as the learning progresses, the movement becomes more automatic, and can be processed based on motor memory without strong dependence of the sensory information. Therefore the possibility has been suggested that the activity of the premotor cortex decreases, and the SMA becomes active in the later learning stage.

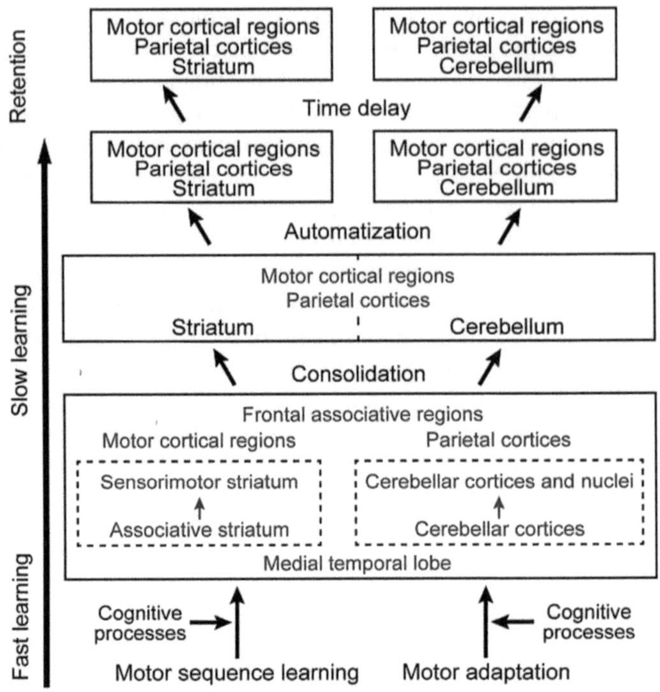

Fig. 4.5 Model of the cerebral plasticity that occurs in both cortico-striatal and cortico-cerebellar systems during motor sequence and adaptation learning (Modified from Doyon and Benali [50])

By comparing the brain activity between learning task of a new sequential movement and an task execution of already-learned sequential movement, Hikosaka et al. [48] proposed that the preSMA is strongly involved in new learning, but that SMA is involved in the execution of sequential movement. Furthermore, Deiber et al. [49] reported that in the associative learning task that associate sensory stimulation with movement, the rostral aspect of the premotor cortex shows greater activation during the early part of skill learning, while the caudal aspect of the premotor cortex becomes more active with learning. Thus, in the learning process of movement, it appears that activation patterns in various brain areas and within the same cortex change. The process of motor learning has been modeled as three stages, fast (early) learning, slow (latter) learning, and period of retention [50] (Fig. 4.5). In the early stage of motor learning, repetition within a single training session induces improvement of performance. At this time, the movement patterns are not established, and it strongly depends on somatosensory information to execute the movements, so it is speculated that sensory input plays an important role for motor learning. Then, the sensory-motor relations are learned and the speed and accuracy of movement improve. Finally, even without further practice of the movement for a long time, its learning performance is retained.

In addition to the cerebral cortex, the cerebellum and basal ganglia are well known to be related to motor learning [48, 50]. In the cerebellum, the Purkinje cell, which generates the sole output in the cerebellum, receives inputs from the climbing fiber and from many parallel fibers originating from the granule cells. The climbing fiber causes strong depolarization of the Purkinje cell. It is hypothesized that when an error in the consequence of the movement arises, this information is transmitted as an error signal by the climbing fiber to the Purkinje cell, and long term depression occurs at the parallel fiber–Purkinje cell synaptic transmission which was related to the error. By repetition of this process, eventually only the synapses which generate the correct movement remain, and an internal model needed for execution of the task is acquired. Thus, it is considered that the error signal from the climbing fiber acts as a "teacher signal" for motor learning. In practice, many studies have pointed out that in the early learning stage for a novel movement, higher activation in a wide area of the cerebellum is observed. It appears that the greater activity change in the early stage might reflect a strong dependence on feedback processing.

Many findings have also revealed that the basal ganglia play an important role in procedural learning and memory. It has been modeled that based on the reward signals sent from the dopaminergic neurons in the substantia nigra, reinforcement learning progresses by coding the difference between actual and predicted rewards [51]. Unlike the supervised learning of the cerebellum in which target motion is presented, only an evaluation about whether or not the results are good is given for this reinforcement learning. This learning process might progress to maximize the future reward. The activation in the caudate nucleus of the basal ganglia was observed during learning of a novel sequence at the motor sequence task, while in the execution of a learned movement, activation of the posterior putamen was involved [52]. It appears that the activated nuclei in the basal ganglia vary with the learning process.

In research on the neural mechanisms of motor learning, two representative experimental paradigms are introduced (Fig. 4.5). One, called adaptation learning, is the type for generating movements in response to changes in the environment. For example, a subject executes target-reaching movement with a robot arm which applies additional torque. The other is called motor sequence learning. One of the examples is finger-tapping task in a four-digit sequence. In an adaptation task, a process of change from sensory information to the generation of modified motor commands is necessary to adapt to environmental perturbations. The process to modify the internal model for minimizing the differences between the desired final state and the current estimated state by repetitive practice is regarded as the adaptation learning. As stated before, this kind of error learning of the internal model is thought to take place in the cerebellum. Recently, Doyon and Benali [50] have proposed a model divided into two learning types of motor sequence and motor adaptation for progressive plastic changes in the brain during the learning of a novel motor task (Fig. 4.5). At the first stage of learning, both motor sequence learning and motor adaptation recruit a wide range of brain areas including motor cortical regions, striatum, and cerebellum in addition to prefrontal, parietal areas and limbic areas. As learning progresses, the cortico-cerebellar system is crucial for consolidating and maintaining in the motor adaptation skill, while the cortico-striatal system is thought to play an important role in the consolidation of motor sequence learning. As described, it has become clear that different parts of the brain, the cerebral cortex and the subcortical regions, are activated depending on the motor task and the stages of learning.

In motor learning, an aspect to prevent the loss of the learned motor skill over time is also important. Interesting research results have been reported on the retention of motor learning. For example, it was reported that if within 4–6 h after learning of a motor task, subjects learned a similar second motor task, the learning of the second task became difficult, and the learning effect of the first motor task became less effective [53, 54]. After 6 h have passed from first task learning, learning a second task does not impair the retention of the first task. These studies indicate that retention of motor learning may be initially susceptible to disruption. There are also research reports that sleep is deeply related to motor memory [55, 56]. It has been shown that sleep can trigger significant performance improvement on a finger movement task, whereas equivalent periods of time during wake provided no significant benefit [56]. Sleep has been implicated in the ongoing process of consolidation after initial acquisition, whereby delayed improvement might be achieved in the absence of additional practice. These kinds of research results are considered important in establishing training protocols for motor learning.

Up to now, the role of the muscles and the central nervous system to execute movement and the involvement of the cerebral cortex and the subcortical regions in motor learning have been introduced with recent research results. The results from motor control and motor learning studies have started to be applied to the motor recovery of motor function disorders by the rehabilitation approach [57]. Motor function recovery also seems to be related to the motor learning mechanism. In practice, the changes of the brain activity involved in motor learning resemble that in motor recovery after brain injury. For the recovery of motor function, it is hoped that the mechanisms of motor learning will become clearer.

4.5 Changes in the Excitability of Neural Pathways During Passive Stepping

4.5.1 Modulation of Corticospinal Tract Excitability

The obstacle to understanding the involvement of the supraspinal centers in human bipedal walking is the difficulty of measurement, but in recent years, research using transcranial magnetic stimulation (TMS) has made advances. TMS is a non-invasive method to generate brief pulse of magnetic fields by a coil placed on the scalp. Each magnetic pulse passes easily through the skull and into the brain, where it induces excitation of neurons. When corticospinal cells are activated by TMS applied to the motor cortex, a contraction of muscles on the contralateral side to the stimulated brain can be evoked. By measuring the amplitude of the motor evoked potential (MEP) in EMG recordings, the excitability of the corticospinal tract can be evaluated [58]. In a previous study regarding TMS applied during human walking, it was observed that the excitability of the corticospinal tract in the gastrocnemius muscle and the tibialis anterior muscle was modulated depending on the phase of walking and almost corresponded to the levels of muscle activity during walking [59]. In addition, Capaday et al. [60] indicated that the corticospinal excitability to the tibialis anterior muscle increased even in the stance phase in which the tibialis anterior muscle was inactive, suggesting that walking-specific changes in the corticospinal excitability occur. In the muscles of the hip joint, TMS at the stance phase elicited hip extension, whereas when stimulation was applied at the initial swing phase it caused the hip flexion [61]. Therefore the corticospinal excitability in the hip muscles is thought to be high in the hip extensors during the stance phase, and in the hip flexors during the swing phase. From these results using TMS, the excitability of the corticospinal tract in the lower limb muscles depends on the phase of locomotion. However, it has not been discussed how the corticospinal pathway acts as motor drives to MNs during locomotion. Petersen et al. [62] applied TMS to the motor cortex at the subthreshold level for the MEP during normal walking, and investigated the effect of TMS on muscle activity in the soleus and tibialis anterior muscles. Since it appears to activate only the inhibitory neurons in the cortex by the weak magnetic stimulation at the subthreshold level [58], it was hypothesized that this weak stimulation might weaken the output from the cortex. Consequently, the activities of both muscles during walking were suppressed by TMS at the subthreshold level. Therefore, the results suggested that the human motor cortex contributes to muscle activity of walking through the corticospinal tract.

During walking, somatosensory information from receptors in the skeletal muscles, the joints and the skin are transmitted to the spinal cord and supraspinal centers [31]. However, it has not been clear whether or not somatosensory input influences the excitability of the corticospinal tract during human walking. Therefore, we conducted experiments using a robotic gait orthosis (Lokomat®, Hocoma AG, Switzerland) developed for locomotion training of locomotor disorders. This gait orthosis provides drives by motors of the hip and knee joint in the exoskeleton under computerized control [63], so that applying the DGO to healthy humans makes it possible to impose passive stepping. Therefore, it is possible to evoke stepping-related sensory information by using the robotic assist without voluntary command for walking. From previous researches, it is considered that of the somatosensory information, afferent inputs from joint and load receptors are important for the generation of the muscle activity during walking and the locomotor recovery by locomotor training [38, 41, 45]. Therefore, with the objective of investigating the effect of load-related sensory inputs on corticospinal excitability, we compared the MEP responses in the lower limb muscles between two body weight loading conditions during passive stepping [64]. The subjects were healthy adults who were instructed to keep their lower limb muscles relaxed during stepping. The body weight unloading conditions of passive stepping were full

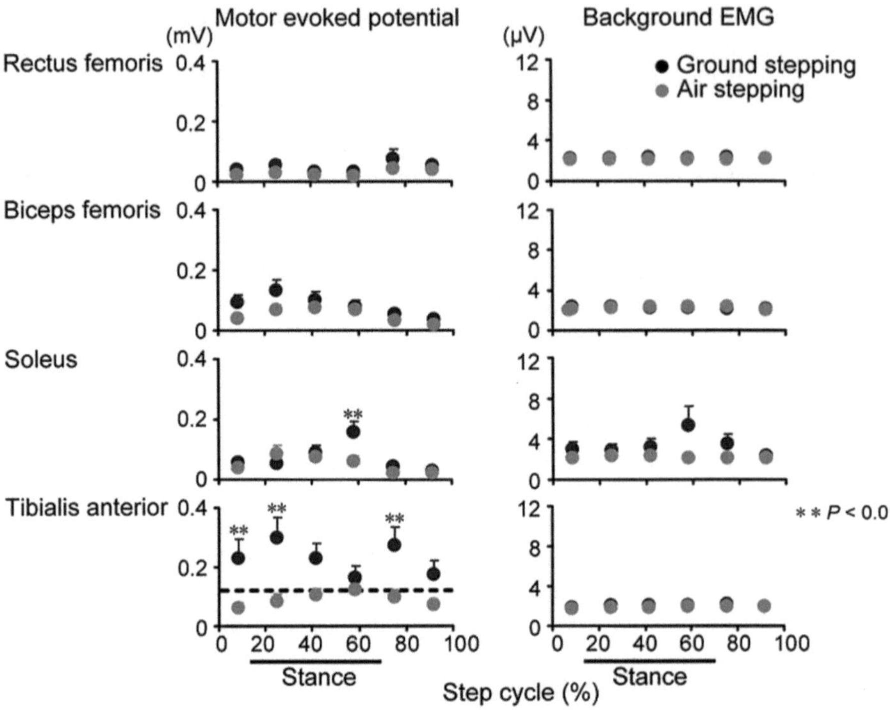

Fig. 4.6 Motor evoked potential and background EMG activity of the lower limb muscles during passive stepping using a robotic gait orthosis (Modified from Kamibayashi et al. [64])

(100 %) body weight unloading (air stepping) and 40 % unloading of body weight (ground stepping) which is close to the level of unloading used in the locomotor training. Because in this experiment a TMS coil was placed on the most appropriate position to evoke MEPs in the tibialis anterior muscle, the MEP amplitude was small in the rectus femoris muscle and the biceps femoris muscle. However, a small MEP modulation was seen in the upper leg muscles across the step cycle (Fig. 4.6). An increase in excitability of the corticospinal tract was seen at the swing phase in the rectus femoris and around initial stance phase in the biceps femoris, and these patterns of modulation were similar to muscle activation patterns in normal walking [65] and previous TMS results during walking [61]. In the tibialis anterior muscle, an increase in MEP amplitude was observed during ground stepping compared to standing (dash line in Fig. 4.6). From the results of a two-way repeated-measure ANOVA, a significant effect of interaction (step condition × step phase) was shown, indicating that the pattern of the MEP modulation differed with or without body weight loading. Compared to air stepping, the MEP amplitude significantly increased in the transition from swing phase to stance phase and in the transition from stance to swing. The facilitation pattern of MEP response during ground stepping resembled that recorded during normal walking in the previous study [59]. Because there were no differences in the movements of the lower limb joints

in the two stepping conditions, it was considered that the increase in the corticospinal excitability of the tibialis anterior muscle during ground stepping might be influenced by load-related afferent inputs. In the evaluation of the background EMG activity at the time of the stimulation by root mean square value, muscle activity was not seen in the rectus femoris, biceps femoris, and tibialis anterior muscles across the step cycle under both stepping conditions (Fig. 4.6). In the soleus muscle, low EMG activity was observed at the late-stance phase of ground stepping. In contrast, the Sol EMG activity during air stepping was not observed. Since simple rhythmic muscle stretching or loading alone does not produce a locomotor EMG activity [45], a combination of locomotor-related sensory inputs would be indispensable to generate this muscle activity. The MEP amplitude in the soleus muscle showed an increase at late-stance phase of ground stepping in parallel with the EMG activation of the soleus muscle during ground stepping. This MEP facilitation is thought to reflect the increased excitability of the MNs to this muscle. In further research, when the input (stimulus intensity)-output (MEP response) relations of the corticospinal tract during passive ground stepping were investigated in more detail, it was clarified that the changes of the corticospinal excitability in the rectus femoris and the biceps femoris muscles depended on the phase of the stepping [66]. Furthermore, the increase in corticospinal excitability of the tibialis anterior muscle was also verified in the same way as the previous research.

4.5.2 Modulation of Spinal Reflex Excitability

A method to investigate the excitability of the monosynaptic reflex pathway during human movement is to evoke the H-reflex by an electrical stimulation to the sensory nerve. During human normal walking, the H-reflex excitability of the soleus muscle is strongly inhibited at the swing phase [24, 67]. However, it was unclear whether the H-reflex excitability shows phase-dependent modulation by substantially reduced descending motor command during passive stepping and whether the load-related sensory inputs elicited during passive stepping also affect the soleus H-reflex excitability. Therefore, in the same way as the TMS experiment, we investigated changes of the H-reflex excitability in the soleus muscle during two passive stepping conditions [68]. Under both conditions, the soleus H-reflexes during passive stepping were significantly inhibited compared to those during standing (Fig. 4.7). The stimulus intensity for the H-reflex was unchanged throughout the recording, since the M-wave amplitude was constant as shown in Fig. 4.7. When comparing between the step phases, the H-reflex was significantly inhibited at the early- and mid-swing phases compared to the stance phase. The modulation pattern during passive stepping resembled that observed during normal walking [24, 67]. Between two stepping conditions, the difference in the H-reflex excitability was not seen, suggesting that the load-related sensory information during passive stepping have little influence on the H-reflex excitability. This reflex

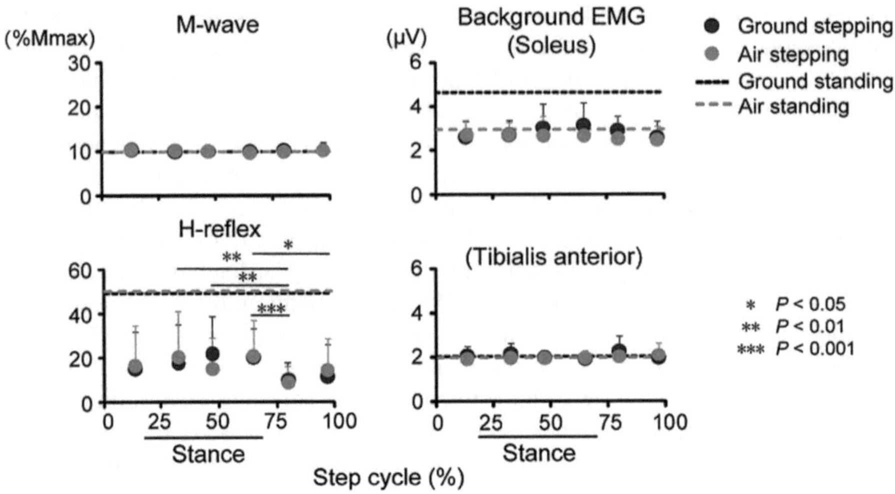

Fig. 4.7 Mean M-wave, H-reflex, and background EMG activity in the soleus and tibialis anterior muscles during passive stepping using a robotic gait orthosis (Modified from Kamibayashi et al. [68])

modulation pattern was observed even in patients with complete spinal cord injury. In this way, since even in passive stepping, the H-reflex inhibition increased during the first half of the swing phase, the source underlying the phase-modulation of the H-reflex during passive stepping might be attributed to the sensory inputs generated by the flexion of the hip and/or knee joints. Next, we investigated the H-reflex excitability during passive stepping in the tibialis anterior muscle. It is known to be difficult to evoke the H-reflex in the tibialis anterior muscle under the condition of no voluntary muscle contraction, but we were able to record it in four healthy subjects. Similar to results in the soleus muscle, in the tibialis anterior muscle, the H-reflex was inhibited by passive stepping when compared to standing posture. Furthermore, by measuring the H-reflex in the flexor carpi radialis muscle, experiments have been done on the influence of sensory input on the H-reflex excitability in the muscle of the upper limb during passive stepping [69]. Also in this muscle, the H-reflex amplitude was smaller during passive stepping than that during standing. As mentioned above, it has become clear that in various muscles of the upper and lower limbs the spinal reflex excitability investigated by using H-reflex might receive inhibitory effects from the afferent inputs generated by the lower limbs during locomotion.

When cutaneous nerves are electrically stimulated in an experiment, it is known that phasic modulation of the cutaneous reflex occurs in the lower limb muscles during normal walking [27, 70]. Similar to the previously-described experiment, using two kinds of passive stepping with different loading, Nakajima et al. [71] induced the cutaneous reflex in the tibialis anterior muscle using stimulation to the tibial nerve. To detect both responses of facilitation and inhibition by the cutaneous reflex, the subjects kept a constant level of the muscle contraction (10 % of the maximum voluntary contraction) in the tibialis anterior muscle during passive stepping. The result showed that while the reflex responses were not modulated during air stepping, the reflex responses were strongly increased during stance-to-swing phase of ground stepping. This modulation pattern of the cutaneous reflex also resembled the results observed in normal walking [70]. Therefore passive stepping causes facilitation in the cutaneous reflex pathways, but as with the excitability in the corticospinal tract, the load-related afferent inputs might have a powerful influence on this pathway.

From the above experimental results, it was found that when load-related information is provided in human passive stepping, the responses by the TMS and cutaneous reflex are modulated in a phase-dependent manner resembling normal walking. The results from the H-reflex measurement in the muscles of upper and lower limbs indicated inhibitory effects during passive stepping compared to standing, but the reflex pathway also showed the same modulation pattern as normal walking. In passive stepping, since the subject did not try to walk voluntarily, it appears the effect of voluntary command was largely reduced. However, by the sensory inputs including the load-related afferents during passive stepping, various neural circuits involved in the locomotion might be activated in the similar way to normal walking. As research into the neural mechanisms of locomotion from human subjects has progressed, the differences of neural control between bipedal and quadrupedal locomotion have become clearer. It was difficult to distinguish the effects from the supraspinal centers and sensory inputs on the excitability of neural pathways during normal walking, but we have obtained new findings using a robot as experimental device. From now on, it is hoped that the accumulation of research results on human locomotion will lead to the development of more effective forms of locomotor rehabilitation.

References

1. Huxley HE (2004) Fifty years of muscle and the sliding filament hypothesis. Eur J Biochem 271:1403–1415
2. Burke RE, Levine DN, Tsairis P, Zajac FE III (1973) Physiological types and histochemical profiles in motor units of the cat gastrocnemius. J Physiol 234:723–748
3. Dietz V (1992) Human neuronal control of automatic functional movements: interaction between central programs and afferent input. Physiol Rev 72:33–69
4. De Luca CJ, LeFever RS, McCue MP, Xenakis AP (1982) Behaviour of human motor units in different muscles during linearly varying contractions. J Physiol 329:113–128
5. Penfield W, Boldrey E (1937) Somatic motor and sensory representation in the cerebral cortex of man as studied by electrical stimulation. Brain 60:389–443
6. Cheney PD, Fetz EE (1985) Comparable patterns of muscle facilitation evoked by individual corticomotoneuronal (CM) cells and by single intracortical microstimuli in primates: evidence for functional groups of CM cells. J Neurophysiol 53:786–804
7. Evarts EV (1968) Relation of pyramidal tract activity to force exerted during voluntary movement. J Neurophysiol 31:14–27

8. Georgopoulos AP, Kalaska JF, Caminiti R, Massey JT (1982) On the relations between the direction of two-dimensional arm movements and cell discharge in primate motor cortex. J Neurosci 2:1527–1537
9. Picard N, Strick PL (1996) Motor areas of the medial wall: a review of their location and functional activation. Cereb Cortex 6:342–353
10. Hoshi E, Tanji J (2007) Distinctions between dorsal and ventral premotor areas: anatomical connectivity and functional properties. Curr Opin Neurobiol 17:234–242
11. Weinrich M, Wise SP, Mauritz KH (1984) A neurophysiological study of the premotor cortex in the rhesus monkey. Brain 107:385–414
12. Rizzolatti G, Fadiga L, Gallese V, Fogassi L (1996) Premotor cortex and the recognition of motor actions. Brain Res Cogn Brain Res 3:131–141
13. Tanji J (1996) New concepts of the supplementary motor area. Curr Opin Neurobiol 6:782–787
14. Roland PE, Larsen B, Lassen NA, Skinhoj E (1980) Supplementary motor area and other cortical areas in organization of voluntary movements in man. J Neurophysiol 43:118–136
15. Shibasaki H, Sadato N, Lyshkow H, Yonekura Y, Honda M, Nagamine T, Suwazono S, Magata Y, Ikeda A, Miyazaki M, Fukuyama H, Asato R, Konishi J (1993) Both primary motor cortex and supplementary motor area play an important role in complex finger movement. Brain 116:1387–1398
16. Aizawa H, Inase M, Mushiake H, Shima K, Tanji J (1991) Reorganization of activity in the supplementary motor area associated with motor learning and functional recovery. Exp Brain Res 84:668–671
17. Boecker H, Dagher A, Ceballos-Baumann AO, Passingham RE, Samuel M, Friston KJ, Poline J, Dettmers C, Conrad B, Brooks DJ (1998) Role of the human rostral supplementary motor area and the basal ganglia in motor sequence control: investigations with H_2 ^{15}O PET. J Neurophysiol 79:1070–1080
18. Shima K, Tanji J (1998) Role for cingulate motor area cells in voluntary movement selection based on reward. Science 282:1335–1338
19. Prochazka A (1989) Sensorimotor gain control: a basic strategy of motor systems? Prog Neurobiol 33:281–307
20. Petersen N, Christensen LO, Morita H, Sinkjær T, Nielsen J (1998) Evidence that a transcortical pathway contributes to stretch reflexes in the tibialis anterior muscle in man. J Physiol 512:267–276
21. Schieppati M (1987) The Hoffmann reflex: a means of assessing spinal reflex excitability and its descending control in man. Prog Neurobiol 28:345–376
22. Capaday C (1997) Neurophysiological methods for studies of the motor system in freely moving human subjects. J Neurosci Methods 74:201–218
23. Zehr EP (2002) Considerations for use of the Hoffmann reflex in exercise studies. Eur J Appl Physiol 86:455–468
24. Capaday C, Stein RB (1986) Amplitude modulation of the soleus H-reflex in the human during walking and standing. J Neurosci 6:1308–1313
25. Capaday C, Stein RB (1987) Difference in the amplitude of the human soleus H reflex during walking and running. J Physiol 392:513–522
26. Brooke JD, Cheng J, Collins DF, McIlroy WE, Misiaszek JE, Staines WR (1997) Sensori-sensory afferent conditioning with leg movement: gain control in spinal reflex and ascending paths. Prog Neurobiol 51:393–421
27. Zehr EP, Stein RB (1999) What functions do reflexes serve during human locomotion? Prog Neurobiol 58:185–205
28. Brooke JD (2004) Somatosensory paths proceeding to spinal cord and brain–centripetal and centrifugal control for human movement. Can J Physiol Pharmacol 82:723–731
29. Barbeau H, Julien C, Rossignol S (1987) The effects of clonidine and yohimbine on locomotion and cutaneous reflexes in the adult chronic spinal cat. Brain Res 437:83–96

30. Orlovsky G, Deliagina T, Grillner S (1999) Neuronal control of locomotion: from mollusc to man. Oxford University Press, New York
31. Rossignol S, Dubuc R, Gossard JP (2006) Dynamic sensorimotor interactions in locomotion. Physiol Rev 86:89–154
32. Grillner S (2011) Control of locomotion in bipeds, tetrapods, and fish. Compr Physiol Supplement 2: Handbook of physiology, the nervous system, motor control, 1179–1236
33. Forssberg H, Grillner S (1973) The locomotion of the acute spinal cat injected with clonidine i.v. Brain Res 50:184–186
34. Mori S, Matsui T, Kuze B, Asanome M, Nakajima K, Matsuyama K (1999) Stimulation of a restricted region in the midline cerebellar white matter evokes coordinated quadrupedal locomotion in the decerebrate cat. J Neurophysiol 82:290–300
35. Drew T, Jiang W, Kably B, Lavoie S (1996) Role of the motor cortex in the control of visually triggered gait modifications. Can J Physiol Pharmacol 74:426–442
36. Hultborn H, Nielsen JB (2007) Spinal control of locomotion–from cat to man. Acta Physiol 189:111–121
37. Dietz V, Colombo G, Jensen L (1994) Locomotor activity in spinal man. Lancet 344:1260–1263
38. Harkema SJ, Hurley SL, Patel UK, Requejo PS, Dobkin BH, Edgerton VR (1997) Human lumbosacral spinal cord interprets loading during stepping. J Neurophysiol 77:797–811
39. Dimitrijevic MR, Gerasimenko Y, Pinter MM (1998) Evidence for a spinal central pattern generator in humans. Ann N Y Acad Sci 860:360–376
40. Nielsen JB (2003) How we walk: central control of muscle activity during human walking. Neuroscientist 9:195–204
41. Van de Crommert HW, Mulder T, Duysens J (1998) Neural control of locomotion: sensory control of the central pattern generator and its relation to treadmill training. Gait Posture 7:251–263
42. Grey MJ, Nielsen JB, Mazzaro N, Sinkjær T (2007) Positive force feedback in human walking. J Physiol 581:99–105
43. Duysens J, Clarac F, Cruse H (2000) Load-regulating mechanisms in gait and posture: comparative aspects. Physiol Rev 80:83–133
44. Faist M, Hoefer C, Hodapp M, Dietz V, Berger W, Duysens J (2006) In humans Ib facilitation depends on locomotion while suppression of Ib inhibition requires loading. Brain Res 1076:87–92
45. Dietz V, Muller R, Colombo G (2002) Locomotor activity in spinal man: significance of afferent input from joint and load receptors. Brain 125:2626–2634
46. Karni A, Meyer G, Jezzard P, Adams MM, Turner R, Ungerleider LG (1995) Functional MRI evidence for adult motor cortex plasticity during motor skill learning. Nature 377:155–158
47. Jenkins IH, Brooks DJ, Nixon PD, Frackowiak RS, Passingham RE (1994) Motor sequence learning: a study with positron emission tomography. J Neurosci 14:3775–3790
48. Hikosaka O, Nakamura K, Sakai K, Nakahara H (2002) Central mechanisms of motor skill learning. Curr Opin Neurobiol 12:217–222
49. Deiber MP, Wise SP, Honda M, Catalan MJ, Grafman J, Hallett M (1997) Frontal and parietal networks for conditional motor learning: a positron emission tomography study. J Neurophysiol 78:977–991
50. Doyon J, Benali H (2005) Reorganization and plasticity in the adult brain during learning of motor skills. Curr Opin Neurobiol 15:161–167
51. Doya K (2000) Complementary roles of basal ganglia and cerebellum in learning and motor control. Curr Opin Neurobiol 10:732–739
52. Jueptner M, Weiller C (1998) A review of differences between basal ganglia and cerebellar control of movements as revealed by functional imaging studies. Brain 121:1437–1449
53. Brashers-Krug T, Shadmehr R, Bizzi E (1996) Consolidation in human motor memory. Nature 382:252–255

54. Shadmehr R, Brashers-Krug T (1997) Functional stages in the formation of human long-term motor memory. J Neurosci 17:409–419
55. Kuriyama K, Stickgold R, Walker MP (2004) Sleep-dependent learning and motor-skill complexity. Learn Mem 11:705–713
56. Walker MP, Brakefield T, Morgan A, Hobson JA, Stickgold R (2002) Practice with sleep makes perfect: sleep-dependent motor skill learning. Neuron 35:205–211
57. Krakauer JW (2006) Motor learning: its relevance to stroke recovery and neurorehabilitation. Curr Opin Neurol 19:84–90
58. Petersen NT, Pyndt HS, Nielsen JB (2003) Investigating human motor control by transcranial magnetic stimulation. Exp Brain Res 152:1–16
59. Schubert M, Curt A, Jensen L, Dietz V (1997) Corticospinal input in human gait: modulation of magnetically evoked motor responses. Exp Brain Res 115:234–246
60. Capaday C, Lavoie BA, Barbeau H, Schneider C, Bonnard M (1999) Studies on the corticospinal control of human walking. I. Responses to focal transcranial magnetic stimulation of the motor cortex. J Neurophysiol 81:129–139
61. Camus M, Pailhous J, Bonnard M (2004) Cognitive tuning of corticospinal excitability during human gait: adaptation to the phase. Eur J Neurosci 20:1101–1107
62. Petersen NT, Butler JE, Marchand-Pauvert V, Fisher R, Ledebt A, Pyndt HS, Hansen NL, Nielsen JB (2001) Suppression of EMG activity by transcranial magnetic stimulation in human subjects during walking. J Physiol 537:651–656
63. Colombo G, Joerg M, Schreier R, Dietz V (2000) Treadmill training of paraplegic patients using a robotic orthosis. J Rehabil Res Dev 37:693–700
64. Kamibayashi K, Nakajima T, Takahashi M, Akai M, Nakazawa K (2009) Facilitation of corticospinal excitability in the tibialis anterior muscle during robot-assisted passive stepping in humans. Eur J Neurosci 30:100–109
65. Winter DA, Yack HJ (1987) EMG profiles during normal human walking: stride-to-stride and inter-subject variability. Electroencephalogr Clin Neurophysiol 67:402–411
66. Kamibayashi K, Nakajima T, Takahashi M, Nakazawa K (2011) Changes in input-output relations in the corticospinal pathway to the lower limb muscles during robot-assisted passive stepping. Conf Proc IEEE Eng Med Biol Soc 2011:4140–4144
67. Simonsen EB, Dyhre-Poulsen P (1999) Amplitude of the human soleus H reflex during walking and running. J Physiol 515:929–939
68. Kamibayashi K, Nakajima T, Fujita M, Takahashi M, Ogawa T, Akai M, Nakazawa K (2010) Effect of sensory inputs on the soleus H-reflex amplitude during robotic passive stepping in humans. Exp Brain Res 202:385–395
69. Nakajima T, Kitamura T, Kamibayashi K, Komiyama T, Zehr EP, Hundza SR, Nakazawa K (2011) Robotic-assisted stepping modulates monosynaptic reflexes in forearm muscles in the human. J Neurophysiol 106:1679–1687
70. Yang JF, Stein RB (1990) Phase-dependent reflex reversal in human leg muscles during walking. J Neurophysiol 63:1109–1117
71. Nakajima T, Kamibayashi K, Takahashi M, Komiyama T, Akai M, Nakazawa K (2008) Load-related modulation of cutaneous reflexes in the tibialis anterior muscle during passive walking in humans. Eur J Neurosci 27:1566–1576

Chapter 5
Movement Disorder and Rehabilitation

Kiyoshi Eguchi and Naoyuki Ochiai

Abstract Impaired motor function affects daily activities in different ways and degrees. For example, dysfunction of the leg causes problems with walking. We here outline the rehabilitation program for disabled people with specific motor system dysfunctions. During the rehabilitation process, it is necessary to pay attention to the part of the body that is functionally impaired as well as to the rest of the body; activities of daily living must also be considered. Various technologies that are being developed in the new field of cybernics can contribute to the rehabilitation of disabled people. In particular, the Hybrid Assistive Limb can improve the walking ability of disabled people with motor dysfunction of the leg.

Keywords Motor function • Activity limitation • Exercise • Rehabilitation

5.1 Introduction

In rehabilitation medicine, we deal with many problems associated with human activities. Human behaviors consist of various mental and physical activities that involve motor function. Here, we focus mainly on movement disorders resulting from nervous and muscular problems and will discuss the possibility to use cybernics technology for rehabilitation. First, in order to facilitate understanding, the body structures and functions associated with human movement will be outlined.

K. Eguchi (✉) • N. Ochiai
Faculty of Medicine, Division of Clinical Medicine, Rehabilitation Department, University of Tsukuba, University of Tsukuba Hospital, Tsukuba, Japan
e-mail: kyeguchi@md.tsukuba.ac.jp

Y. Sankai et al. (eds.), *Cybernics: Fusion of human, machine and information systems*,
DOI 10.1007/978-4-431-54159-2_5, © Springer Japan 2014

5.2 Body Structures and Functions Associated with Human Movement

To understand in more detail the items outlined here, it is advisable to refer to textbooks on physiology, kinesiology, and biomechanics.

The ultimate body part that generates movement is the musculoskeletal system. The bones are organs that support forms of each body part. Although the bones appear static, their components actually are under constant metabolic activity. The bones play an important role in phosphorus and calcium metabolism, which is regulated by several hormones, vitamin D metabolites, vitamin K, etc. Mechanical stimuli elicited by loading and movement also play an essential role in this metabolism. Movement of the body requires the articular structures. Between the contact surfaces of a joint, the hyaline cartilage and synovial fluid containing glycosaminoglycan allow smooth movement. Regarding joint function, excellent mobility is important for the upper limbs. For the lower limbs, supporting body weight is as important as mobility.

Movement itself is generated by striated muscles, which are also called skeletal muscles. The skeletal muscles, which are attached to the different bones at points called origin and insertion, contract to move the joints between these bones and generate movement. There are also biarticular muscles that cross 2 joints and contribute to an efficient control of movement. Movement varies depending on the muscles involved and fixation of the limbs. Some interesting examples are as follows: The gastrocnemius muscles located in the lower limbs function to bend the knee joint. When the positions of the ankle and hip joints are fixed as in the standing position, the muscles contribute to the extension of the knee joint. The muscles bending the fingers, such as the superficial and deep flexor muscles, cross 2 or more joints between the origin and insertion points. In order to exert strong force to hold an object, the wrist joint, one of the joints between the origin and insertion points, should be positioned in dorsiflexion.

Energy to contract the striated muscles is produced by the hydrolysis of adenosine triphosphate (ATP), which is supplied by the metabolism of glucose and fatty acid. These reactions require oxygen. Oxygen deficiency initiates anaerobic metabolism, but major reactions become sluggish under anaerobic conditions. To continue active muscle activities, the respiratory and circulatory systems should supply sufficient oxygen. The contracting cells of muscle tissue are multinucleated and elongated as fibers, called muscle fibers. One spinal motoneuron innervates many muscle fibers. A group consisting of one spinal motoneuron, which is called an alpha motor neuron, and all the corresponding muscle fibers it innervates conform a motor unit. This motor unit receives input signals controlled by the upper center and causes the contraction of muscles.

Signals of muscle contraction are detected by unique intramuscular and extramuscular receptors. Within muscles, there are special muscle fibers with receptors that perceive muscle length and its change rate. Outside of the muscles, the receptors in tendons arranged in tandem with muscle fibers perceive the tension generated by muscle contraction. These signals from muscles are transmitted to the spinal cord by sensory neurons and also rapidly transmitted through the central nervous system.

In the central nervous system, the afferent nervous system transmitting input signals from muscles and the efferent nervous system transmitting output signals to muscles are connected at various levels, causing a phenomenon called reflex. Furthermore, various networks, some of which form loops, function to control movement, including control of posture. Cutaneous, visual, auditory, and equilibrium senses also participate in the control of movement via afferent input signals. So that humans can program movements, control executed movements, and learn to perform more accurate and skillful movements, the spinal cord forms various networks with brain areas, such as the cerebral cortex, basal ganglia, thalamus, cerebellum, and brainstem. Regarding the function of the nervous system associated with movement and muscles, refer to Part II. 4 Motor Control and Learning.

5.3 Movement Disorders

When spinal motoneurons, which are the final common pathway of the nervous system for the generation of movement, and peripheral nerves or neuromuscular junctions and muscles themselves are damaged, muscular atrophy occurs and muscle strength decreases. As a result, effort to move joints generates only weak torques. When there is damage of the descending pathway from the cerebral motor cortex at levels upstream of motoneurons the patient shows complex symptoms generally called spastic paralysis. In case of acute onset, flaccid paralysis occurs in the early stage, and then an enhancement of the stretch reflex gradually becomes evident. Muscle tone is often increased with passive movements; besides, the degrees and patterns of increased muscle tone vary depending on the extent of the nervous system damaged. If an injury blocks all descending pathways of the nervous system that generates movement, only a reflex will generate movement. If the injury is partial, voluntary movement will be restricted. As muscle strength decreases, moving each muscle separately often becomes difficult. Several muscles are simultaneously activated in particular combination, and an intended movement occurs in a certain level of a deformed pattern involving several joints of the affected limb. Typically, possible movements degenerate into those emphasizing either flexion or extension. Regarding the hands and fingers, it becomes difficult to individually bend and stretch fingers. This phenomenon often becomes apparent especially during the recovery process. Along with recovery, separate movement of each joint gradually becomes possible. In the last stage of recovery, movement speed becomes normal. As a possible mechanism to cause these phenomena in the central nervous system the relatively lower center where signals from the higher center decrease may generate movements similar to intended movements in compensation for a few descending input signals and coarse control. In other words, the lower center relatively close to the periphery in the central nervous system, such as the spinal cord, is hypothesized to free the functions restricted in normal conditions and compensate the decrease in signals. This hypothesis is also a concept called hierarchical representation, which originates from the hypothesis proposed by Jackson [1] in the 19th century. It is considered that recovery may be at least partially attributable to plasticity of neural networks. However, the associations between injury sites in the central nervous system, ranging from the cerebrum to the spinal cord, and symptoms have not been completely elucidated as yet. In clinical neurology, no quantitative method to determine the severity of this phenomenon has yet been established. In clinical practice, assessment methods proposed by Brunnström [2] and Fugl-Meyer [3] are used for treating patients with cerebrovascular disorder in several countries, including Japan.

Other movement disorders resulting from central nervous system disorder include those considered to be a disorder of the motor control system such as ataxia, involuntary movement and impairment of postural reflexes, disorders of programming movements, and a combination of several disorders. These movement disorders attributable to central nervous system disorder are sometimes referred to as narrowly-defined movement disorder.

For people to move smoothly, it is necessary that muscles, bones, joints, heart, lungs, endocrine and metabolic systems, etc., function properly as well as the peripheral and central nerves including autonomic nerves. Moreover, the body structures and functions can be maintained in appropriate conditions by adequately moving the body. While excessive movement results in dysfunction due to overuse, insufficient movement results in dysfunction due to disuse. Especially, the latter is important in terms of its easy susceptibility, thus prophylactic measures are considered necessary starting from the acute phase of many injuries and diseases. Dysfunction due to disuse is also a risk factor for sarcopenia [4], an age-related muscular atrophy that is less reversible. However, because the difference between overuse and disuse is small in some diseases characterized by pathological conditions which mainly involve inflammation or rapidly progressing degeneration, determination of the most appropriate amount of activity may require careful considerations. The dysfunction due to disuse has been called disuse syndrome [5]. In recent years, because life in the space, where there is almost no load of gravity, causes problems similar to disuse, new studies on its prevention are being conducted.

5.4 Technology to Collect Data on Movement of the Body

In order to solve problems of human body movements with Cybernics Technology, data on the movements should be collected and analyzed. In recent years, there has been outstanding progress in the development of technologies to noninvasively visualize and analyze the internal structures and functions of the body. Improvements in the usage of strong magnetic field, ultrasound, optical wavelength, near-infrared light, X-ray, radioactive isotopes, etc. have allowed examining the morphology of deep body structures, their changes, blood flow, blood oxygen saturation, etc. Their use also allows assessing local or systemic metabolism of specific substances. These technologies are helpful for assessing lesion sites and pathological conditions in people with a disease.

Important data directly associated with movements include changes in joint angles, generation of torque, and changes in pressure load of the sole. Based on these data, it is possible to know the state of the lower limbs during walking. Biological reactions, which reflect the reaction of the whole body to a load, can be noninvasively determined from vital signs, such as pulse, heart rate, blood pressure, and respiratory rate, as well as peripheral arterial oxygen saturation and analysis of expired gas for oxygen uptake and expiratory quotient. Neural and muscular activities can be partially detected as electrical or magnetic activities from the skin surface. Examples include electrocardiogram, electromyogram mainly using compound muscle action potential, electroencephalogram, magnetocardiogram, and magnetoencephalogram. Weak reactions have been determined by averaging several measurements; moreover, for laboratory examinations, reactions may be recorded by stimulating a part of the body with electricity or a magnetic field. When the central nervous system is examined, it should be kept in mind that patterns between divergence and convergence and between facilitation and inhibition of transmitted "signals" vary in the course of reactions to stimulation. Deep electrical activities can be detected by inserting recording electrodes at appropriate positions, even though invasive. Based on these data, movements and their disorder can be objectively assessed and measured to analyze their physiological and pathophysiological mechanisms. Studies on technologies to assess the will of people are also being conducted, with the aim of developing a brain machine interface (BMI). Regarding the above, refer to Part III. 13 Electroneurophysiology and Brain Functional Imaging for Brain-Machine-Interface.

5.5 Rehabilitation for Movement Disorders

The aim of rehabilitation of disabled people is to achieve the most appropriate life that can be possible for them. The aim of rehabilitation for those with movement disorders is the same. The classification of life functions and disabilities by the World Health Organization (Fig. 5.1) [6] indicates issues that should be solved by rehabilitation. The problems of physical and psychological functions and physical structures are called impairments, which include disorder of motor function. Difficulty in tasks and daily activities performed by individuals are called activity limitations, to which difficulty in walking and self-care corresponds. A problem due to involvement in life situations is a participation restriction.

If impairment of physical functions can be relieved by treatment, overall life functions will be improved in many cases. Impairment of motor function is often treated by exercising the impaired movement itself. In order to increase muscle strength, exercise with a resistive load equal to or exceeding that experienced in

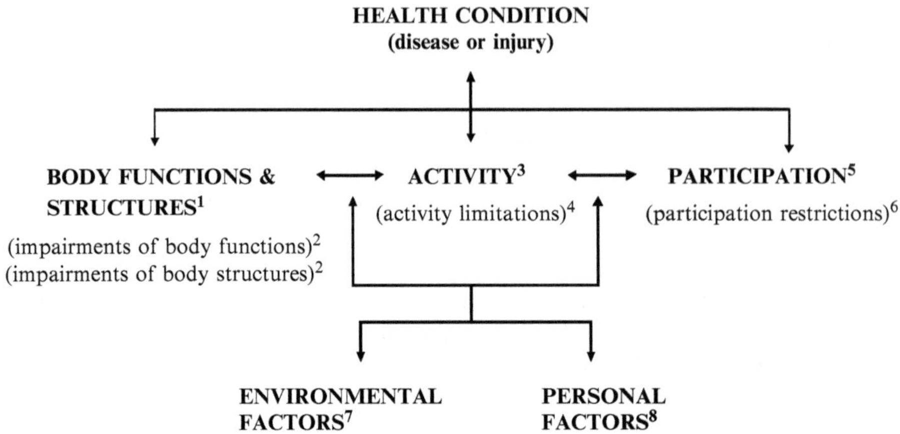

Fig. 5.1 Basic concept of international classification of functioning, disability and health
[1] Body functions are the physiological functions of body systems (including psychological functions). Body structures are anatomical parts of the body such as organs, limbs and their components.
[2] Impairments are problems in function or structure as a significant deviation or loss.
[3] Activity is the execution of a task or action by an individual.
[4] Activity limitations are difficulties an individual may have in executing activities.
[5] Participation is involvement in a life situation.
[6] Participation restrictions are problems an individual may have to be involved in life situations.
[7] Environmental factors make up the physical, social, and attitudinal environment in which people live and conduct their lives.
[8] Personal factors include lifestyle, habits, social background, education, life events, race/ethnicity, sexual orientation and assets of the individual

daily living is usually performed with muscles targeted for increasing muscle strength. Electric stimulation has been used as an adjunct procedure, and recently, there is a procedure in which antagonist muscles are contracted by electric stimulation to create a resistive load [7]. Moreover, the mechanism of muscle hypertrophy and reactions of the musculoskeletal system to external stimuli have been elucidated, leading to the development of procedures that restrict the blood flow in muscles [8] and procedures that use vibration stimulation [9] for increasing muscle strength and volume. In order to efficiently perform muscle strength exercise, the speed of movement and the range of joint motion are crucial. Muscle strength is most efficiently generated at the speed and joint angle within those repeatedly used in muscle strength exercise. In the case of exercise aiming at improving endurance, sustained movements are performed with a lower load and for longer time than in an exercise aiming at increasing muscle strength. Moreover, heart rate, blood pressure and expired gas are monitored in order to control the intensity of movements. The anaerobic metabolic threshold estimated by analysis of expired gas indicates the intensity of movement effective for improving endurance, being one of the indices of physical fitness.

As for exercise aiming at relieving movement disorders resulting from central nervous system disorder, movements necessary for activities targeted for improvement are often repeated many times, instead of performing resistance exercise aiming at increasing muscle strength. Several procedures to facilitate difficult movements and to inhibit movements deviating from normal are proposed. Brunnström is one of the researchers who proposed such a procedure in the 1960s based on her experiences [2]. Motor learning theories, as well as estimated plasticity of the brain, should be considered when an exercise program is designed. Patients with ataxia often maintain muscle strength although muscle tone is decreased. A resistive load expected to increase proprioceptive input stabilizes movements of these patients at least temporarily and improves movement coordination. Regarding some symptoms of parkinsonian syndrome, especially repetitive movements such as walking, externally presented rhythm may be effective to attain a relief of symptoms.

However, even without the interventions described above, physical functions may change to relieve impairment spontaneously, as daily living activities constantly involves moving of the body. To demonstrate the medical significance of the effects of therapeutic approaches, double-blind randomized controlled trials should be conducted. In fact, there are only a few therapeutic approaches in which the recommended procedure significantly relieves impairment due to central nervous system disorder. The reasons for this are at least partially as follows: A trial with a control group receiving no intervention for a long period is ethically almost impossible. Because of effects of daily physical activities, the difference with the control group may be actually small under ordinary trial protocols. Moreover, patterns of impairment vary in patients with central nervous lesions. Thus, an extremely large-scale trial involving a large number of patients is required to reveal statistical significance. Such a large-scale trial is difficult to conduct.

On the other hand, repetitive practice of a movement that is a daily living task while using compensatory procedures may lead to an adjustment of the body to adapt the movement and further reduce the activity limitation even though assessment of the impairment does not reveal clear improvement. Statistical analysis of rehabilitation treatment effects is often performed focused on efficiency for improvement of activity. In the actual rehabilitation process, even with a high possibility to relieve impairment, achieving relief often requires a long period. There are also some cases of impairment that cannot be solved by the current medical care but must be treated, such as rehabilitation after amputation of the upper or lower limb. Thus, in the field of rehabilitation, much effort is devoted to reduce activity limitation by compensation. If no reduction of activity limitation for a long period leads to a prolonged state of the reduced quantity of daily activities, there may be a risk for impairment due to disuse spreading to the whole body in addition to the impairment causing the limitation. On the contrary, for example in a lower-limb amputee, wearing a prosthetic limb does not change the state of impairment but solves activity limitation due to difficulty in walking by a compensatory procedure. If this results in improved independence and increased activities, the overall physical condition may improve. Even in case of local impairment of the musculoskeletal system, goals can be achieved efficiently by practicing a movement after immediately reducing the activity limitation by a compensatory procedure, in addition to local treatment including exercise. As exercise aiming to relieve physical dysfunction originating from the central nervous system, tasks included in activities of daily living are used, and walking is often used for treatment of movement disorder of the lower limbs. Compensatory procedures include the use of walking aids, such as a cane, and orthoses.

In recent years, devices to assist human movements targeted for compensation have been developed using robot technology. It is expected that both physical functions and activities can be more efficiently improved by inducing preferable movements with such devices and by repeatedly practicing the movements. One example of such devices is the Hybrid Assistive Limb (HAL), developed as a wearable robot that recognizes and assists human movements based on data on bioelectric signal related to muscle activities, joint angles, ground reaction force, etc. (For details of the development background and mechanism of HAL, refer to Part II. 2 Wearable Robot Technology.) Generally, orthoses used to compensate dysfunction of the lower limbs partially restrict joint movement in order to increase strength and stability of the lower limbs. On the other hand, while HAL is worn for walking, it assists movements of the hip and knee joints with actuators and induces movements in which these joints follow nearly normal tracks. Inducing movement in this way can also be expected to add haptic feedback effects.

In the first stage of assessing the effects of exercise using HAL, we conducted walking-based exercise wearing HAL in seven patients with chronic cerebral stroke and six patients with chronic spinal cord disorder who had walking disability due to at least moderate lower limb paralysis but who could walk using a walking aid, such as a cane, or orthoses (Fig. 5.2). The subjects performed the exercise approximately twice a week for a total of 16 sessions. During each session lasting approximately 1 h, the subjects repeated the exercise for a total of approximately 20–30 min. Before and after a series of 16 sessions, 10-m free walking with the same walking aid or orthoses used in daily living was assessed. The mean walking speed improved by 20 % or more in both patient groups. Although this study involved patients in the chronic phase, the results suggested that statistically significant differences were likely to be demonstrated by increasing the number of subjects. Moreover, assessment of balance showed slight improvement. These results showed that, although wearing and removing HAL require help, it can be used as an auxiliary device for walking exercise at institutions providing rehabilitation treatment. At present, we are analyzing which factor of the functions associated with walking improves walking ability by what mechanism. In part, the improvement may be attributable to changes in functions of muscles and the nervous system associated with movement of the lower limbs. However, in patients with differences in lesion site and extent, complications, amount of movement in daily living, etc., the degree and type of impairment vary, and factors for improving physical functions also differ. In the field of rehabilitation, walking is considered as a part of activities of daily living. The walking exercise using HAL might have improved one aspect of the ability to perform this activity. The improvement in walking speed

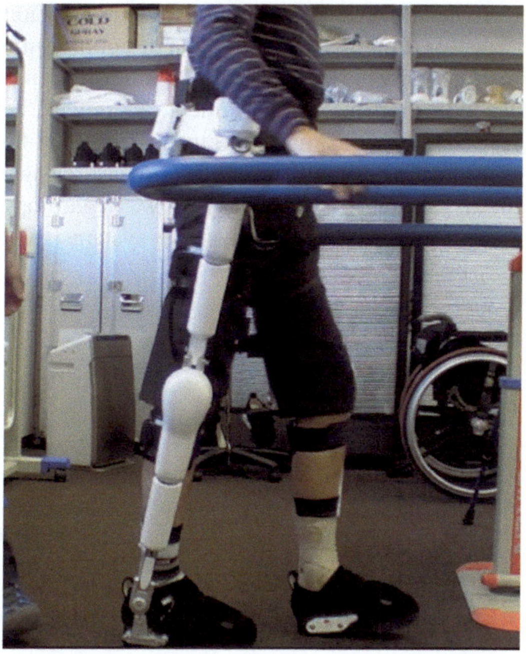

Fig. 5.2 Walking exercise using HAL

means a possible increase of the walking distance during the same period. If endurance is improved by repetition, it will be easy to increase daily walking time and distance. By establishing a good cycle, the effects of walking can be expected to spread out to the whole body including the musculoskeletal, cardiopulmonary, and metabolic systems.

At present, the majority of robots developed to assist walking exercise cannot be moved from installation sites. If HAL, which moves as its wearer walks, is developed into a robot that disabled people can use in their activities of daily living in the future, activity limitations can be reduced. Depending on physical conditions, HAL can be expected to be useful to improve impaired physical functions during such activities.

If an interface that more closely connects the brain and a device is developed, devices that more directly recognize the will of people can be developed to assist movement. A prosthetic hand is an example of devices that are desired to adopt such BMI. If weight of a prosthetic limb can be reduced, it will be easier to add parts to the limb than exoskeleton. Moreover, if a wearable exoskeleton robot assisting movement can be controlled, it might be possible for paretic limbs whose functional recovery is difficult to attain to be moved by will through the exoskeleton robot. In the future, with advances in technology such as the application of BMI to these robots, even patients in a "locked-in" state who cannot express their will on their own may become able to resume activities.

In rehabilitation, resolution of participation restrictions may be the ultimate issue, for it involves equalization of opportunities for social participation. In people with movement disorder, limited mobility remarkably restricts social participation depending on their environment. Moreover, depending on purposes of traveling, assistance for information transmission may be helpful. If the costs of individual assistance do not surpass those of measures against activity limitation, the demand for an assistance system may grow. Regarding environmental intervention, development and installation of various systems and assistant devices that can be shared may be necessary.

References

1. Jackson JH (1884) The Croonian lectures on evolution and dissolution of the nervous system. Br Med J 51(1214):660–663
2. Sawner KA, LaVigne JM (1992) Brunnstrom's movement therapy in hemiplegia. A neurophysiological approach, 2nd edn. JB Lippincott, Philadelphia
3. Fugle-Meyer AR, Jääskö L, Leyman I, Olsson S, Steglind S (1975) The post-stroke hemiplegic patient I. A method for evaluation of physical performance. Scand J Rehab Med 7:13–31
4. Cruz-Jentoft AJ, Baeyens JP, Bauer JM, Boirie Y, Cederholm T, Landi F, Martin FC, Michel JP, Rolland Y, Schneider SM, Topinková E, Vandewoude M, Zamboni M, European Working Group on Sarcopenia in Older People (2010) Sarcopenia: European consensus on definition and diagnosis: report of the European Working Group on Sarcopenia in Older People. Age Aging 39:412–423
5. Bortz WM (1984) The disuse syndrome. West J Med 141:691–694
6. World Health Organization (2001) International classification of functioning disability and health. World Health Organization, Geneva
7. Yanagi T, Shiba N, Maeda T, Iwasa Y, Umezu Y, Tagawa Y, Matsuo S, Nagata K, Yamamoto T, Basford JR (2003) Agonist contractions against electrically stimulated antagonists. Arch Phys Med Rehabil 84:843–848
8. Takarada Y, Takazawa H, Sato Y, Takebayashi S, Tanaka Y, Ishii N (2000) Effects of resistance exercise combined with moderate vascular occlusion on muscular function in humans. J Appl Physiol 88:2097–2106
9. Lau RW, Liao LR, Yu F, Teo T, Chung RC, Pang MY (2011) The effects of whole body vibration therapy on bone mineral density and leg muscle strength in older adults: a systematic review and meta-analysis. Clin Rehabil 25:975–988

Chapter 6
Regenerative Medicine for Spinal Cord Injury Using Olfactory Mucosa Autografts

Koichi Iwatsuki and Toshiki Yoshimine

Abstract The central nervous system has limited regenerative capacity, and functional restoration of the damaged system is difficult. Treatment is still limited to cerebrospinal protection after injury and reconstruction of neural networks by rehabilitation. In case of incomplete spinal cord injury, neural networks can be reconstructed because nerve tissues remain at the site of the injury. However, in case of complete spinal cord injury, all scaffolds for reconstruction of neural networks are lost. Thus, functional recovery through rehabilitation cannot be expected. At present, enhancement of residual function is the only treatment approach. Regarding spinal cord injury, expectations have been placed on regenerative medicine using stem cells including induced pluripotent stem cells, which have recently captured attention. However, regenerative medicine using stem cells is effective only during the acute-to-subacute phase, a period before scar tissues are formed in the injured spinal cord. Regenerative medicine using stem cells is completely ineffective in the chronic phase. In case of planning treatment for chronic-phase spinal cord injury, it is necessary to supply scaffolds where neuronal axons can grow to form neural networks, neurons, and neurotrophic factors for growth and protection of neuronal axons. In other words, all of the three elements, i.e., scaffolds, neurons, and neurotrophic factors are necessary. In addition, transplantation including these three elements requires avoiding ethical problems and immunological rejection. These conditions are not satisfied by cell transplantation, but by tissue transplantation, particularly by autologous tissue transplantation. The olfactory mucosa contains olfactory nerves associated with olfaction and is an extracranial region with exceptionally active nerve regeneration. The mucosa, which is embryologically derived from the central nerve as primordium, contains

K. Iwatsuki (✉) • T. Yoshimine
Department of Neurosurgery, Osaka University Medical School, Suita, Japan
e-mail: kiwatsuki@nsurg.med.osaka-u.ac.jp

Y. Sankai et al. (eds.), *Cybernics: Fusion of human, machine and information systems*,
DOI 10.1007/978-4-431-54159-2_6, © Springer Japan 2014

stem cells, olfactory ensheathing cells that have axonal growth effects, and various neurotrophic factors. The mucosa is endoscopically resectable and spontaneously regenerates after resection. Because the olfactory mucosa allows active nerve regeneration under physiological conditions, it is considered useful as a scaffold for neuronal axon regeneration. We conducted an animal study and then a human clinical study on treatment of chronic spinal cord injury using olfactory mucosa autografts. At the end of 2011, this treatment was designated as an advanced medical treatment.

Keywords Spinal cord injury • Olfactory mucosa • Regeneration

6.1 Introduction

Olfactory mucosa autografts for complete paraplegic patients with chronic-phase spinal cord injury were first performed by Lima et al. at Egas-Moniz Hospital in Lisbon, Portugal, in 2001 [1, 2]. Olfactory mucosa is the only extracranial region where nerve regeneration is observed under physiological conditions [3]; the mucosa contains olfactory ensheathing cells (OEC) and neural stem cells that contribute to the repair of spinal cord injury [4]. Especially, because an autologous graft can be endoscopically harvested from the nasal cavity of the patient [5], neither immunological rejection nor ethical problems become an issue. We have been performing this procedure since 2007 in Japan, and are currently investigating its safety and efficacy.

6.2 History of Experimental Studies on Spinal Cord Injury

In the late 1970s, transplantation of fetal nerve tissue was introduced as an experimental therapy for central nerve injury. In a model of brain injury, neurons arising from an embryonic graft and neurotransmitters secreted from the injured region in the host brain, which indicated enhanced axonal growth and functional recovery, were confirmed [6]. Because fetal nerve tissue contains neurons, the mechanism of neuronal axonal restoration based on this transplantation procedure was attributed to formation of bidirectional synaptic connections between neurons contained in the transplanted tissue and the host spinal cord [7]. This discovery gave a new direction to basic studies on spinal cord injury towards clinical practice. However, this procedure could not be applied in humans because, as transplantation for one patient with spinal cord injury required 10–15 fetuses, the procedure was ethically unacceptable. Then, neural stem cells or embryonic stem (ES) cells contained in fetal tissue attracted attention.

Many therapies using stem cell transplantation to treat spinal cord injury are under investigation, and great expectations are placed especially on induced pluripotent stem (iPS) cells and ES cells. On the other hand, survival of transplanted stem cells is low in cell-based therapies including stem cells. It has been revealed that many of them die within 24 h after transplantation [8]. In recent studies, development of scaffolds for survival of these cells is a major trend of research [9].

6.3 Acute and Chronic Phases of Spinal Cord Injury

The pathological conditions of spinal cord injury in the acute-to-subacute and chronic phases are completely different. Thus, treatment strategies in each phase also differ.

In the injured spinal cord, cells are destroyed, and both nerve fibers and blood vessels are sheared. This is the so-called primary injury, followed by the secondary cytotoxic injury, such as inflammation [10]. However, inflammatory responses after the primary injury that are considered the secondary injury are reported to be important for repair [11]. There are ongoing studies to clarify the cytokines or cells associated with exacerbation of pathological conditions or repair in the acute phase [12].

The injury site loses neurons and, in the chronic phase after the secondary injury, is covered by glial scar tissue that is unlikely to allow axonal regeneration [13]. Thus, treatment in the chronic phase requires replenishment of neurons, facilitation of axonal growth, reduction of glial scar tissue that inhibits axonal regeneration and improvement of the spinal microenvironment that inhibits spontaneous axonal regeneration [14, 15]. In other words, it is necessary to create the conditions that favor the formation of scaffolds for axonal growth [1].

6.4 Cell Transplantation Therapy in the Acute-to-Subacute Phase

Regarding transplantation therapy using stem cells, such as ES and iPS cells, or using neural cells differentiated from these stem cells, functional recovery owing to remyelination of axons, etc. has been reported, and there are great expectations concerning the use of stem cells [16, 17]. Geron Corporation, an American entrepreneurial venture, developed a therapy for spinal cord injury using human ES cells, which was approved by the Food and Drug Administration of the United States in 2010. Although this therapy was performed in the first case in October 2010, Geron recently withdrew from its development. Regarding the use of human ES cells in clinical studies or treatment in Japan, neither safety issues nor ethical problems, similar to those concerning aborted fetuses, have been solved. Because human iPS cells derived from autologous cells are associated with fewer ethical problems, studies aiming at clinical application of iPS cells are being vigorously conducted. However, their mechanism to produce effects is considered to be basically the same as that of ES cells. The effects of iPS cells may be limited to the first 8 days after injury.

Bone marrow stromal cells contain abundant neurotrophic factors that have neuroprotective effects, [18] and clinical studies have been conducted in several countries for a long period. The clinical studies on transplantation of bone marrow stromal cells in the acute-to-subacute phase conducted in South Korea and Czechoslovakia demonstrated neurological functional recovery [19–21]. In Japan, bone marrow stromal cells were transplanted into three patients with acute-phase spinal cord injury at Kansai Medical University Hospital. No serious adverse event has been reported until now. Further development of the technique is expected.

In these clinical studies, bone marrow stromal cells were transplanted into patients in the acute-to-subacute phase of the lesion. Because this phase corresponds to a period when some spontaneous recovery may be possible even in cases with complete paraplegia, the efficacy of the cell transplantation is difficult to discuss. However, the future progress of several studies is expected.

6.5 Transplantation Therapy in the Chronic Phase

In the chronic phase of spinal cord injury, death of neurons, rupture of neuronal axons, and glial scar occur. Thus, replenishment of neurons, axonal growth factors for neural network construction, and scaffolds for axonal growth, are necessary. Many investigators have confirmed that, if peripheral nerves or cultured Schwann cells are transplanted, central neuronal axons will grow in the transplant as a permissive scaffold. Cheng et al. resected spinal cord segments of adult rats and bridged the gaps with several intercostal nerve grafts with the aim to reduce an inhibitory environment [22]. Transplantation of OEC performed by Li et al. was also an attempt to reduce the inhibitory effect of the environment [23]. Thus, three factors consisting of cells that can replenish lost neurons, axonal growth factors, and scaffolds permissive for axonal growth are necessary in the chronic phase.

6.5.1 Neural Stem Cells

Although neural stem cells can serve for replenishment of neurons, simply transplanted stem cells cannot survive for a long period [24]. However, recent studies have revealed that, if the local microenvironment at the spinal cord injury is improved, nerves and axons can regenerate [7, 25]. Transplanted neural stem cells not only differentiate into neural cells but also secrete various and numerous factors that facilitate axonal growth [26]. Transplantation of neural stem cells is promising in terms of cell replenishment and axonal growth. However, it has been revealed that transplantation of neural stem cells alone cannot exert a sufficient regenerative effect without improvement of the local microenvironment at the spinal cord injury [26].

6.5.2 *Olfactory Ensheathing Cells (OEC)*

The olfactory system that extends from the olfactory mucosa to the olfactory bulb of the central nervous system is an exceptional tissue where nerves and axons regenerate under physiological conditions throughout nearly the entire life [3]. This exceptional neuroregenerative effect is attributed mainly to neural stem cells and OEC contained in the olfactory mucosal epithelium [27]. Of these cells, OEC are cells that have axonal growth effects in the chronic phase of spinal cord injury [28]. Unlike oligodendrocytes in the central nervous system or Schwann cells in peripheral nerves, OEC can extend neuronal axons from the olfactory nerves at the periphery to the olfactory bulb at the center [27, 29]. Unlike Schwann cells, it has been revealed that adult OEC extend axons from retinal ganglion cells which are classified as central nerves [30], and that OEC cocultured with hippocampal neurons better integrate with astrocytes as compared to OEC cocultured with Schwann cells [31]. OEC have a protective action on extended axons against axonal inhibitory factors in adult central nerves [29]. OEC transplanted into the injured spinal cord secrete abundant axonal growth factors and form a scaffold for axonal growth [23, 32]. In addition, it has been revealed that OEC promote myelination of axons to improve nerve conduction velocity [33, 34] and regenerate the transected descending axonal pathway to restore function [23, 35]. Furthermore, OEC infiltrate the glial scar tissue to some extent and secretevarious neurotrophic factors and adhesion molecules to facilitate axonal growth [32]. Mackay-Sim et al. at Griffith University, transplanted OEC into six patients with chronic-phase spinal cord injury, and reported that no serious adverse event occurred during 3 years after transplantation [28]. In this clinical study, neurological functional recovery was observed in one patient.

6.5.3 *Olfactory Mucosa*

Because the spinal cord is a naturally inhibitory environment for axonal growth [14, 15], formation of scaffolds is necessary for the survival of transplanted stem cells and axonal growth [1, 9]. The olfactory mucosa contains neural stem cells that can replenish neurons and OEC that exert a neuronal axonal growth action; thus, neurons actively regenerate in the olfactory mucosa. Based on these findings, the olfactory mucosa itself would be useful as a scaffold of regeneration of neuronal axons [3]. Basic studies using rats have also confirmed the usefulness of the olfactory mucosa [36, 37]. The olfactory mucosa may be an ideal graft to treat chronic-phase spinal cord injury [1, 2].

6.6 Olfactory Mucosa Transplantation to Treat Spinal Cord Injury

According to autologous olfactory mucosa transplantation to treat spinal cord injury in the chronic phase, that is at least 6 months after spinal cord injury (Fig. 6.1a), the mucosa is endoscopically removed and cut into small pieces (Fig. 6.1b). After the intramedullary scar tissue at the injury site is removed (Fig. 6.1c), the pieces of olfactory mucosa are transplanted into the cavity left by the scar tissue (Fig. 6.1d).

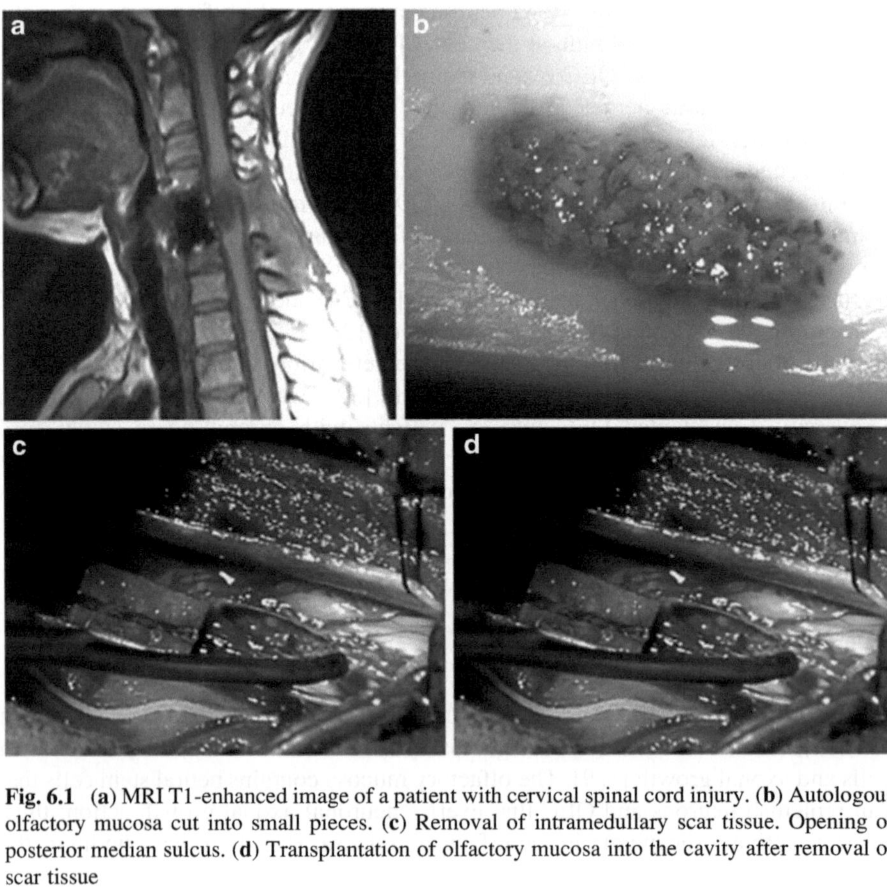

Fig. 6.1 (**a**) MRI T1-enhanced image of a patient with cervical spinal cord injury. (**b**) Autologous olfactory mucosa cut into small pieces. (**c**) Removal of intramedullary scar tissue. Opening of posterior median sulcus. (**d**) Transplantation of olfactory mucosa into the cavity after removal of scar tissue

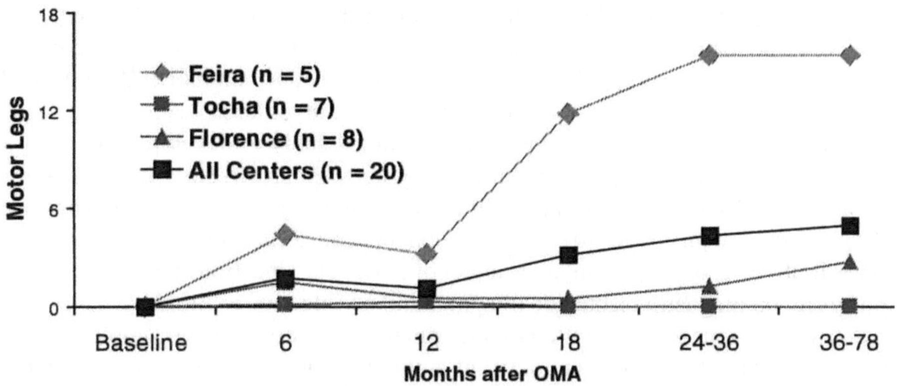

Fig. 6.2 ASIA motor legs scores and WISCI and FIM after OMA with rehabilitation at individual centers (A) ASIA motor legs scores at given times after OMA. After preoperative rehabilitation (mean = 8 months; range = 1–27 months), all 20 patients had a motor leg scores of 0. The greatest improvement after OMA was the primarily paraplegic patients receiving rehabilitation at SS (◆) with 5/5 patients improving, some improvement primarily in tetraplegics at GC (▲) with 4/8 patients improving, and no improvement (7/7 patients) in the primarily tetraplegics at RP (□) [38]

Although the scar tissue is just partially removed not to damage normal spinal cord tissue, sufficient opening of the posterior median sulcus is necessary along the cephalocaudal axis of the injury site for bridging the gap in the spinal cord [1, 2]. Lima et al. performed autologous olfactory mucosa transplantation in 20 patients with chronic-phase spinal cord injury that caused complete motor paralysis of both lower limbs; there were 17 men and 3 women whose ages ranged from 19 to 37 years. The patients underwent intensive rehabilitation. After a follow-up period of 12–45 months after the operation (mean: 27.7 months), American Spinal Injury Association (ASIA) classification scores improved from A to C in six patients, from B to C in three patients, and from A to B in two patients. Electromyography (EMG) of lower limb muscles revealed voluntary contractions in 15 patients. Furthermore, Lima et al. reported that improvement in bladder function test results was achieved in five patients (Fig. 6.2). All patients recovered olfaction, and recovery was achieved within 2 months after the operation in 95 % of the patients. Regarding adverse events, subcutaneous accumulation of spinal fluid was observed in three patients, all of which resolved naturally or after a simple suture. In one patient, hypersensitive enteritis was observed 1 year after the operation and reported to have persisted for 5 years. This event is considered to be visceral neuropathic pain. Moreover, another patient concomitantly developed bacterial meningitis caused by methicillin-resistant Staphylococcus aureus, which was cured with vancomycin. However, the ASIA classification score worsened from B to A. Two months later, it improved to B again [1, 2].

The team at Detroit Medical Center provided a similar rehabilitation program to 38 patients who underwent olfactory mucosa transplantation and 22 patients without transplantation. Although no statistically significant difference was observed, the team reported that motor function improved in 58 % of the patients with transplantation, versus 27 % of those without transplantation (The 26th Annual National Neurotrauma Society Symposium held in July 2008).

Since 2002, we have been conducting a clinical study to develop therapies for functional recovery of injured spinal cord by autologous olfactory mucosa transplantation. The inclusion criteria are: at least a 6-month period after the occurrence of spinal cord injury, age 40 years or younger, complete motor paralysis of the lower limbs of class A or B in the Frankel or ASIA classification, a 3-cm or shorter injury site on magnetic resonance imaging, and no infection in the nasal cavity. As of April 2010, four patients with thoracic spinal cord injury causing complete motor paralysis of both lower limbs underwent autologous olfactory mucosa transplantation: two patients on February 7–8, 2008, 1 on July 17, 2009, and 1 on March 19, 2010. In these four patients, there has been neither infection nor development of a malignant neoplasm associated with this procedure. Although hyposmia, headache, and pain at the site of the spinal cord injury occurred as adverse events in some patients, all events resolved without progressing to a serious condition. There has been no safety problem that would affect the continuation of the study. EMG revealed waveforms generated from the lower rectus abdominis muscle, paraspinal muscle, and tensor fasciae latae muscle in one of the four patients and EMG waveforms generated from the lower rectus abdominis muscle in another patient. Moreover, EMG waveforms were generated from the quadriceps femoris muscle in one of the two remaining patients. Lima et al. emphasize the importance of providing long-term rehabilitation in combination with olfactory mucosa transplantation. They discuss that recovery cannot be expected by olfactory mucosa transplantation or rehabilitation alone, and that rehabilitation for remodeling of skeletal muscles, blood vessels, and nerves is necessary. Although the ideal type of rehabilitation remains unknown, Lima et al. especially advocate the importance of walking rehabilitation with weight bearing that is called brain-initiated overground nonrobotic/nonweight supported training (BIONT) [1, 2].

6.7 Conclusion

Regarding spinal cord injury, there is evidence that combination therapy using transplantation with other factors is more effective than cell-based transplantation therapy alone [39, 40]. It may be difficult to achieve success using a single factor, such as specific cells. Olfactory mucosa is an ideal transplantation tissue at present because it contains the cells, axonal growth factors, and provides a scaffold for regeneration. Because reconstructed nervous tissue obtained by transplantation is not natural, remodeling of skeletal muscles, blood vessels, and reconstructed neural networks is necessary. Thus, rehabilitation after transplantation is very important.

References

1. Lima C, Escada P, Pratas-Vital J et al (2009) Olfactory mucosal autografts and rehabilitation for chronic traumatic spinal cord injury. Neurorehabil Neural Repair 24:10–22
2. Lima C, Pratas-Vital J, Escada P et al (2006) Olfactory mucosa autografts in human spinal cord injury: a pilot clinical study. J Spinal Cord Med 29:191–203; discussion 204–196
3. Farbman AI (1994) Developmental biology of olfactory sensory neurons. Semin Cell Biol 5:3–10
4. Murrell W, Feron F, Wetzig A et al (2005) Multipotent stem cells from adult olfactory mucosa. Dev Dyn 233:496–515
5. Winstead W, Marshall CT, Lu CL et al (2005) Endoscopic biopsy of human olfactory epithelium as a source of progenitor cells. Am J Rhinol 19:83–90
6. Anderson DK, Howland DR, Reier PJ (1995) Fetal neural grafts and repair of the injured spinal cord. Brain Pathol 5:451–457
7. Bregman BS, Coumans JV, Dai HN et al (2002) Transplants and neurotrophic factors increase regeneration and recovery of function after spinal cord injury. Prog Brain Res 137:257–273
8. Laflamme MA, Chen KY, Naumova AV et al (2007) Cardiomyocytes derived from human embryonic stem cells in pro-survival factors enhance function of infarcted rat hearts. Nat Biotechnol 25:1015–1024
9. Samadikuchaksaraei A (2007) An overview of tissue engineering approaches for management of spinal cord injuries. J Neuroeng Rehabil 4:15
10. Rowland JW, Hawryluk GW, Kwon B et al (2008) Current status of acute spinal cord injury pathophysiology and emerging therapies: promise on the horizon. Neurosurg Focus 25:E2
11. Pereira JE, Costa LM, Cabrita AM et al (2009) Methylprednisolone fails to improve functional and histological outcome following spinal cord injury in rats. Exp Neurol 220:71–81
12. Ankeny DP, Popovich PG (2009) Mechanisms and implications of adaptive immune responses after traumatic spinal cord injury. Neuroscience 158:1112–1121
13. Filbin MT (2003) Myelin-associated inhibitors of axonal regeneration in the adult mammalian CNS. Nat Rev Neurosci 4:703–713
14. Mukhopadhyay G, Doherty P, Walsh FS et al (1994) A novel role for myelin-associated glycoprotein as an inhibitor of axonal regeneration. Neuron 13:757–767
15. Schwab ME, Caroni P (1988) Oligodendrocytes and CNS myelin are nonpermissive substrates for neurite growth and fibroblast spreading in vitro. J Neurosci 8:2381–2393
16. Keirstead HS, Nistor G, Bernal G et al (2005) Human embryonic stem cell-derived oligodendrocyte progenitor cell transplants remyelinate and restore locomotion after spinal cord injury. J Neurosci 25:4694–4705
17. Nistor GI, Totoiu MO, Haque N et al (2005) Human embryonic stem cells differentiate into oligodendrocytes in high purity and myelinate after spinal cord transplantation. Glia 49:385–396
18. Parr AM, Tator CH, Keating A (2007) Bone marrow-derived mesenchymal stromal cells for the repair of central nervous system injury. Bone Marrow Transplant 40:609–619
19. Sykova E, Homola A, Mazanec R et al (2006) Autologous bone marrow transplantation in patients with subacute and chronic spinal cord injury. Cell Transplant 15:675–687
20. Tator CH (2006) Review of treatment trials in human spinal cord injury: issues, difficulties, and recommendations. Neurosurgery 59:957–982; discussion 982–957
21. Yoon SH, Shim YS, Park YH et al (2007) Complete spinal cord injury treatment using autologous bone marrow cell transplantation and bone marrow stimulation with granulocyte macrophage-colony stimulating factor: Phase I/II clinical trial. Stem Cells 25:2066–2073
22. Cheng H, Cao Y, Olson L (1996) Spinal cord repair in adult paraplegic rats: partial restoration of hind limb function. Science 273:510–513
23. Li Y, Field PM, Raisman G (1997) Repair of adult rat corticospinal tract by transplants of olfactory ensheathing cells. Science 277:2000–2002

24. Okada S, Ishii K, Yamane J et al (2005) In vivo imaging of engrafted neural stem cells: its application in evaluating the optimal timing of transplantation for spinal cord injury. Faseb J 19:1839–1841
25. Fawcett JW (1998) Spinal cord repair: from experimental models to human application. Spinal Cord 36:811–817
26. Han SS, Kang DY, Mujtaba T et al (2002) Grafted lineage-restricted precursors differentiate exclusively into neurons in the adult spinal cord. Exp Neurol 177:360–375
27. Raisman G (1985) Specialized neuroglial arrangement may explain the capacity of vomeronasal axons to reinnervate central neurons. Neuroscience 14:237–254
28. Mackay-Sim A, Feron F, Cochrane J et al (2008) Autologous olfactory ensheathing cell transplantation in human paraplegia: a 3-year clinical trial. Brain 131:2376–2386
29. Doucette R (1990) Glial influences on axonal growth in the primary olfactory system. Glia 3:433–449
30. Leaver SG, Harvey AR, Plant GW (2006) Adult olfactory ensheathing glia promote the long-distance growth of adult retinal ganglion cell neurites in vitro. Glia 53:467–476
31. van den Pol AN, Santarelli JG (2003) Olfactory ensheathing cells: time lapse imaging of cellular interactions, axonal support, rapid morphologic shifts, and mitosis. J Comp Neurol 458:175–194
32. Kafitz KW, Greer CA (1999) Olfactory ensheathing cells promote neurite extension from embryonic olfactory receptor cells in vitro. Glia 25:99–110
33. Lu J, Feron F, Mackay-Sim A et al (2002) Olfactory ensheathing cells promote locomotor recovery after delayed transplantation into transected spinal cord. Brain 125:14–21
34. Smith PM, Lakatos A, Barnett SC et al (2002) Cryopreserved cells isolated from the adult canine olfactory bulb are capable of extensive remyelination following transplantation into the adult rat CNS. Exp Neurol 176:402–406
35. Ramon-Cueto A, Plant GW, Avila J et al (1998) Long-distance axonal regeneration in the transected adult rat spinal cord is promoted by olfactory ensheathing glia transplants. J Neurosci 18:3803–3815
36. Aoki M, Kishima H, Yoshimura K et al (2010) Limited functional recovery in rats with complete spinal cord injury after transplantation of whole-layer olfactory mucosa: laboratory investigation. J Neurosurg Spine 12:122–130
37. Iwatsuki K, Yoshimine T, Kishima H et al (2008) Transplantation of olfactory mucosa following spinal cord injury promotes recovery in rats. Neuroreport 19:1249–1252
38. Lima C et al (2010) Olfactory mucosal autografts and rehabilitation for chronic traumatic spinal cord injury. Neurorehabil Neural Repair 24(1):10–22
39. Nikulina E, Tidwell JL, Dai HN et al (2004) The phosphodiesterase inhibitor rolipram delivered after a spinal cord lesion promotes axonal regeneration and functional recovery. Proc Natl Acad Sci U S A 101:8786–8790
40. Pearse DD, Pereira FC, Marcillo AE et al (2004) CAMP and Schwann cells promote axonal growth and functional recovery after spinal cord injury. Nat Med 10:610–616

Part III
Next-Generation Interface

Chapter 7
Augmented Human Technology

Kenji Suzuki

Abstract In order to create a future society where assisted lifestyles will become widely available, we need technology that will support, strengthen, and enhance limited human capabilities. The supports for both physical and cognitive functions are definitely needed for the future rehabilitation and physical exercise. In this chapter, a cognitive neuroscience approach for realizing augmented human technology in order to enhance, strengthen, and support human cognitive capabilities is described. Wearable devices allow the subject high mobility and broaden the spectrum of environments in which bodily motion and physiological signal recognition can be carried out. In this scenario, augmented human technology is regarded as a wearable device technology that enhances human capabilities, particularly cognitively assisted action and perception.

Keywords Wearable device • Bioelectrical signal processing • Biofeedback • Kinematic and physiological cues • Biomechanical analysis

7.1 Introduction

Biomechanical analysis of human movement has been undertaken in various fields to aid the comprehension and evaluation of essential human motions. In the fields of sports and medical rehabilitation, biomechanics has recently being considered to be an indispensable field of study. In particular, electromyography (EMG) is extensively used as an effective way of understanding human muscle dynamics. An electromyogram provides a real-time representation of muscle activity and is commonly used to improve performance in electrophysiological studies and rehabilitation. Although existing methods provide some benefits, they still have

---

K. Suzuki (✉)
Center for Cybernics Research/Faculty of Engineering,
Information and Systems, University of Tsukuba, Tsukuba, Japan
e-mail: kenji@ieee.org

Y. Sankai et al. (eds.), *Cybernics: Fusion of human, machine and information systems*,
DOI 10.1007/978-4-431-54159-2_7, © Springer Japan 2014

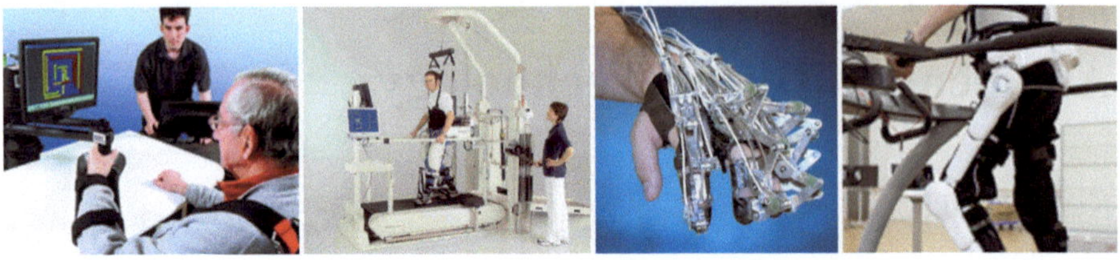

Fig. 7.1 Rehabilitation robots: The rehabilitation of deficits in sensory motor function may not suppress the cause, and hence, rehabilitation robots/wearable devices may lead the brain to find new solutions

drawbacks with respect to spatial and time consistency, which are important elements of biofeedback. In other words, simultaneous understanding of the relationship between muscle activity and body motion is difficult and requires appropriate equipment and suitable training of the subject.

Neuromuscular rehabilitation with biofeedback is important for individuals with disabilities in order to learn motor function. Because of the plasticity of the brain, repetitive actions can help the brain, spinal cord, and nervous system to work together to re-route the signals that were interrupted by strokes, injuries, and other illnesses. Different robotic approaches are aimed at providing robot-aided sensorimotor stimulation and additional sensorimotor training of the paralyzed or paretic upper/lower limb delivered by a robotic-device-enhanced motor outcome [1].

For example, MIT-MANUS [2] was introduced as a pilot system to investigate the potential applications of using robots to support the neuro-rehabilitation of the motor function of the upper limb, as illustrated in the leftmost image of Fig. 7.1. Further, LOKOMAT has been used to help people whose ability to walk has been impaired by a stroke, spinal cord or brain injury, or neurological or orthopedic condition to learn to walk again [2, 3]. On the other hand, the full-body exoskeleton-type robot, robot suit Hybrid Assistive Limb (HAL), that has been developed to support a physically challenged person's daily life can help elderly and disabled people. The HAL has already been used as an assistive tool for neuro-rehabilitation [4–6].

In addition to such robotic approaches, biofeedback technology has been widely used since the 1960s and the action-perception and sensory-motor coordination have been studied extensively to treat certain medical conditions and improve human performance. The following standard definition of biofeedback has been formulated by leading professional organizations [7].

> Biofeedback is a process that enables an individual to learn how to change physiological activity for the purposes of improving health and performance. Precise instruments measure physiological activity such as brainwaves, heart function, breathing, muscle activity, and skin temperature. These instruments rapidly and accurately "feed back" information to the user. The presentation of this information—often in conjunction with changes in thinking, emotions, and behavior—supports desired physiological changes. Over time, these changes can endure without continued use of an instrument.

Table 7.1 Key issues related to augmented human technology

Key issues	Related technology
Biofeedback on the body	Motion measurement (sensory inputs) Signal processing Modality conversion (mapping) Output (wearable or portable device)
Real-time response and coherence	A media technology to support and enhance human cognitive capabilities Multisensory feedback
Kinematic and physiological cues	Bioelectrical signals and electro-physiology can be obtained from the human skin in daily life Understanding muscle dynamics

In this chapter, a cognitive neuroscience approach for realizing augmented human technology in order to enhance, strengthen, and support human cognitive capabilities is described. Wearable devices allow the subject high mobility and broaden the spectrum of environments in which bodily motion and physiological signal recognition can be carried out. In this scenario, augmented human technology is regarded as the wearable device technology that enhances human capabilities, particularly cognitively assisted action and perception. The key issues related to augmented human technology can be summarized in Table 7.1.

In studies related to augmented human technology, the coherence of how similar in time and frequency the two signals, i.e., sensory input and outcomes, are plays an important role. Coherence training is needed for the coupling or connection between the brain and the motor functions. The salient temporal features and frequency characteristics of these physiological signals are mapped into visual or sound features by compact and lightweight wearable devices. These devices allow people to get visual or auditory feedback based on muscle tension while preserving the property of the original signal.

From various studies, it is considered that these feedbacks are sufficient for displaying the amount of and change in bodily motion and muscle activity, and wearable devices are appropriate in different situations. In principal, the rehabilitation of deficits in a sensory motor function may not suppress the cause but may lead the brain to find new solutions. Neuromuscular retraining with biofeedback is very useful for patients in learning new motor controls. Moreover, qualitative and affective characteristics such as facial expressions are important in several different domains.

7.2 Related Works

It is known that there are visual, auditory, and somatosensory spatial representations in the superior colliculus [8]. In recent years, sonification and visualization have attracted attention, as they enable an intuitive understanding of muscle activity. Visualization is effective for presenting multichannel muscle activity information, thereby facilitating an easy understanding of the interaction between

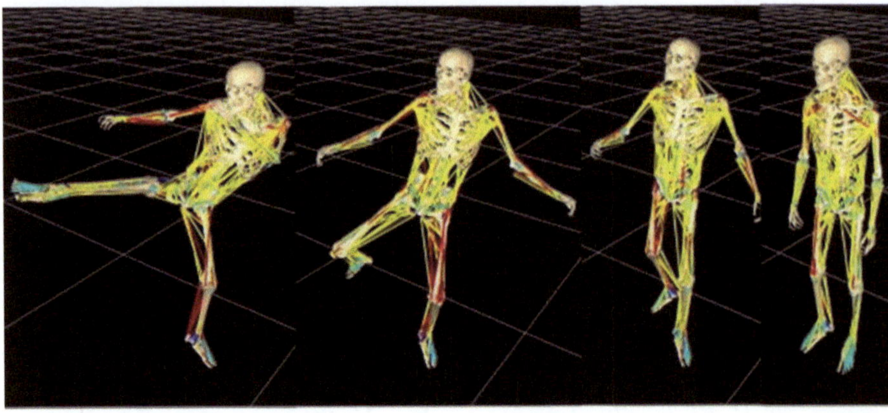

Fig. 7.2 Somatosensory computation for a man-machine interface from motion capture data and a musculoskeletal human model [8]

multiple muscles, whereas sonification is an effective method of presenting the variation in muscle activity with respect to time. For instance, Nakamura et al. [9] and Delp et al. [10] developed a graphical interface for visualizing musculoskeletal geometry. Mixed reality is also an effective visualization method that combines actual human motion and the corresponding muscle activity as a color variation on the display [11]. Although these methods are aimed at providing an intuitive understanding of muscle activity, they require an LCD display or large-scale equipment such as a motion capture device, thereby limiting the range of the application considerably.

In addition to visual and auditory display, multisensory feedback has recently been paid attention to with the aid of advanced technologies. For example, Narumi et al. [12] investigated the illusion-based "Pseudo-gustation" method for changing the perceived taste of food by using a wearable device, which allows users to change the perceived taste on the basis of the effect of the cross-modal interaction of vision, olfaction, and gustation. Hamanaka et al. [13] proposed a headphone-type interface with auditory feedback according to the wearer's head direction. When the user changes his orientation and directs it to different musical instruments one at a time, different auditory feedback is given to the user. Several haptic devices were invented, and some are commercially available.

On the other hand, in addition to typical sensory processing such as visual, auditory, olfactory, taste, and haptics, several approaches have attempted to recognize human affective and emotional performance. For instance, as a wearable approach for facial expression recognition, an example of this is the use of displacement sensors attached to the facial skin, as in MIT's Expression Glasses [14]. SixthSense [15] is an attempt to overlap the virtual world onto human reality. A camera and a small projector allow the user to demonstrate a bi-directional feedback loop: a person's physical experience and information from computing devices are fed into both worlds. As shown in Figs. 7.2, 7.3 and 7.4, these kinds of

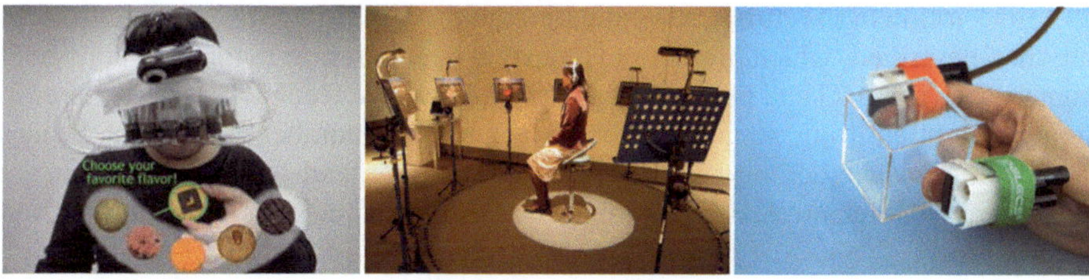

Fig. 7.3 Wearable devices for enhancing human capabilities: not only visual feedback, auditory, olfactory and haptic display are developed so far

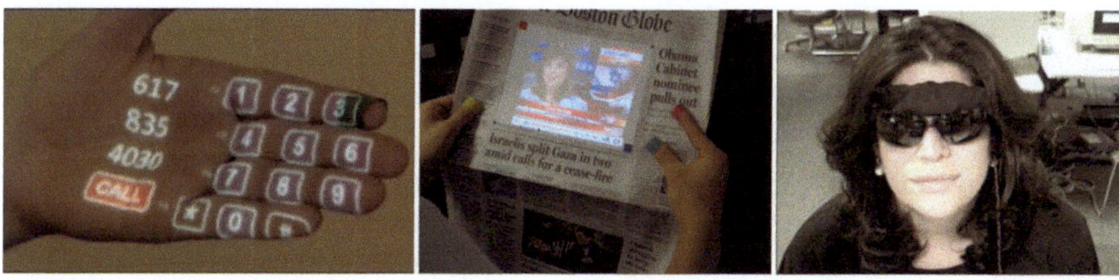

Fig. 7.4 SixthSense (*left and center*). A wearable gestural interface to combine the virtual and physical world. Expression Glasses (*right*). A wearable approach for facial expression recognition

works are also regarded as augmented reality (AR) [16] or mixed reality (MR) [17]. Wearable devices are often used in these works and are successfully employed in various domains.

Several technologies are used for detecting human intentions, such as physiological measurement and analysis of bodily motion. In addition to traditional sensing components for movement sensing and the recognition of body posture and motion [18], bioelectrical signals such as EMG and pulse waves are often used in the related works. As EMG signals are electrical signals, they propagate to and from neighboring muscles in a phenomenon called crosstalk [19]. Taking this into account, it is advised that electrodes be placed away from the front of the face. However, crosstalk has a critical drawback: The signals from all facial muscles, even those not involved in facial expressions, are propagated. Further, even during a single facial expression, the signals from all contracted muscle fibers are detected simultaneously as a mixed signal. Some attempts have been made to overcome the problem of distal detection in the upper extremities. In one case, crosstalk was used for successfully predicting finger movements from signals measured distally on the arm.

Tsenov et al. [20] used an independent component analysis (ICA) to separate the acquired signals on a person's arm into their independent components for better classification. Naik et al. [21] used both ICA and an artificial neural network (ANN) to classify hand and finger movements.

In the following sections, several case studies with different wearable devices are then described, which are not only capable of measuring human physiological signals such as EMG and pulse but also designed to give feedbacks to the wearer in terms of light-emitting, sound, and robotic actuators. A number of different devices for reading muscle activity, bodily motion, heart rate, and facial expressions are presented with the potential applications to assistive technology, rehabilitation, and entertainment.

7.3 Case Studies

7.3.1 BioLights: Visual EMG Biofeedback

A wearable interface is developed, which allows users to perceive muscle activity in an intuitive manner while providing an unrestricted system [22]. Muscle activity or muscular tension is visualized on the surface of the body in the shape and position of the muscle in real time; this interface aids an intuitive understanding of multichannel muscle activity. It is designed as a wearable, thin, and light interface device, which enables a wide range of uses. Several experiments were conducted to evaluate the system performance. In addition, an experiment was conducted to investigate the possible applications of the interface to neuro-rehabilitation; this experiment involved the use of the interface in combination with an exoskeleton.

Figure 7.5 shows an overview of the developed interface. It is focused on the rectus femoris, biceps femoris, and semitendinosus of both legs because these muscles contribute to the following basic movements of the lower limbs: extension, flexion, internal rotation, and external rotation. The developed interface consists of three modules: (i) measurement module, (ii) control module, and (iii) display module. Disposable electrodes and an amplifier are installed in the measurement module, and signal processing and filtering are conducted via the control module. These modules and all other equipment are installed and sewn onto a pair of sports pants. Two muscle-activity visualization systems are developed in this case study:

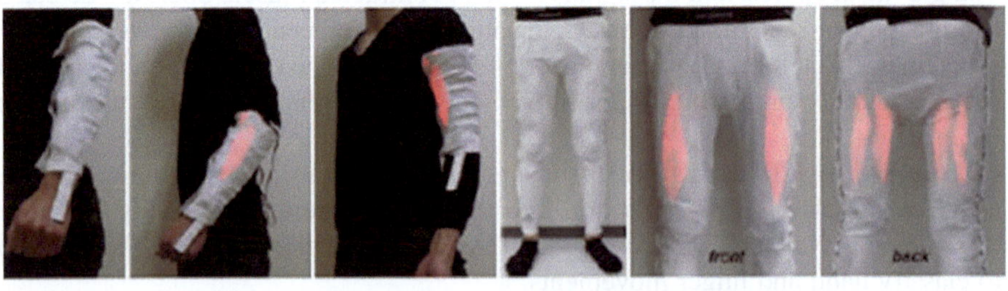

Fig. 7.5 BioLights: light emitting wear for visualizing upper and lower-limb muscle activity

the maximum voluntary contraction (%MVC) visualization system and the muscular tension visualization system.

The interface is intended to be wearable and is hence designed using stretch fabric. For developing the display module, a light-emitting stretch fabric is utilized, which is composed of a warp of numerous optical fibers and a woof of nylon threads. The light-emitting surface is designed in accordance with the shape of the muscle for an intuitive understanding of the muscle activity. Scratching on the optical fibers creates a slightly coarse surface from which light is emitted in the arbitrary shape of the muscle. Consequently, it appears as if the user's muscles are glowing red. In order to enhance the brightness, two super luminosity LEDs are used as light sources for each muscle; these LEDs generate sufficient brightness for the glow to be identified even under fluorescent light. Several buttonhooks sewn onto the side of the garments allow the user to slip these garments on and off easily. Small bend sensors are positioned at the knee and hip joints to measure the angle variation associated with physical exertion. These sensors are also used for calculating the muscular tension by utilizing a biomechanics model. The total weight of the wearable interface is 1.1 kg, which enables users to use it without feeling restricted or experiencing difficulty in movement.

Maximum voluntary contraction (%MVC) is used in this system as the degree of muscle activity. The calibration process is mandatory before using the interface. In this case study, the signal captured under resting conditions and maximum voluntary conditions is considered to be 0 % and 100 %, respectively. A microprocessor is used as a controller, and a Lipo-battery, as the power source. This system realizes unrestricted muscle-activity visualization. The EMG signal is acquired through a 12-bit A/D converter operating at 1 kHz. A full-wave rectifier, band-path, and comb filter are used for reducing artifacts and noise. After integral processing, the signal undergoes PWM for lighting the LEDs. The brightness is corrected using an exponential function by considering the logarithmic characteristics of human vision. This system's properties can be modified by changing the number of integrations and the maximum PWM value. An increase in these values results in an improvement of the resolution and realizes a relatively smooth light emission. On the other hand, a decrease in these values improves the response time of the system. The former is considered effective for rehabilitation, and the latter, for sports training.

On the other hand, because muscular tension is indispensable for analyzing the interaction between multichannel muscles, the visualization of %MVC depends only on the activity of each muscle, while muscular tension reflects the interaction between muscles, i.e., the difference between muscle forces. A muscular-tension visualization system is then developed by utilizing a modified Hill-Stroeve model [23, 24], which is a simplified version of the model proposed by Winters and Stark [25]. The knee and hip joint angles (obtained from the bend sensors positioned at each joint) and the EMG signal of the lower-limb muscles are used as the data for the models.

As the possible applications in the field of neurorehabilitation were clearly demonstrated as illustrated in Fig. 7.6, the developed interface is currently used at

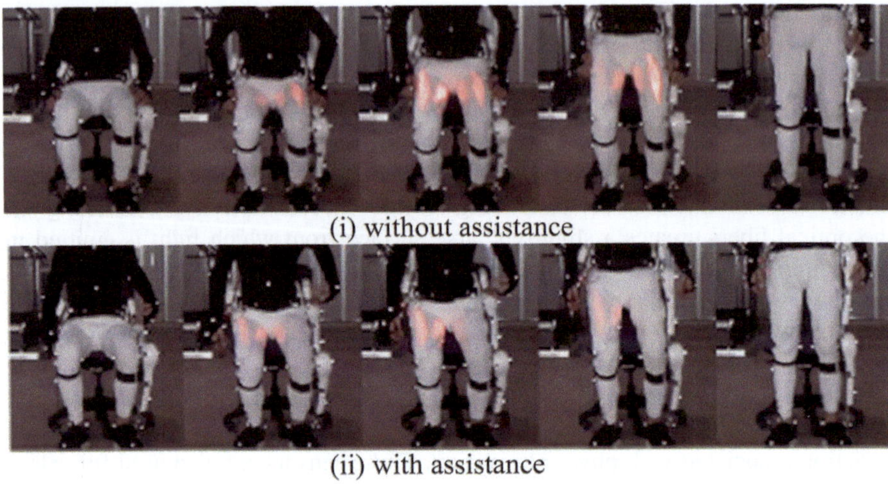

Fig. 7.6 BioLights: differences in muscle activity during squatting motion, (i) without and (ii) with assistance

the clinical trials. The effectiveness in allowing users to perceive muscle activity in both static and dynamic states is verified throughout the study. A notable feature of the developed interface is that the activity of the target muscles can be observed in real time at the position of the muscle by the wearer as well as by other observers. It is believed that this interface has various applications in the fields of sports and rehabilitation; it enables better coaching and a better relationship between patients and physical therapists. For the visualization of multichannel muscle activities, the interference of each muscle EMG must be considered in future systems. This sort of wearable approach for visualizing human physiological signals provides a new tool for biofeedback devices. In addition to EMG signals, other biosignals such as heartbeats can be considered for a further implementation of the device.

7.3.2 *BioTones: Auditory EMG Biofeedback*

In order to directly convert human movement to sound, a wearable device that generates sounds on the basis of bioelectrical signals, particularly surface EMG, is developed [26] as shown in Fig. 7.7. There are some studies [27, 28] on the sound generation from EMG signals in the field of computer music. Some biomedical studies [29–31] employed EMG feedback delivered in the auditory mode as a physiological indicator. However, they focused very little on the kinds of the sound and the usability as a device. Thus, a useful wearable tool is proposed, which is available even for use in daily life, on the basis of the auditory biofeedback method. This novel technology can be of assistance in preventive healthcare, rehabilitation, and sports training, among others.

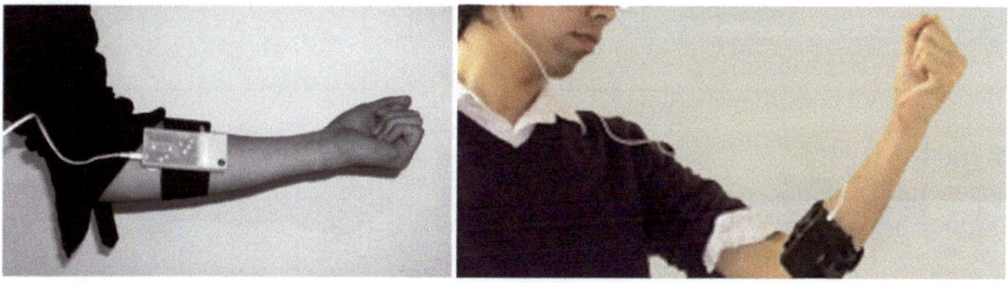

Fig. 7.7 BioTones: A wearable device for converting a person's bioelectrical signals on the basis of electromyogram signals into audio sounds. The device is capable of extracting the signals and generating audio sounds. The users can simply listen to the generated sound by using normal headphones

In the proposed method, the salient features of an EMG signal are mapped onto sound features by a wearable device that is capable of obtaining the EMG signal and creating an audio signal. This device allows people to obtain auditory feedback from muscle tension while preserving the property of the original signal. The proposed approach is suitable for several applications such as biofeedback treatment, sports training, and entertainment. In particular, an application to the biofeedback treatment for migraine headaches and tension headaches is considered.

The electromyogram monitor is used for monitoring human neuromuscular function as the visualization of muscular activities. The monitor is widely used for not only medical purposes but also the analysis of muscular activities observed during exercise and considered in the field of sports science. However, there are several critical problems in terms of visual feedback: (i) people are forced to stay in front of the monitor, and (ii) multiple EMG signals are displayed using traditional monitors because of the complexity of the signal features although the principle feature is the activity level. On the other hand, the auditory feedback is also effective for showing the change in and the characteristics of the bioelectrical signals caused by the muscular activity. Sound has three basic characteristics: loudness, pitch, and timbre. Not only the control of loudness and pitch but also timbre control makes it possible to represent a variety of muscular activity.

BioTones consists of a pair of disposable electrodes, a bioelectric amplifier, a microprocessor, a digital signal processor, and an audio amplifier. This enables it to extract bioelectrical signals and generate audio signals. The user can listen to the generated sounds simply through a normal headphone system. The developed prototype is designed to measure the bioelectrical signals on the surface of the flexor carpi radialis muscle. This muscle of the human forearm is used for flexing and abducting the hand. The device is fixed to the forearm with a tightened belt.

There are several mapping rules in accordance with the target application. There are two features of bioelectrical signals: level and frequency characteristics as well as sound features. Direct mapping is regarded as the direct correspondence between bioelectrical and audio signals in terms of the level and frequency. On the other hand, cross mapping is regarded as the alternation of the level and frequency characteristics between bioelectrical and audio signals. This device does not aim

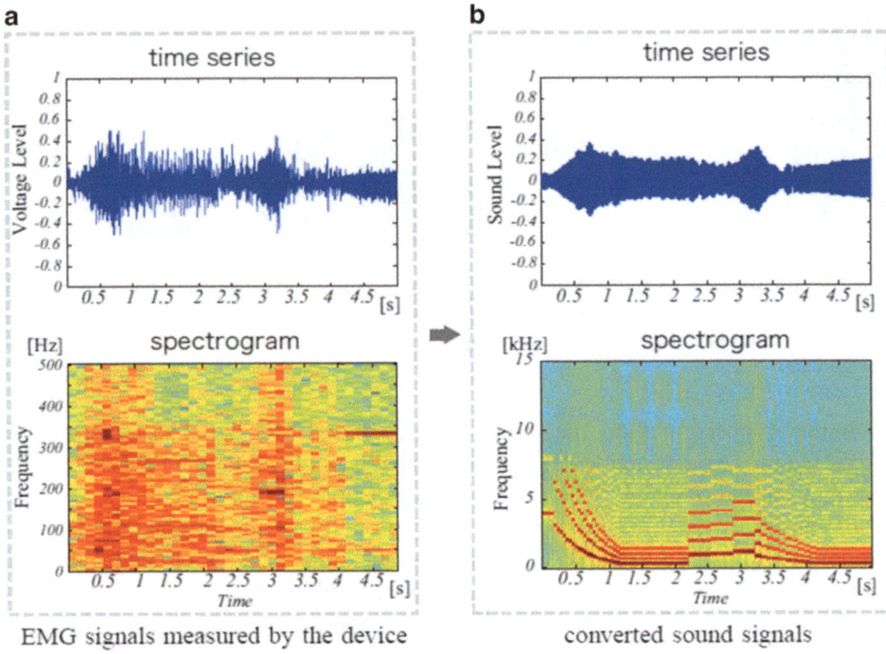

Fig. 7.8 Examples of bioelectrical and audio signals: (**a**) a bioelectrical signal, and (**b**) the converted audio signal. Signal conversion is performed by two types of mappings: direct mapping and cross mapping

to extract the salient features of bioelectrical signals but to preserve the original features as much as possible. The purpose of these mappings is to represent a variety of the muscular activity by a variety of sound features. Examples of bioelectrical and audio signals are shown in Fig. 7.8.

A wearable device for EMG auditory biofeedback is introduced, which allows the wearer to cognize the muscles' activity using a compact and lightweight device. Moreover, the characteristics of auditory stimuli are evaluated as biofeedback compared to common visual biofeedback. From the experimental results, it can be seen that the auditory feedback is appropriate for displaying the amount of and change in muscle activity. It is considered that the auditory feedback device can be used easily in different situations, such as in the office, while moving, and while playing sports, because it does not require any display unit. Furthermore, the sound conversion with varying loudness, frequency, or rhythm conversion can be used as an alternative to solve the complexity of showing several muscle activities simultaneously, which is not easy by common visual biofeedback. The system can be extended for multiple-channel auditory biofeedback. The advantage of putting multiple BioTones on the body and listening in parallel to multiple channels will be investigated. A device with a built-in speaker has already been developed. Multiple channels can be implemented by giving each device a different pitch by using loudness conversion.

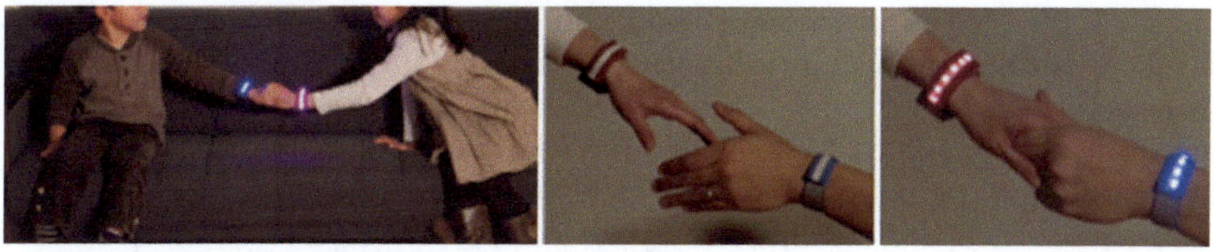

Fig. 7.9 Enhanced touch: This wearable device with electrodes senses touch and identifies other users. Six full-color LEDs are installed in the bracelet, which light up when a handshake occurs

This novel method of sonification is an alternative to the visualization technique. It should be noted that the temporal and pressure resolution is higher than the visual perception because of the characteristics of auditory perception. The wearable device benefits a wide range of users because people can obtain auditory feedback solely by wearing it and listening to sound at any time and place, even in transit or while walking.

7.3.3 Enhanced Touch: Physical Touch and Haptic Biofeedback

Haptic modality is often used for human communication. In this case study, a novel bracelet-type device has been developed for sensing physical contact among people in order to support direct communication between people by inducing touch with appropriate visual feedback [32]. The device detects and records the touch of users when they simply wear the device on their wrists as illustrated in Fig. 7.9.

Physical touch is a fundamental element of human communication, and several benefits and positive effects of such touch have been reported in the communication and therapeutic domain, such as Positive Touch and Deep Touch Pressure [33]. The typical symptoms of autism among children include avoidance of direct touch with other people and the tendency to engage in lone activities. Some studies have reported that the training of touch by therapists contributes to the alleviation of these symptoms. Thus far, human coders have attempted to observe their activity via recorded video, but this is not an objective measure and is time consuming for checking all the touches among people in a session. Measuring the time of touching, partner, and frequency are desirable data, but there is no practical equipment for this purpose. Similar technology is used for an instrumental device [34], but users needed to grasp and hold the same device together.

The communication technology based on a body area network [35] is used in order to detect touching between people and communication through the human body. This technology is known as an alternative solution of communication between humans and objects. Since the information is transferred via the human body, it can be utilized for sensing physical contact among people. The developed device is used for sensing touches and identifying others, which can be performed by the wearable device with electrodes. The six full-color LEDs are installed in the bracelet, which light up when a handshake occurs. The pair of electrodes is located on the inside of the case so as to fit the wrist. The device communicates with another device using a specific protocol. The received conducted signal is first amplified and demodulated, and then handled by the microprocessor. Every microprocessor attempts to transmit a synchronous signal at random intervals within 10 ms in order to detect if touching has occurred and to synchronize with the other device.

Several visual effects are programmed to visualize not only the physical touch but also the touching condition such as the duration of physical touch and the history of past touching. For example, color blending is implemented for effective visual feedback to show the duration of touching. A unique color—from the three primary colors (red, green, and blue)—is assigned to each device.

When a user wears the device and touches another person with the developed device on both their hands, the LEDs of both devices light up with the corresponding unique color. During the handshake, the two different colors change and are then blended gradually as long as the touching lasts. In other words, the degree of color blending represents the duration of the touching. The LED colors in the two devices are changed to the same color. This manner of lighting allows the proposed method to measure the duration of physical contact along with the device's ability to identify other devices.

The devices for sensing human contact can be used recognizing a social network based on physical contact. The bracelet-type device lights up—with a different color for each—when the wearer shakes hands with another wearer. Not only the contact sensing but also the electrical communication is used for identifying and sharing the device ID. It is considered that the proposed device can provide a novel playful interaction method between humans. It is also planned to verify if the device contributes to motivating touching among users by lighting LEDs or by playing interactive social games. This technology can be used for supporting and enhancing the experiences on play and social interaction among people by using playful devices. The device mediates between humans without missing the fundamental properties of human activities. This is a cyber-physical system of measuring and presenting human physical activities such as physical contact, spatial movement, and facial expressions, where the psychological and social aspects of human activities can also be enhanced.

7.3.4 HOTARU: Visual Biofeedback Based on Heartbeats

The heartbeat is one of the fundamental vital signs of human beings. As the heart beats independently of any nervous or hormonal influences, the rhythm of the heart gives an important signal from the body. In addition to the rhythm of the heart, the heartbeat is regulated by the autonomic nervous system.

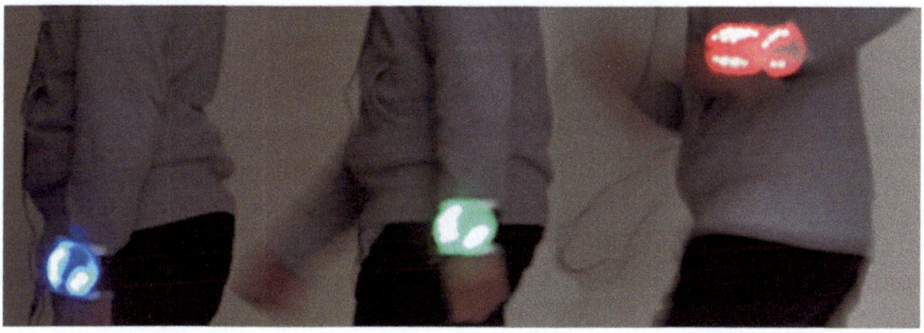

Fig. 7.10 HOTARU ("firefly" in Japanese): a conceptual image of using the developed device

In this case study, a novel method of heartbeat tracking is proposed and a wearable device to visualize the heart beat, named HOTARU ("firefly" in Japanese), is developed [36]. A number of systems and devices for heartbeat measurement exist, which can be used for measuring heart function or exercise volume and as a psychological barometer for measuring stress or relaxation. However, since the measurement of biological signals is not stable because of several unexpected noises, the user is asked to firmly attach the sensor, for example, the electrode, and to keep quiet during the measurement of the heartbeat rate. Fast Fourier transform (FFT) is used as the traditional method of measuring the heartbeat rate, while the signals with unexpected noises in the measured signal are ignored.

A wearable device is developed to indicate the heartbeat in real time with a different color of LED. The color changes according to the heartbeat rate and blinks in synchronization with the heartbeat pulse. The developed system cannot only track the heartbeat but also interpolate it from the noisy signals in real time. The heartbeat is extracted from the original signal of the photoplethysmographic (PPG) sensor, which contains the noise delivered by body movement or other unexpected causes. In the proposed method, when the system cannot determine the heartbeat, because of the sensor's alignment or a temporary lack of pulse, the heartbeat is interpolated on the basis of the past signal and the linear prediction algorithm.

The developed device consists of a microprocessor, LED displays, and a PPG sensor that can measure the heartbeat pulse by using optical absorptance of the human body. The user is asked to attach the PPG sensor that is a clip-type interface on the ear and to wear a bracelet-type interface with LEDs on his/her wrist. The brightness of the LEDs changes in sync with the heartbeat and their color corresponds to the heartbeat rate (HBR). As shown in the left image of Fig. 7.10, blue implies that the HBR is less than 60, green means that the HBR is from 60 to 80, and red implies that the HBR is more than 80.

Traditionally, the measurement of the heartbeat is focused on the heartbeat pulse itself, but the tracking accuracy depends upon the environment. It is usually not stable because of the noise, and the users are asked to rest during the measurement. The intervals of the heartbeat pulse are at a low frequency from approximately 0.5 to 2.0 Hz, and these intervals are assumed not to change rapidly. However, precise intervals are difficult to recognize from the measured signals by using only peak detection because of the noises, which are usually impulse noise and look like the heartbeat pulse. FFT is used for their analysis.

A novel method of heartbeat tracking is then implemented. The pattern matching is carried out between the measured signal ***P***(x,t) and the ideal heartbeat pulse ***Pc***(x), which is prepared in advance. The cross-correlation *z*(x,t) is calculated with a fixed time window, which is the same as the length of the ideal heartbeat pulse. The matching result z is expected to be a periodic signal, and it is synchronized with the real heartbeat pulse. The computational cost to obtain the coefficients of all possible cross-correlation values is very high and not suitable for real-time calculation; hence, only limited coefficients are used in this process. In addition, in order to reduce the computational cost, the cross-correlation values are obtained only at a certain time, which is estimated using the linear prediction process.

Then, a modified peak detection algorithm is employed by combining a Kalman filter to predict the intervals of the heartbeat, which is based on the linear prediction and uniform distribution function. Assuming that these intervals do not change rapidly, the next heartbeat interval can be estimated from the transition of the previous several intervals. Further, the center value of the probability density function (PDF) is solely used for the detection of the peak candidate in ***P***. The peaks are detected within the *z* time range of reliability on the basis of this PDF.

This wearable device opens new experiences among users to understand each other's physiological status during day-to-day activities for presenting the current heartbeat in a different color. The LED lights up in sync with the heartbeat, and the color changes according to the calculated HBR. The developed device allows users to freely move and play without attaching the sensor or electrode firmly. Potential applications include tools for children to promote social interaction. The user testing with several people is planned. The sound feedback according to the heartbeat pulse for computer games and VR avatar will also be implemented.

7.3.5 Head Orientation Sensing for Cognitively Assisted Locomotion

From the point of view of support for motion and locomotion, it is quite important to consider not only the lower limbs but also the gaze and the head because they are tightly coupled with the gait behavior during human locomotion. In addition, qualitative and affective characteristics such as facial expressions are important in several different domains. In this section, a head-mounted wearable device for detecting the head orientation is described in order to utilize kinematic cues during human locomotion.

Mobility aids such as manual and electric wheelchairs are widely used by people with reduced mobility. Such equipment allows elderly and disabled people to support their mobility needs. In addition, robotic-assisted locomotion such as

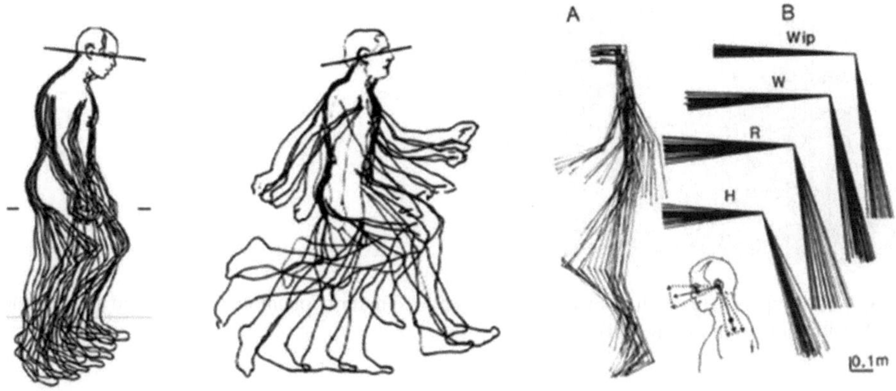

Fig. 7.11 *Head stabilization*: Physiology of perception and action during various locomotor tasks in humans [37, 38]

exoskeletons has received a considerable amount of attention in recent years because of its potential use not only as a mobility aid but also for locomotion training.

It is known that the head is turned toward the future walking direction during natural human locomotion, and this head anticipation and changes in gaze direction occur according to the path [37–39] as illustrated in Fig. 7.11. The head direction thus anticipates the future body trunk direction and the walking direction. Along with body balance and posture, the human head orientation plays an important role in the prediction of the walking direction and future motions such as standing and sitting.

In this case study, a novel wearable device is proposed for the measurement of the head orientation and position, which can be applied to extend the existing mobility aids. The wearable device can provide important cues for predicting the future walking direction and behavior by observing the head direction and the difference between this direction and the body trunk direction. The developed device, which can be easily worn and removed, measures the head orientation and position irrespective of the location and enables the prediction of the future walking direction in real time for assisted locomotion, such as exoskeleton robots and wheelchairs. It is also designed to be small and lightweight for long-term comfortable use.

Head Anticipation Measurement in Natural Walking: It is known that during human locomotion, the gaze turns first, the head turns next, and then the body direction follows sequentially, and finally, the walking direction changes. By observing this head anticipation, one can predict the future walking direction. An experiment is conducted to detect the head anticipation by using the developed device and evaluate the detection accuracy by using a motion capture system.

The subjects were asked to walk naturally to form 8-shaped trajectories in the $2.5 \times 3.0\ m^2$ measurement space of the motion capture system. There were no visual cues except the lines indicating the end of the measurement space. One trial consisted of two laps of walking, and each subject was asked to perform three trials. The subjects were three adults, and their ages were 24, 25, and 30 years.

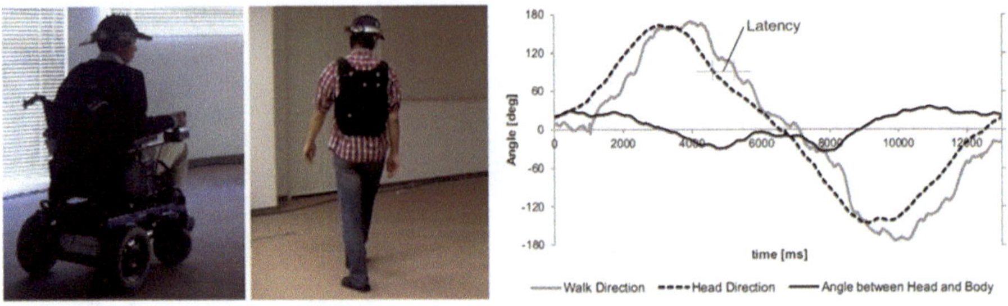

Fig. 7.12 Experiments with an electric wheelchair and natural locomotion (*right*) and an example of head anticipation during walking

Figure 7.12 indicates that the head angle against the body, as measured by the developed device is summed with the body angle measured by the motion capture system. The average latency time and its standard deviation from the head to the walking direction measured by the developed device was 687(196) ms, and the one measured by the motion capture system was 707(178) ms.

The measurement accuracy of the developed device was evaluated using the motion capture system. The head anticipation latency to the walk/locomotion direction during natural walking and during wheelchair locomotion with the developed device was also measured; the latency was 687 ms in the case of walking and 694 ms in the case of wheelchair locomotion. Therefore, it was verified that it is possible to use the developed device for predicting the direction of walking/wheelchair locomotion.

This is a novel wearable device for the measurement of the head orientation on the basis of both the inertia sensors and the optical marker tracker without accumulated errors, which is designed for robot-assisted locomotion, particularly, the prediction of the direction of walking/wheelchair locomotion. Cognitively assisted locomotion is a new approach to lower-limb exoskeleton control based on head and gaze motor behavior. Using behavioral analysis and cognitive neuroscience findings based on head and gaze tracking, we developed a head-mounted measurement device for sensing the head orientation. This study included the analysis of patients who recovered their locomotor skills at cognitive and meta-cognitive levels, such as biofeedback, mood influence, self-consciousness, and confidence, rather than at mechanical levels.

7.3.6 *Face Reader: Reading Facial Expressions for Affective Feedback*

In the previous sections, the sensing and recognition of body posture and motion were mainly described. In addition to sensing movement, the valence and intensity of affective reactions play an important role in human interactions. In particular,

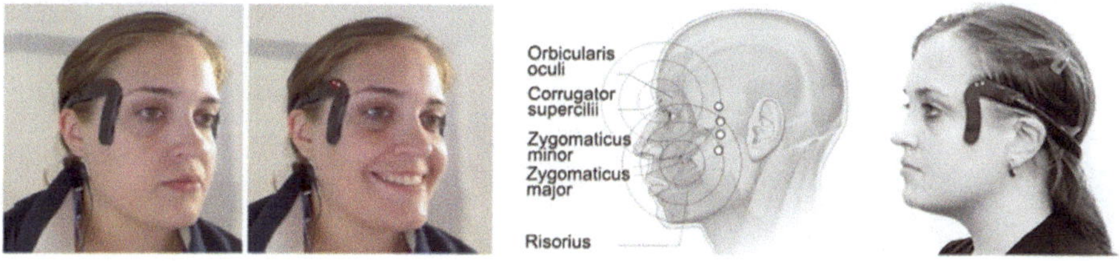

Fig. 7.13 *Face Reader*: This is a device for reading facial expressions on the basis of bioelectrical signals and the model of EMG signal propagation (Modified from, electrode position, and proposed interface device)

facial expressions play a significant role in the exchange of interpersonal information by providing additional information about the emotional state or intention of the person displaying them [40]. Thus far, several approaches have been followed in order to read emotions automatically from the face. The most traditional approach to recognizing emotional facial expressions uses video and photographic cameras and subsequently computer vision algorithms to identify facial expressions. Another approach for facial expression recognition is a wearable approach. However, to date, no reliable and unobtrusive interfaces to read facial expressions and display them for a long time have been developed.

In this case study, the use of the facial bioelectrical potentials captured on areas on the side of the face is proposed in order to obtain information about facial expressions. Because of the mixed nature of crosstalk, it is necessary to transform the sampled signal. A classification method is introduced by combining two techniques: ICA to transform the signals into independent components and ANN to accurately identify facial expressions.

This is a novel method for reading expressions on the human face through an unobtrusive wearable device by applying computational methods to bioelectrical signals captured on the side of the face. In contrast to the previous approaches, the proposed approach offers robustness against occlusion, changing lighting conditions, and changing facial angles. Electrode locations were carefully selected on the basis of the facial displacement and physiology in order to capture usable signals without covering or inhibiting the expressions. The captured signals were considered a mixture of distal electromyographic signals and other biological signals and were used for achieving a personal, pattern-based identification of the facial expressions. More than 90 % accuracy of facial expression recognition of a "smile" and more than 85 % of both the "smile" and the "frown" were ascertained using this method even when presented with crosstalk from other muscles. Figure 7.13 shows the developed wearable device, called Face Reader, which cannot only identify emotional facial expressions in real time but also display them in a continuous manner.

The goal of this research is to develop an emotional communication aid to improve human-human and human-system interactions through an emotion reading system that can recognize the subject's emotions in real time and can display the

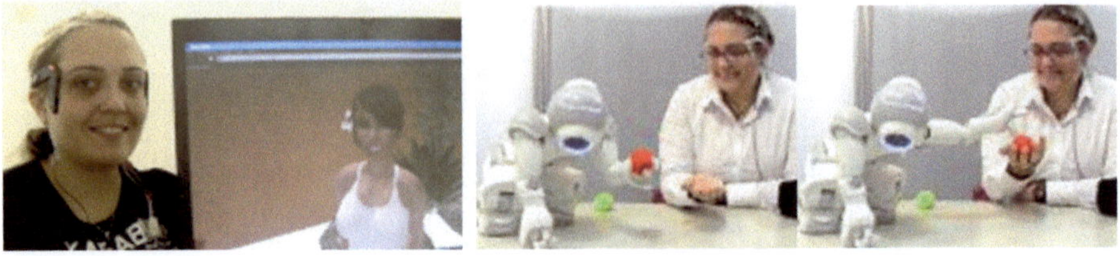

Fig. 7.14 *Smiling Avatar (right) and Emotionally Assisted Interaction*: Emotion reader is used for controlling an avatar and a humanoid robot

output in different formats. Further, it must be unobtrusive to the user and not inhibit expressions; it should also work in any environment irrespective of the changing lighting conditions and the changing positions of the subject.

Face Reader [41] has applications in several areas, particularly in therapy and assistive technology. Further, it can aid the visually impaired in the following manner: the listener can perceive the speaker's facial expressions through alternative forms of communication such as audio or vibro-tactile stimulation. Another application lies in increasing the quality of life for patients suffering from facial paralysis, where the signals obtained from the healthy side of the face can be used for controlling a robot mask that produces an artificial smile on the paralyzed side [42]. Because it is an unobtrusive wearable device, it can be used outside the laboratory for continuous expression detection in environments where cameras are not supported or where subjects require high mobility.

For example, Face Reader can be used in human-computer emotional interactions for diverse types of agents, such as animating an on-screen avatar or for emotion-based coaching of a robot [43] by using facial expressions. Figure 7.14 shows examples of potential applications of the device.

7.4 Conclusions

In this chapter, a cognitive neuroscience approach for realizing augmented human technology by using several wearable devices in order to enhance, strengthen, and support human cognitive capabilities was described. Different physiological signals and human kinematic and physiological characteristics were considered throughout the presented case studies.

In addition to augmented human technology (ATH), human enhancement technologies (HETs) were regarded as techniques that could be used not only for treating illness and disability but also for enhancing human characteristics and capacities. Several approaches using the developed wearable devices were attempted. As biomedical sciences and enhancement technologies progress, new ethical and social implications should be considered [44]. Thus far, many such enhancement technologies have already become widely available, for example, cosmetic surgery for aesthetic enhancement. Future enhancement technologies include those related to genetics, pharmacology, cognitive functions, and longevity.

In order to create a future society where assisted lifestyles will become widely available, we need technology that will support, strengthen, and enhance limited human capabilities. The supports for both physical and cognitive functions are definitely needed for future rehabilitation and physical exercise because the rehabilitation of deficits in sensory motor functions may not suppress the cause but may lead the brain to find new solutions.

References

1. Volpe BT, Krebs HI, Hogan N, Edelstein L, Diels C, Aisen M (2000) A novel approach to stroke rehabilitation – robot-aided sensorimotor stimulation. Neurology 54(10):1938–1944
2. Hogan N, Krebs HI, Charnnarong J, Srikrishna P, Sharon A (1992) MIT-MANUS: a workstation for manual therapy and training. In: IEEE international workshop on robot and human communication. Tokyo, Japan, pp 161–165
3. Krewer C, Heller S, Husemann B, Mller F, Koenig E (2007) Effects of locomotion training with assistance of a robot-driven gait orthosis in hemiparetic patients after stroke: a randomized controlled pilot study. Stroke 38:349–354
4. Wirz M, Zemon DH, Rupp R, Scheel A, Colombo G, Dietz V, Hornby TG (2005) Effectiveness of automated locomotor training in patients with chronic incomplete spinal cord injury: a multicenter trial. Arch Phys Med Rehabil 86(4):672–680
5. Suzuki K, Mito G, Kawamoto H, Hasegawa Y, Sankai Y (2007) Intention-based walking support for paraplegia patients with robot suit HAL. Adv Robot 21(12):1441–1469
6. Tsukahara A, Kawanishi R, Hasegawa Y, Sankai Y (2010) Sit-to-stand and stand-to-sit transfer support for complete paraplegic patients with robot suit HAL. Adv Robot 24 (11):1615–1638
7. Association for Applied Psychophysiology and Biofeedback (2008) http://www.aapb.org/
8. Wallace MT, Wilkinson LK, Stein BE (1996) Representation and integration of multiple sensory inputs in primate superior colliculus. J Neurophysiol 76(2):1246–1266
9. Nakamura Y, Yamane K, Suzuki I, Fujita Y (2004) Somatosensory computation for man-machine interface from motion capture data and musculoskeletal human model. IEEE Trans Robot 21(1):58–66
10. Delp SL, Loan JP, Hoy MG, Zajac FE, Topp EL, Rosen JM (1990) An interactive graphic-based model of the lower extremity to study orthopaedic surgical procedures. IEEE Trans Biomed Eng 37(10):757–767
11. Murai A, Kurosawa K, Yamane K, Nakamura Y (2009) Computationally fast estimation of muscle tension for realtime bio-feedback. In: Annual international conference of the IEEE EMBS. Minnesota, US, pp 6546–6549
12. Narumi T, Nishizaka S, Kajinami T, Tanikawa T, Hirose M (2011) Meta cookie+: an illusion-based gustatory display. Lecture notes in computer science, vol 6773/2011. Springer, pp 260–269
13. Hamanaka M, Lee S (2006) Sound scope headphones: controlling an audio mixer through natural movement. In: 2006 international computer music conference. New Orleans, USA, pp 155–158
14. Scheirer J, Fernandez R, Picard W (1999) Expression glasses: a wearable device for facial expression recognition. In: CHI '99 extended abstracts on human factors in computing systems, pp 262–263

15. Mistry W, Maes P (2009) SixthSense–a wearable gestural interface. In: SIGGRAPH Asia 2009, Emerging Technologies. Yokohama
16. Azuma RT (1997) A survey of augmented reality. Presence 6(4):355–385
17. Tamura H, Yamamoto H, Katayama A (2001) Mixed reality: future dreams seen at the border between real and virtual worlds. IEEE Comput Graph Appl Mag 21(6):64–70
18. Zeng H, Zhao Y (2011) Sensing movement: microsensors for body motion measurement. Sensors 11:638–660
19. Fridlund A, Cacioppo JT (1986) Guidelines for human electromyographic research. Psychophysiology 23:567–589
20. Tsenov G, Zeghbib A, Palis F, Soylev N, Mladenov V (2008) Visualization of an on-line classification and recognition algorithm of EMG signals. J Univ Chem Technol Metall 43(1):154–158
21. Naik G, Kumar D, Singh V, Palaniswam M (2006) Hand gestures for HCI using ICA of EMG. In: HCSNet workshop on the use of vision in human-computer interaction, vol 56, Canberra, Australia
22. Igarashi N, Suzuki K, Kawamoto H, Sankai Y (2010) BioLights: light emitting wear for visualizing lower-limb muscle activity. In: Annual international conference of the IEEE EMBS. Buenos Aires, Argentina, pp 6393–6396
23. Stroeve S (1999) Impedance characteristics of a neuromusculoskeletal model of the human arm I. posture control. Biol Cybern 81:475–494
24. Hill A (1938) The heat of shortening and the dynamic constants of muscle. Royal Soc Lond B126:136–195
25. Winters JM, Stark L (1985) Analysis of fundamental human movement patterns through the use of in-depth antagonistic muscle models. IEEE Trans Biomed Eng 32(10):826–839
26. Tsubouchi Y, Suzuki K (2010) BioTones: a wearable device for EMG auditory biofeedback. In: Annual international conference of the IEEE EMBS, Buenos Aires, Argentina, pp 6543–6546
27. Knapp RB, Lusted HS (1990) A bioelectric controller for computer music applications. Comput Music J 14:42–47
28. Atau T (2000) Musical performance practice on sensor-based instruments, trends in gestural control of music. Science et Musique 14:389–405
29. Budzynski TH, Stoyva JM (1969) An instrument for producing deep muscle relaxation by means of analog information feedback. J Appl Behav Anal 2:231–237
30. Epstein LH, Hersen M, Hemphill DP (1974) Music feedback in the treatment of tension headache: an experimental case study. J Behav Ther Exp Psychiatry 5(1):59–63
31. Alexander AB, French CA, Goodman NJ (1975) A comparison of auditory and visual feedback in biofeedback assisted muscular relaxation training. Soc Psychophysiol Res 12:119–124
32. Iida K, Suzuki K (2011) Enhanced touch: a wearable device for social playware. In: ACM 8th advances in computer entertainment technology conference. doi:10.1145/2071423.2071524
33. Pardew EM, Bunse C (2005) Enhancing interaction through positive touch. Young Except Child 8(2):21–29
34. Baba T, Ushiama T, Tomimatsu K (2007) Freqtric drums: a musical instrument that uses skin contact as an interface. In: International conference on new interfaces for musical expression, New York, USA, pp 386–387
35. Zimmerman TG (1996) Personal area networks: near-field intrabody communication. IBM Syst J 35(3/4):609–617
36. Suzuki K, Iida K, Shimokakimoto T (2012) Social playware for supporting and enhancing social interaction. In: 17th international symposium on artificial life and robotics. Oita, Japan, pp.39–42
37. Pozzo T, Berthoz A, Lefort L (1990) Head stabilization during various locomotor tasks in humans. I. Normal subjects. Exp Brain Res 82:97–106
38. Pozzo T, Berthoz A, Lefort L, Vitte E (1991) Head stabilization during various locomotor tasks in humans. II. Patients with bilateral peripheral vestibular deficits. Exp Brain Res 85:208–217

39. Kadone H, Bernardin D, Bennequin D, Berthoz A (2010) Gaze anticipation during human locomotion – top-down organization that may invert the concept of locomotion in humanoid robots. Int Symp Robot Hum Interact Commun 19:587–592
40. Ekman P, Friesen WV, Ellsworth P (1982) What emotion categories or dimensions can observers judge from facial behavior? In: Ekman P (ed) Emotion in the human face. Cambridge University Press, Cambridge
41. Gruebler A, Suzuki K (2010) Measurement of distal EMG signals using a wearable device for reading facial expressions. In: Annual international conference of the IEEE EMBS. Buenos Aires, Argentina, pp 4594–4597
42. Jayatilake D, Suzuki K (2012) Robot assisted facial expressions with segmented shape memory alloy actuators. Int J Mech Autom 1(3/4):224–235
43. Gruebler A, Berenz V, Suzuki K (2012) Emotionally assisted human-robot interaction using a wearable device for reading facial expressions. Adv Robot 26(10):1143–1159
44. Gems D (1999) Enhancing human traits: ethical and social implications. Nature 396:222–223

[illegible]

Chapter 8
Haptic Interface and Cybernics

Hiroo Iwata

Abstract This chapter presents work carried out in projects to develop haptic technologies, including finger/hand manipulation and locomotion. It is well known that the sense of touch is indispensable for understanding the real world. The last decade has seen significant advances in the development of haptic interfaces. Nevertheless, methods for implementing haptic interfaces are still in the trial-and-error stages. Compared with visual and auditory displays, haptic interfaces are not frequently used in everyday life. This paper introduces some of the issues and solutions with regard to haptic interfaces identified in the past 18 years of research conducted by the author.

Keywords Haptics • Force • Locomotion • Computer–human interaction

8.1 Introduction

It is well known that the sense of touch is indispensable for understanding the real world. The use of force feedback to enhance computer–human interaction has often been discussed. A haptic interface is a feedback device that generates a sensation perceived by the skin and muscles, including a sense of touch, weight, and rigidity. Compared with ordinary visual and auditory sensations, haptics is difficult to synthesize. Visual and auditory sensations are assimilated by specialized organs, the eyes and ears. On the other hand, a sensation of force can occur at any part of the human body and is therefore inseparable from actual physical contact. These characteristics have led to many difficulties when developing a haptic interface. Thus, we have to focus on the specific part of the body where haptic sensation is dominant in human activities.

H. Iwata (✉)
Faculty of Engineering, Information and Systems, University of Tsukuba, Tsukuba, Japan
e-mail: iwata@kz.tsukuba.ac.jp

Y. Sankai et al. (eds.), *Cybernics: Fusion of human, machine and information systems*,
DOI 10.1007/978-4-431-54159-2_8,

First, the fingers and hand are essential for object manipulation. Many haptic interfaces have been built for hand–object interaction, of which exoskeletons and pen-based haptic interfaces are the most popular, although these have difficulties with respect to natural interaction.

The other important part for haptic sensation is the foot. Walking on foot is the most intuitive way to move about. It is well known that the sense of distance and orientation is much better when walking than when riding in a vehicle. Some locomotion interfaces have been proposed, but it is difficult to mimic natural walking using hardware.

This chapter discusses major issues in the implementation of effective haptic interfaces. Solutions to the issues are provided with reference to the history of the author's research activity.

8.2 Mechanism of Haptics and Methods for Haptic Feedback

8.2.1 Somatic Sensation

A haptic interface generates synthetic stimulation for somatic sensation, including proprioception and skin sensation. Proprioception is complemented by the mechanoreceptors of the skeletal articulations and muscles. There are three types of joint position receptors: free nerve endings, and Ruffini and Pacinian corpuscles. Ruffini corpuscles detect static force, whereas the function of Pacinian corpuscles is to measure the acceleration of the joint angle. Position and motion of the human body is perceived by these receptors. Force sensation is perceived by the mechanoreceptors of muscles: muscle spindles and Golgi tendons. These receptors detect contact forces applied by an obstacle in the environment.

Skin sensation is perceived by the mechanoreceptors and thermoreceptors of the skin. The sense of touch is evoked by these receptors. Mechanoreceptors of the skin are classified into four types: Merkel disks, and Ruffini, Meissner, and Pacinian corpuscles. These receptors detect the edges of an object, skin stretch, velocity, and vibration, respectively.

8.2.2 Proprioception and Haptic Interfaces

A haptic interface is a mechanical device that generates a reaction force from virtual objects. Research on haptic interfaces has recently grown rapidly, although the technology is still in a state of trial-and-error. There are several approaches for implementing haptic interfaces.

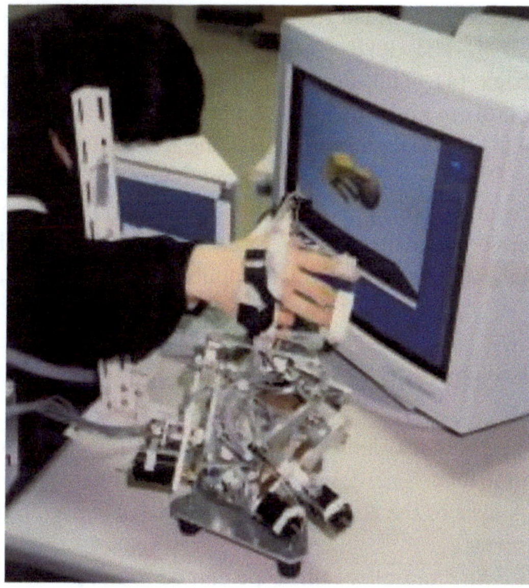

Fig. 8.1 Desktop force display

8.2.2.1 Exoskeleton Type Haptic Interface

An exoskeleton is a set of actuators attached to the hand or body. In the field of robotics research, exoskeletons have often been used as master-manipulators for teleoperations. However, most master-manipulators require a large amount of hardware and therefore have a high cost, which restricts their application areas. Compact hardware is necessary for use in human–computer interactions. The first example of a compact exoskeleton suitable for desktop use was proposed in 1990 [1]. The device applies force to the fingertips as well as the palm. Figure 8.1 shows an overall view of the system.

Lightweight and portable exoskeletons have also been developed. Burdea used small pneumatic cylinders to apply a force to the fingertips [2].

8.2.2.2 Tool-Handling Haptic Interface

A tool-handling force display is the easiest way to realize force feedback. The configuration of this type of interface is similar to that of a joystick. Unlike the exoskeleton, a tool-handling force display does not need to be fitted to the user's hand. Although it cannot generate a force between the fingers, it still has practical advantages.

A typical example of this category is the pen-based force display [3]. A pen-shaped grip is supported by two pantographs with three degree of freedom (DOF) providing six DOF force/torque feedback. Another example of this type is the Haptic Master, which was demonstrated at the Edge venue at SIGGRAPH 1994. The device has a ball-shaped grip to which six DOF force/torque is fed back [4]. This device employs a parallel mechanism in which a top triangular platform and a base triangular platform are connected by three sets of pantographs. This compact hardware has the ability to carry a large load.

Massie and Salisbury developed the PHANToM, which includes a three DOF pantograph [5]. A thimble with a gimbal is connected to the end of the pantograph, enabling a three DOF force to be applied to the fingertips. The PHANToM has become one of the most popular commercially available haptic interfaces.

8.2.2.3 Object-Oriented Haptic Interface

The object-oriented type of force display is a radical idea for the design of a haptic interface. The device moves or deforms to simulate the shapes of virtual objects. A user of the device can physically make contact with the virtual object through its surface.

An example of this type can be found in the work of Tachi et al. [6]. Their device consists of a shape approximation prop mounted on a manipulator. The position of the fingertip is measured, and the prop moves to provide a contact point for the virtual object. McNeely proposed an idea referred to as "Robotic Graphics" [7], which is similar to Tachi's method. Hirose developed a surface display that creates a contact surface using a 4×4 linear actuator array [8]. The device simulates an edge or a vertex of a virtual object.

8.2.2.4 Passive Prop

A passive input device equipped with force sensors is an alternative approach for constructing haptic interfaces. Murakami and Nakajima used a flexible prop to manipulate a 3D virtual object [9]. The force applied by the user is measured, and the deformation of the virtual object is determined based on the applied force. Sinclair developed a force sensor array to measure pressure distribution [10]. These passive devices allow users to interact using their bare fingers. However, since these devices have no actuators, they cannot represent the shape of virtual objects.

8.2.3 Proprioception and Full-Body Haptics

One of the new frontiers for haptic interface research is full-body haptics, which includes foot haptics. Force applied to the whole body plays a very important role in locomotion. The most intuitive way to move about in the real world is by walking

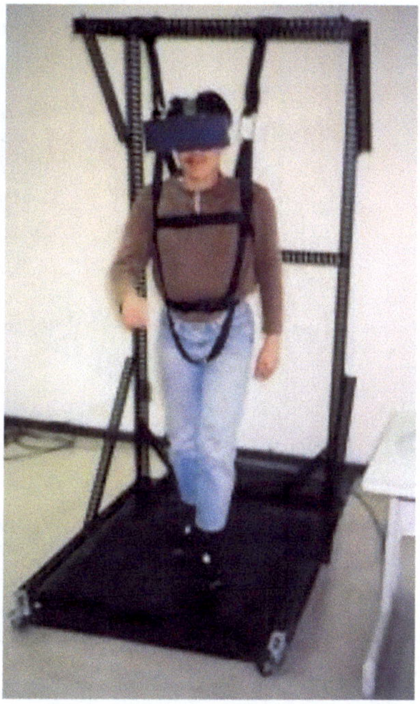

Fig. 8.2 First prototype of the Virtual Perambulator

on foot. A locomotion interface is a device that provides the sense of walking while the walker's body remains localized in the real world. Several approaches have been proposed for realizing locomotion interfaces.

8.2.3.1 Sliding Device

The project, called the "Virtual Perambulator", was aimed at developing a locomotion interface using a specialized sliding device [11]. The primary objective of the first stage was to enable the walker's feet to change direction. Controlling steering bars or joysticks is not as intuitive as locomotion. The first prototype of the Virtual Perambulator was developed in 1989 [12]. An overview of the apparatus is shown in Fig. 8.2. A user of the system wore a parachute-like harness and omni-directional roller skates, with the walker's torso fixed to the framework of the system by the harness. An omni-directional sliding device was used to change the direction of the feet. Specialized roller skates equipped with four casters were developed to enable two-dimensional motion. The walker could freely move his/her feet in any direction. Motion of the feet was measured by an ultrasonic range detector. From the results of these measurements, an image of the virtual space was projected in the head-mounted display corresponding to the motion of the walker. The direction of locomotion in virtual space was determined by the direction of the walker's step.

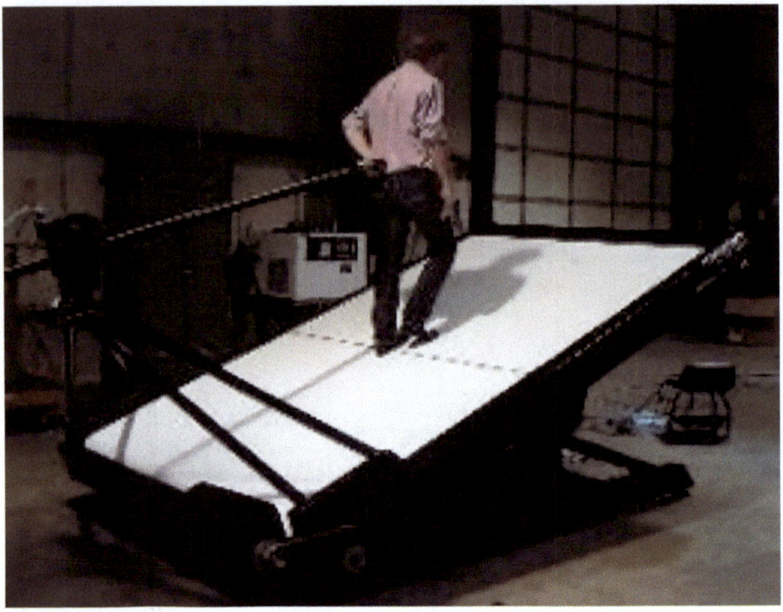

Fig. 8.3 Treadport

8.2.3.2 Treadmill

A simple device for virtual walking is the treadmill, ordinarily used for physical fitness. An application of this device to a virtual building simulator was developed at the University of North Carolina [13]. This treadmill has a steering bar similar to that of a bicycle. A treadmill equipped with a series of linear actuators underneath the belt was developed at ATR [14]. The device, known as the GSS, simulates the slope of virtual terrain. The Treadport developed at the University of Utah is a treadmill combined with a large manipulator connected to a walker [15]. The manipulator provides gravitational force while the walker negotiates a slope. Figure 8.3 shows the Treadport.

The omni-directional treadmill employs two perpendicular treadmills, one inside the other. Each belt comprises approximately 3,400 separate rollers, woven together in a mechanical fabric. The motion of the lower belt is transmitted by the rollers to the walker. This mechanism enables omni-directional walking [16].

8.2.3.3 Foot Pad

A foot pad applied to each foot is an alternative implementation of a locomotion interface. Two large manipulators driven by hydraulic actuators were developed at the University of Utah and applied as a locomotion interface. These manipulators are attached to a walker's feet. The device is called BiPort [http://www.sarcos.com]. The manipulators can mimic ground viscosity in a virtual environment (VE). A similar device, developed at the Cybernet Systems Corporation, uses two three DOF motion platforms for the feet [17]. These devices, however, have not been evaluated or applied in a VE.

8.2.3.4 Pedaling Device

In the battlefield simulator for the NPSNET project, a unicycle-like pedaling device is used for locomotion in a virtual battlefield [18]. A user of the system changes direction by twisting at the waist.

The OSIRIS, a simulator for night-vision battle, utilizes a stair stepper device. A player changes direction by controlling the joystick or twisting at the waist.

8.2.3.5 Gait Recognition for Walking

Slaters et al. proposed locomotion in VEs by "walking in place." They recognized the walking gait using a position sensor and neural network [19].

8.2.4 Skin Sensation and Tactile Display

The technology for creating tactile displays that stimulate skin sensation is well known and has been applied to communication aids for the blind as well as master systems for teleoperations. A sense of vibration is relatively easy to generate, and a substantial amount of work has been done on using vibration displays [20, 21]. A micro-pin array has also been used for tactile displays and has enabled the provision of a communication aid for the blind in the form of a teletaction system [22, 23]. It has the ability to convey texture or 2D-geometry [24].

The micro-pin array looks similar to an object-oriented force display, but it can only create skin sensation. The stroke distance of each pin is short, so the user cannot feel the 3D-shape of a virtual object directly. The main objective of tactile displays is to convey a sense of the fine texture of an object's surface. Recent research on tactile displays has focused on selective stimulation of mechanoreceptors in the skin. As mentioned at the beginning of this section, there are four types of mechanoreceptors in the skin: Merkel disks, and Ruffini, Meissner, and Pacinian Corpuscles. By stimulating these receptors selectively, various tactile sensations such as roughness or slip can be presented. Micro air jets [25] and micro electrode arrays [26] are used for selective stimulation.

8.3 Technologies for Finger/Hand Haptics

8.3.1 Desktop Force Display

Our research into haptic interfaces began in 1986. The first step was the use of an exoskeleton. In the field of robotics research, exoskeletons have often been used as master-manipulators for teleoperations. Virtual reality systems in the 1980s employed a conventional master-manipulator [1]. However, most master-manipulators require a large amount of hardware and therefore have a high cost, which restricts their application areas. Compact hardware is needed to use them in human–computer interactions. We therefore proposed the concept of a desktop force display with the first prototype developed in 1989. The device is a compact exoskeleton for desktop use [2]. Figure 8.1 depicts an overall view of the desktop force display.

Force sensation contains six-dimensional information: three-dimensional force and three-dimensional torque. The core element of the force display is a six DOF parallel manipulator. The main design feature of parallel manipulators is an octahedron, known as the "Stewart platform". This mechanism consists of an upper triangular platform and a base triangular platform connected by six length-controllable cylinders. This compact hardware has the ability to carry a large load. The structure, however, has some practical disadvantages in terms of the small working volume and lack of backdrivability (reduction of friction) of the mechanism. In our system, three sets of parallelogram linkages (pantographs) are employed instead of linear actuators. Each pantograph is driven by two DC motors, each of which is powered by a pulse width modulation amplifier. The top end of the pantograph is connected to a vertex on the top platform by a spherical joint. This mechanical configuration has the same advantages as the octahedron mechanism, but the pantograph mechanism improves the working volume and backdrivability of the parallel manipulator. The inertia of the moving parts of the manipulator is so small that compensation is not needed.

The working space of the center of the top platform is a spherical volume with a diameter of approximately 30 cm. Each joint angle of the manipulator is measured by potentiometers, with 1 % linearity. The maximum load of the manipulator is 2.3 kg, which is more than that of a typical hand.

The top platform of the parallel manipulator is fixed to the palm of the operator by a U-shaped attachment, which enables the operator to move the hand and fingers independently. Three actuators are set coaxially with the first joint of the thumb, forefinger, and middle finger of the operator, respectively, with the last three fingers working together. DC servo motors are employed for each actuator.

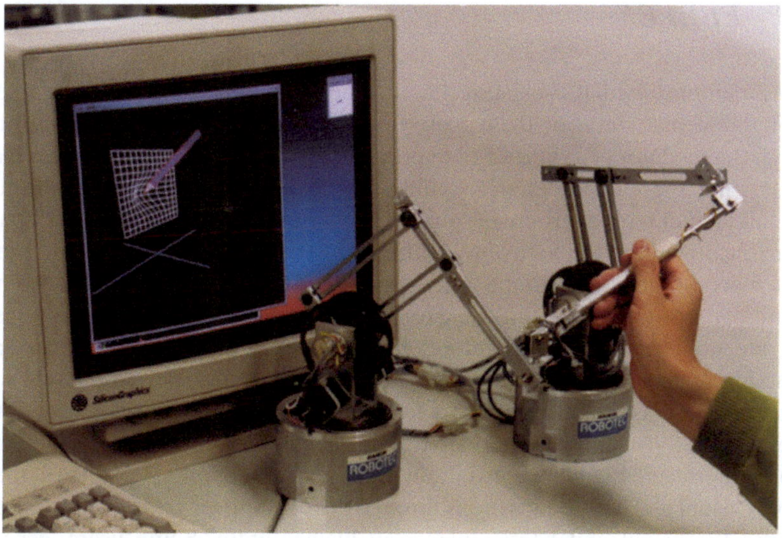

Fig. 8.4 Pen-based force display

8.3.2 Pen-Based Force Display

Exoskeletons are cumbersome for users to put on and take off. This disadvantage restricts practical use of force displays. Tool-handling methods for implementing a force display do so without a glove-like device. A pen-based force display is proposed as an alternative device [2]. A six DOF force reflective master manipulator with a pen-shaped grip has been developed. All users are familiar with the use of pens in their everyday life. Moreover, people use spatulas or rakes to model solid objects. These devices have stick-shaped grips similar to that of a pen. As such, a pen-based force display can easily be applied to the design of 3D shapes.

The human hand has the ability to perform six DOF motion in a 3D space. In the case where a six DOF master manipulator is built using serial joints, each joint must support the weight of the upper joints. This characteristic enforces the need for large hardware in the manipulator. We used a parallel mechanism to reduce the size and weight of the manipulator. The pen-based force display employs two three DOF manipulators. Both ends of the pen are connected to these manipulators. The total number of DOF of the force display is six. Three DOF force and three DOF torque are applied to the pen. An overall view of the force display is shown in Fig. 8.4. Each three DOF manipulator is composed of a pantograph link. Through this mechanism, the pen is free from the weight of the actuators.

8.3.3 FEELEX

Having demonstrated the existing haptic interfaces to a number of people, the author found that some of them were unable to fully experience virtual objects through the medium of synthesized haptic sensation. There seem to be two reasons for this. First, these haptic interfaces allow the user to touch the virtual object only at a single point or a group of points. These contact points are not spatially continuous, owing to the hardware configuration of the haptic interfaces. The user feels a reaction force through the grip or thimble. By using Velcro bands attached to specific parts of the user's fingers, exoskeletons provide more contact points, but these are not continuous. Therefore, these devices fail to recreate the natural interaction sensation when compared with manual manipulation in the real world.

The second reason that some users fail to perceive the sensation is related to the combination of visual and haptic displays. A visual image is usually combined with a haptic interface by using a conventional CRT or projection screen. Thus, the user receives visual and haptic sensations through different displays, and therefore has to integrate the visual and haptic images in his/her brain. Some users, especially elderly people, have difficulty in integrating this process.

Considering these problems, a new interface device has been developed as part of the "FEELEX" project, where the word FEELEX is derived from a conjunction of "feel" and "flex." The major goals of this project are:

i. To provide a spatially continuous surface that enables users to feel virtual objects using any part of their fingers or even the whole palm; and
ii. To provide visual and haptic sensations simultaneously using a single device that does not require the user to wear any extra apparatus.

A new configuration for a visual/haptic display was designed to achieve these goals. Figure 8.5 illustrates the basic concept of the FEELEX. The device is composed of a flexible screen, an array of actuators, and a projector. The flexible screen is deformed by the actuators to simulate the shape of virtual objects. An image of the virtual objects is projected onto the surface of the flexible screen. Deformation of the screen converts the 2D image from the projector into a solid image. This configuration enables the user to touch the image directly using any part of the hand. The actuators are equipped with force sensors to measure the force applied by the user. The hardness of the virtual object is determined by the relationship between the measured force and its position on the screen. If the virtual object is soft, a large deformation is caused by a small applied force.

8.3.3.1 FEELEX 1

The FEELEX 1, developed in 1997, was designed to enable double-handed interaction using the whole palm. Therefore, the optimum size of the screen was determined to be 24 cm $\times$ 24 cm. The screen is connected to a linear actuator array

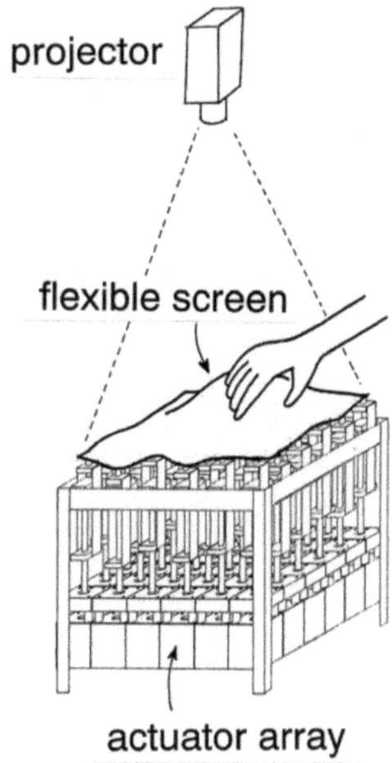

Fig. 8.5 Basic design of the FEELEX

that deforms its shape. Each linear actuator is composed of a screw mechanism driven by a DC motor. The screw mechanism converts the rotation of an axis of the motor to linear motion of a rod. The motor must generate both motion and a reaction force on the screen. The diameter of the smallest motor that can drive the screen is 4 cm.

Therefore, a 6×6 linear actuator array can be set under the screen. The deformable screen is made of a rubber plate and a white nylon cloth, with the thickness of the rubber being 3 mm. Figure 8.6 shows an example of the device.

The screw mechanism of the linear actuator has a self-locking function that maintains its position while the motor is off. With a hard virtual wall, it is difficult to simulate tool-handling force displays. Considerable motor power is required to generate the reaction force from the virtual wall, and this often leads to uncomfortable vibrations. The screw mechanism does not suffer from this problem. A soft wall can be represented by the computer-controlled motion of the linear actuators based on the data from the force sensors. A force sensor is set at the top of each linear actuator, with two strain gauges used as the force sensor. The strain gauge detects small displacements of the upper end of the linear actuator caused by the force applied by the user. The position of the upper end of the linear actuator is measured by an optical encoder connected to the axis of the DC motor. The maximum stroke of the linear actuator is 80 mm, and the maximum speed is 100 mm/s.

The system is controlled via a PC. The DC motors are interfaced by a parallel I/O unit, and the force sensors are interfaced by an A/D converter unit. The force sensors provide interaction with the graphics. The position and strength of the force applied by the user are detected by a 6×6 sensor array. The graphics projected onto the flexible screen are changed according to the measured force.

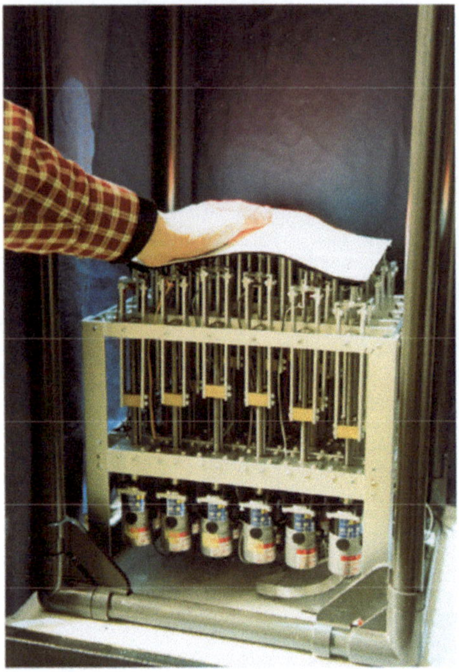

Fig. 8.6 Overview of the FEELEX 1

8.3.3.2 FEELEX 2

The FEELEX 2 was designed to improve the resolution of the haptic surface. To determine the resolution of the linear actuators, we considered the situation where a medical doctor palpates a patient. Results of interviews with several medical doctors confirmed that they usually recognize a tumor using their index, middle, and third fingers. The size of a tumor is estimated by comparing it to the width of their fingers, i.e., two-fingers or three-fingers large. Thus, the distance between the axes of the linear actuators should be smaller than the width of a finger. Considering the above, the distance was set at 8 mm. This 8-mm resolution enables the user to hit at least one actuator when touching any arbitrary position on the screen. The size of the screen is 50 mm $\times$ 50 mm, which allows the user to touch the surface using three fingers.

To realize 8-mm resolution, a piston-crank mechanism was employed for the linear actuator. Since the motor is much larger than 8 mm, it should be placed at a position offset from the rod. The piston-crank mechanism can easily achieve this offset position. Figure 8.7 illustrates the mechanical configuration of the linear actuator. A servo-motor from a radio-controlled car was used as the actuator. The rotation of the axis of the servo-motor is converted to linear motion of the rod by a crank-shaft and linkage. The stroke of the rod is 18 mm, and the maximum speed is 250 mm/s. The maximum torque of the servo-motor is 3.2 kg-cm, which applies a 1.1-kgf force at the top of each rod. This force is sufficient for palpation using the fingers.

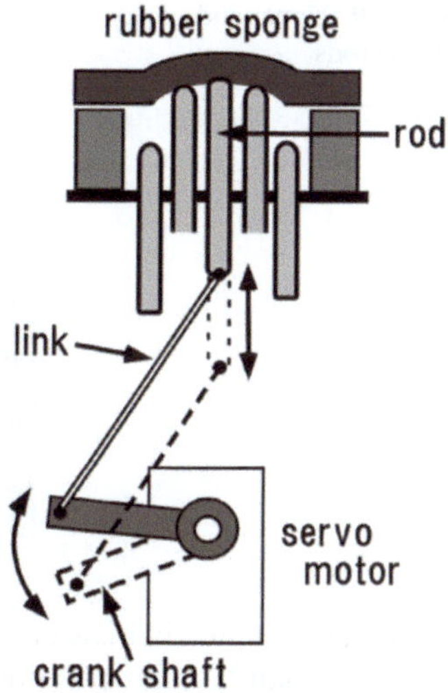

Fig. 8.7 Piston-crank mechanism

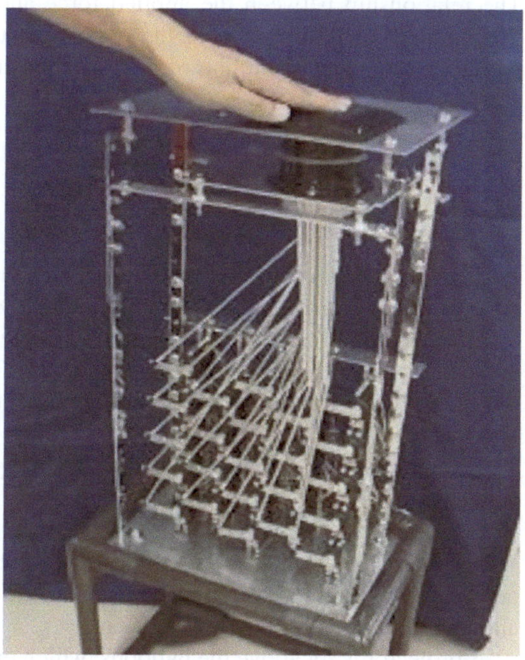

Fig. 8.8 Image of the FEELEX 2

The flexible screen is supported by 23 rods, with the servo-motors set remotely from the rods. A picture of the FEELEX 2 is shown in Fig. 8.8, in which the 23 separate sets of piston-crank mechanisms are clearly visible.

Figure 8.9 shows the upper ends of the rods. The photo was taken while the flexible screen was off. The diameter of each rod is 6 mm. A strain gauge cannot be placed on top of a rod because of its small size. Thus, the electric current going to

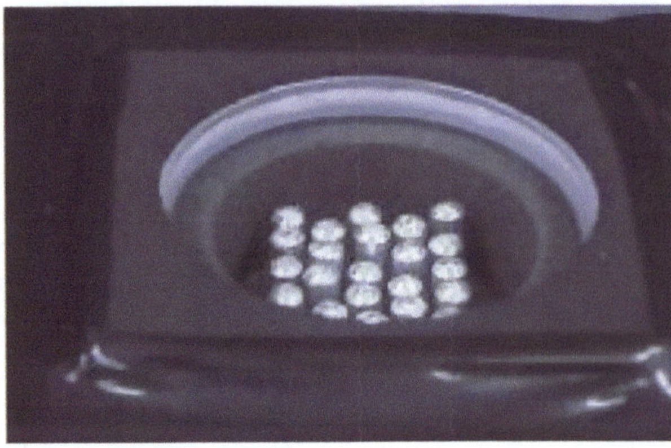

Fig. 8.9 Upper ends of the rods

each servo-motor is measured to estimate the force. The servo-motor generates a force to maintain the position of the crank-shaft. When the user applies a force to the rod, the electric current to the motor increases to balance the force. The relationship between the applied force and the electric current is measured. The applied force at the top of the rods is calculated using data from the electric current sensor. The resolution of the force sensing capability is 40 gf.

8.3.4 Volflex

A major limitation of the FEELEX is that it cannot display the side or rear view of a virtual object. To overcome this limitation, we designed a volumetric object-oriented haptic interface. The Volflex is a new haptic interface that provides the user with a physical 3D surface for interaction. The device is composed of a group of air balloons, which constitute the interaction surface. These balloons are arranged in a body-centered cubic lattice, with a tube connected to each balloon. The volume of each balloon is controlled by an air cylinder. The tubes are connected to each other by springs. This mechanical flexibility enables an arbitrary shape for the interaction surface. Each air cylinder is equipped with a pressure sensor that detects the force applied by the user. Based on the pressure data, the device is programmed to perform like clay, although unlike real clay, the Volflex allows the user to "undo" an operation.

A projector is set above the balloons, which projects an image onto the surface of the device, and not onto the user's hand. We developed a mechanical rotary shutter that separates the projector and camera. The camera captures the user's hand, which is eliminated from the projected image. Figure 8.10 shows an overall view of the Volflex.

Virtual clay is one of the ultimate goals of interactive techniques in 3D graphics. Digital tools for 2D paint applications are considered to be mature technology.

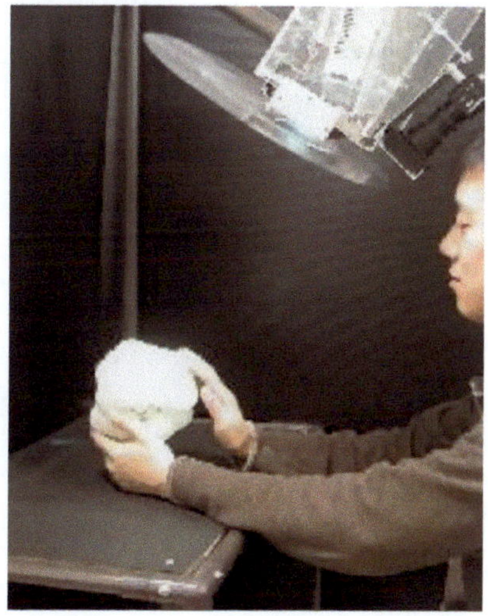

Fig. 8.10 View of the Volflex

On the other hand, tools for 3D shape manipulation are still in the early stages of development. Shape design of a 3D object is one of the major application areas for haptic interfaces, as it requires good haptic sensations.

The Volflex provides an effective interface device for manipulation of virtual clay by using a lattice of air balloons. 2D paint tools are popular and a digital picture is easy to draw. The Volflex is a new digital tool for creating 3D shapes, which has the potential to revolutionize methods for industrial design. Designers use their palms or the joints of their fingers to deform clay models when carrying out rough design tasks. The Volflex has the ability to support such natural manipulation.

The Volflex is not only a tool for 3D shape design, but also an interactive work of art. The physical properties of a virtual object can be designed by programming controllers for the balloons. The projected image can also be designed. The combination of the haptic and visual displays provides a new platform for interactive sculpture.

8.4 Technologies for Full-Body Haptics

8.4.1 Torus Treadmill

8.4.1.1 Basic Design of the Torus Treadmill

The key principle in a treadmill-based locomotion interface is to make the floor move in a direction opposite to that of the walker. The motion of the floor cancels the displacement of the walker in the real world. The major problem in treadmill-based locomotion interfaces is to allow the walker to change direction.

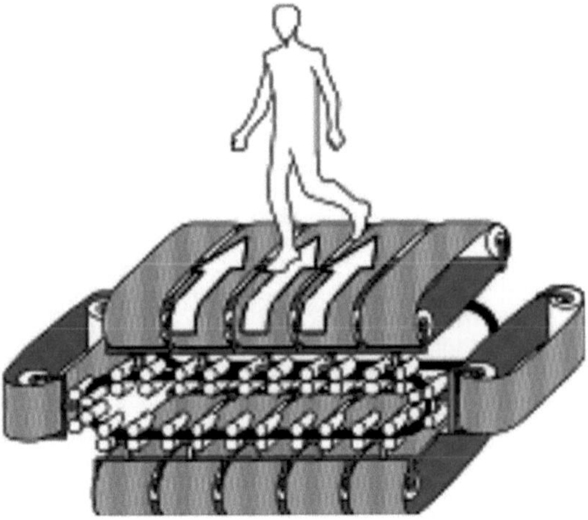

Fig. 8.11 Structure of Torus Treadmill (X motion)

An omni-directional active floor enables a virtually infinite area. To realize an infinite walking area, geometric configuration of an active floor must be chosen. A closed surface driven by actuators has the ability to create an unlimited floor. The following requirements for implementation of the closed surface must be considered.

i. The walker and actuators must be placed outside the surface.
ii. The walker area must be a planar surface.
iii. The surface must be constructed from a material with very little stretch.

The shape of the closed surface is generally a surface with holes. If the number of holes is zero, the surface is a sphere, which is the simplest infinite surface. However, the walking area of the sphere is not a planar surface. A very large diameter is required to create a planar surface on a sphere, which restricts implementation of the locomotion interface.

A closed surface with one hole like a doughnut is called a torus. A torus can be implemented by a group of belts, which create a planar surface for the user to walk on. A closed surface with more than one hole cannot create a planar walking surface. Thus, the torus is the only form suitable for a locomotion interface.

8.4.1.2 Mechanism and Performance

The Torus Treadmill was implemented by a group of belts connected to each other [27]. Figures 8.11 and 8.12 illustrate the basic structure of the Torus Treadmill. Twelve treadmills are employed in the Torus to move the walker along in the X-direction. These 12 treadmills are connected side by side and driven in a perpendicular direction. This motion moves the walker along in the Y-direction.

Figure 8.13 shows an overall view of the apparatus. The 12 treadmills are connected to four chains and mounted on four rails. The chain drives the walker

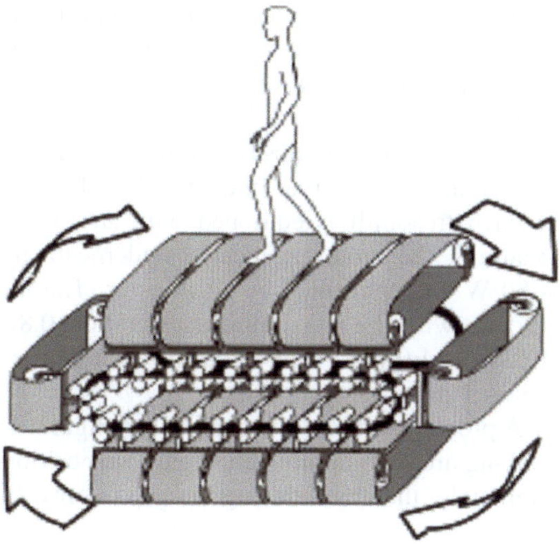

Fig. 8.12 Structure of Torus Treadmill (Y motion)

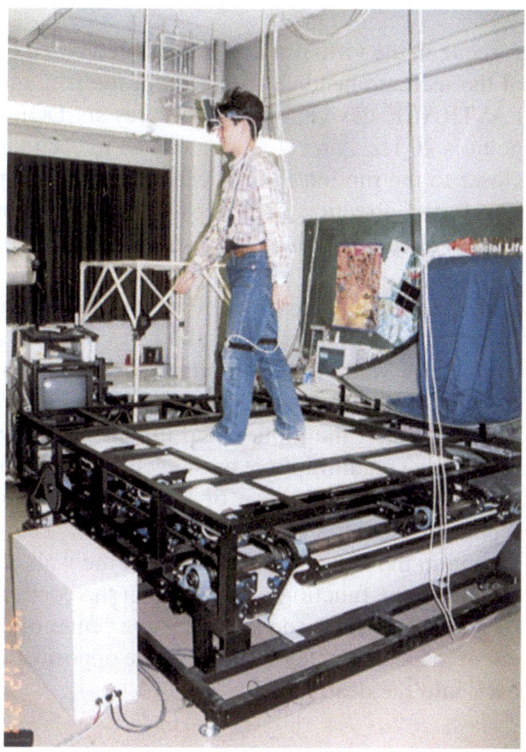

Fig. 8.13 Torus Treadmill

along in the Y-direction. The rail supports the weight of the treadmills and the walker. An AC motor is used to drive the chains. The power of the motor is 200 W and controlled by an inverter. The maximum speed of rotation is 1.2 m/s and the maximum acceleration is 1.0 m/s^2. The deceleration caused by friction is 1.5 m/s^2. Frequency characteristics are limited by a circuit protector of the motor driver with the maximum switching frequency 0.8 Hz.

Each treadmill is equipped with an AC motor. To reduce the length of the treadmill, the motor is located underneath the belt. The power of each motor is 80 W and controlled by an inverter. The maximum speed of each treadmill is 1.2 m/s with the maximum acceleration 0.8 m/s^2. The deceleration caused by friction is 1.0 m/s^2. The width of each belt is 250 mm and the overall walkable area is 1 m $\times$ 1 m.

A problem with this mechanical configuration is the gap between the belts in the walking area. To minimize the gap, we positioned the driver unit of each treadmill alternately, thereby reducing the gap to only 2 mm.

8.4.1.3 Control Algorithm for the Torus Treadmill

A scene in the virtual space is generated based on the results of the motion tracking of the feet and head. The motion of the feet and head is measured by a Polhemus FASTRACK device, which measures six DOF motion. The sampling rate at each point is 20 Hz. A receiver is attached to each knee; we could not place the sensors closer to the motion floor because the steel frame distorts the magnetic field. The length and direction of a step is calculated from the data from the sensors. The user's viewpoint in the virtual space moves according to the length and direction of the steps.

To keep the walker in the center of the walking area, the Torus Treadmill must be driven according to the walker. A control algorithm is required to achieve safe and natural walking. From our experience with the Virtual Perambulator project, the walker should not be connected to a harness or mechanical linkages, since such devices restrict the motion and inhibit natural walking. The control algorithm for the Torus Treadmill must be safe enough to allow removal of the harness from the walker. In the final stage of the Virtual Perambulator Project, we succeeded in replacing the harness with a hoop frame. The walker could walk freely and turn around in the hoop, which supported the walker's body, while the feet moved. We simulated the function of the hoop in the control algorithm for the Torus Treadmill by placing a circular dead zone in the center of the walking area. If the walker steps out of the area, the floor moves in the opposite direction so that the walker is carried back into the dead zone.

8.4.2 *GaitMaster*

8.4.2.1 Methods for Presenting Uneven Surfaces

One of the major research issues in locomotion interfaces is the presentation of uneven surfaces. Locomotion interfaces are often applied to simulations of buildings or urban spaces. These spaces usually include stairs. A walker should be provided with a sense of ascending or descending stairs. Moreover, in certain applications of locomotion interfaces, such as training simulators or entertainment devices, rough terrain must also be represented.

Presentation of a virtual staircase was tested in the early stages of the Virtual Perambulator project. A string, connected to the roller skate on each foot, was pulled by a motor. When ascending stairs, the front foot of the walker was pulled up. When the walker descended the stairs, the back foot was pulled up. However, this method was not successful because of instability.

Later, a six DOF motion platform was applied to the final version of the Virtual Perambulator, with the user supported by a hoop frame. The walker stood on the top plate of the motion platform. Pitch and heave motion of the platform was used. If the walker stepped forward to climb a step, the pitch angle and vertical position of the floor increased. After completing the climbing motion, the floor returned to the neutral position. If the walker stepped forward to go down a step, the pitch angle and vertical position of the floor decreased. This inclination of the floor was intended to present a height difference between the feet, while the heave motion was intended to simulate vertical acceleration. However, this method failed in simulations of stairs mainly because the floor was flat.

A possible method for creating a height difference between the feet is the application of two large manipulators. The BiPort is a typical implementation of this method. A four DOF manipulator driven by hydraulic actuators is connected to each foot. The major problem with this method, however, is how to enable the manipulators to trace the turning motion of the walker. When a walker turns around, the two manipulators interfere with each other.

The Torus Treadmill provides natural turning motion. A walker on the Torus Treadmill can physically turn about on the active floor. Turning motion using the feet plays a major role in the performance of human spatial recognition. Vestibular and proprioceptive feedback is essential to the sense of orientation [28]. The Torus Treadmill can be modified to simulate uneven surfaces. If we install an array of linear actuators on each treadmill, an uneven floor can be realized by controlling the length of each linear actuator. However, this method is almost impossible to implement, because a very large number of linear actuators are required to cover the surface of the torus-shaped treadmills, and the control signals for each actuator must be transmitted wirelessly.

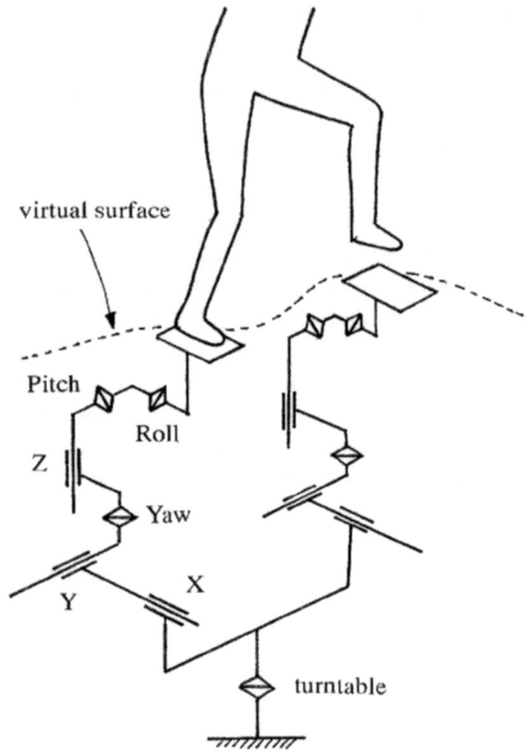

Fig. 8.14 Basic design of the GaitMaster

8.4.2.2 Basic Design of the GaitMaster

A new locomotion interface that simulates an omni-directional uneven surface has been designed. The device is called the "GaitMaster." The core elements of the device are two six DOF motion-bases mounted on a turntable. Figure 8.14 illustrates the basic configuration of the GaitMaster.

A walker stands on the top plate of the motion-base. Each motion-base is controlled to trace the position of the foot, while the turntable is controlled to trace the orientation of the walker. The motion of the turntable prevents interference between the two motion-bases.

The X and Y motion of the motion-base traces the horizontal position of the feet and cancels the motion thereof by moving in the opposite direction. The rotation around the yaw axis traces the horizontal orientation of the feet, while the Z motion traces the vertical position of the feet and cancels its motion. The rotation around the roll and pitch axis simulates inclination of the virtual surface.

Fig. 8.15 Canceling the ascending motion

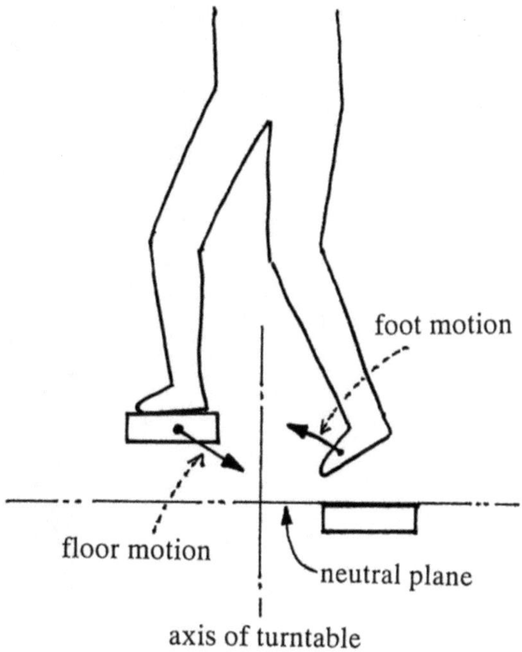

8.4.2.3 Control Algorithm for the GaitMaster

The control algorithm must maintain the position of the walker in the neutral position of the GaitMaster, and thus the motion-platforms must cancel the motion of the feet. The procedure for this cancellation is explained below.

i. Suppose the right foot is at the forward position and the left foot is at the backward positon while walking.
ii. As the walker steps forward on the left foot, the weight of the walker is transferred to the right foot.
iii. The motion-platform of the right foot goes backward according to the displacement of the left foot, so that the central position of the walker is maintained.
iv. The motion-platform of the left foot follows the position of the left foot. When the walker finishes stepping forward, the motion-platform supports the left foot.

If the walker goes up or down stairs, a similar procedure can be applied. The vertical motion of the feet is canceled using the same principal. The vertical displacement of the forward foot is canceled according to the motion of the backward foot, so that the central position of the walker is maintained at a neutral height. Figure 8.15 illustrates the method for canceling the ascending motion.

The turntable rotates so that the two motion-platforms can trace the rotational motion of the walker. If the walker changes walking direction, the turntable rotates to trace the orientation of the walker. The orientation of the turntable is determined

Fig. 8.16 GaitMaster

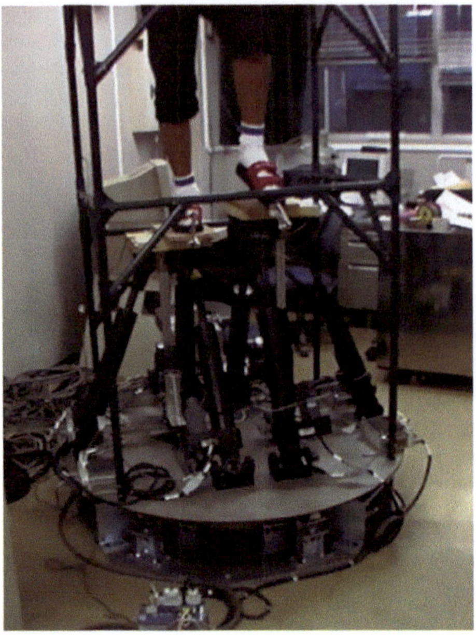

according to the direction of the feet. The turntable rotates so that its orientation is at the middle of the feet. The walker can physically turn around on the GaitMaster using this control algorithm for the turntable.

8.4.2.4 Prototype GaitMaster

Figure 8.16 illustrates the prototype GaitMaster. To simplify the mechanism of the motion-platform, the surface of the virtual space was defined as a set of planar surfaces. Most buildings and urban spaces can be simulated without inclination of the floor. Thus, we can ignore the roll and pitch axis of the motion-platforms. Each platform in the prototype GaitMaster is composed of three linear actuators on top of which a yaw joint is mounted. We disassembled a six DOF Stewart platform and created two XYZ stages. Three linear guides are applied to support the orientation of the top plate of the motion-platform. The load of each motion-platform is approximately 150 kg. A rotational joint around the yaw axis is mounted on each motion platform. The joint is equipped with a spring that moves the feet to the neutral direction.

The turntable was developed using a large DD motor with a maximum angular velocity of 500 deg/sec. Connected to each foot is a three DOF goniometer, which measures the back-and-forth and up-and-down motion, as well as the yaw angle. The control algorithm mentioned in the previous section was implemented and successfully realized the presentation of virtual stairs.

8.4.3 *Robot Tile*

8.4.3.1 CirculaFloor Project

Locomotion interfaces often require bulky hardware, since they have to carry the user's whole body. Moreover, the hardware is not easy to reconfigure to improve its performance or to add new functions. Considering these issues, the goals of the CirculaFloor project are twofold.

i. Develop compact hardware for the creation of the infinite surface for walking.

The major disadvantage of existing locomotion interfaces is their difficult installation. We need to solve the position for demonstration at SIGGRAPH.

ii. Develop a scalable hardware architecture for future improvement of the system.

Another disadvantage of existing locomotion interfaces is the inherent difficulty in improving the system. We need to design a new hardware architecture that allows us to upgrade the actuation mechanism easily or to add new mechanisms for the creation of uneven surfaces.

To achieve these goals, we designed a new configuration for a locomotion interface using a set of omni-directional movable tiles. Each tile is equipped with a holonomic mechanism that achieves omni-directional motion. An infinite surface is simulated by circulating the movable tiles. The motion of the feet is measured by position sensors. The tile moves in an opposite direction to the measured direction of the walker to cancel the motion of the step. The position of the walker is fixed in the real world by this computer-controlled motion of the tiles. The circulation of the tiles has the ability to cancel the displacement of the walker in an arbitrary direction. Thus, the walker can freely change direction while walking. Figure 8.17 shows an overall view of the CirculaFloor.

The CirculaFloor is a new method that incorporates features of both the treadmill and footpad. It creates an infinite omni-directional surface by using a set of movable tiles. The combination of tiles provides a sufficient area for walking, and thus precision tracing of the foot position is not required. Moreover, it has the potential to create an uneven surface by mounting an up-and-down mechanism on each tile.

8.4.3.2 Method for Creating an Infinite Surface

The current method of circulating the movable tiles is designed to satisfy the following conditions. (i) Two of the movable tiles are used to pull the user back to the center of the dead zone. (ii) The rest of the movable tiles are used to create a new surface in front. (iii) Each tile is moved the shortest distance to the next destination, while avoiding collisions with the other tiles. (iv) The control program allocates all destinations to the tiles, and determines when the tiles reach their destinations. (v) To simplify the algorithm, the tiles do not rotate according to the

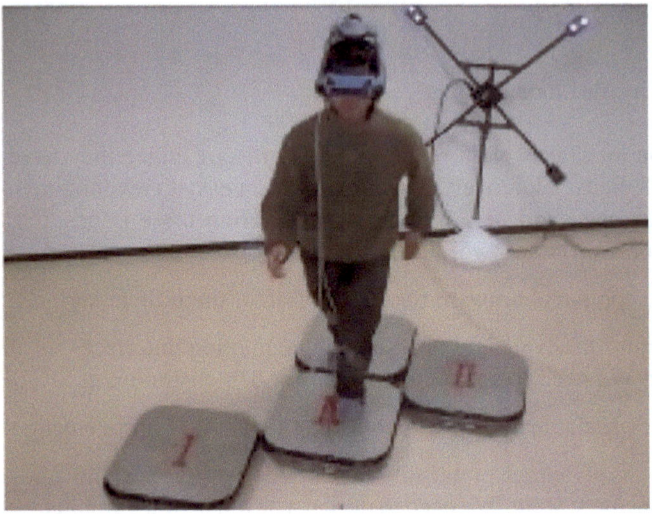

Fig. 8.17 CirculaFloor

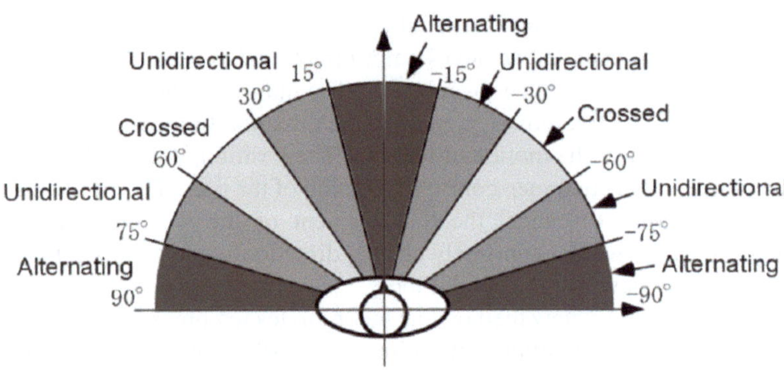

Fig. 8.18 Pulling-back modes corresponding to the walking direction

walking direction. Considering the above conditions, the circulation method is varied according to the walking direction. Three modes, "alternating circulation", "unidirectional circulation", and "cross-circulation" have been designed corresponding to the direction (Fig. 8.18).

Alternating circulation (Fig. 8.19): This mode is adopted for directions between ±15° and ±75–105°. The tiles used to create a new front surface (white-colored tiles in Fig. 8.19) move around to the front of the tiles for alternatively pulling back (in Fig. 8.19, gray-colored tiles) from the left (Path-1)/right (Path-2) sides.

Unidirectional circulation (Fig. 8.20): This mode is adopted for directions between ±15–30° and ±60–75°. The tiles used to create a new front surface move around in a unidirectional circulation to the right/left front of the tiles involved in pulling back.

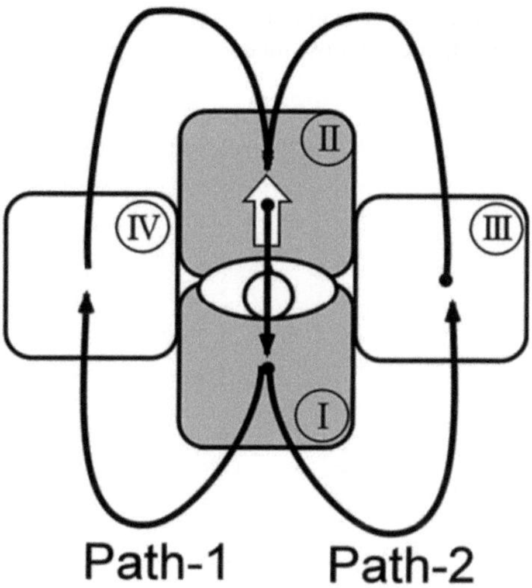

Fig. 8.19 Circulation of movable tiles in alternating mode

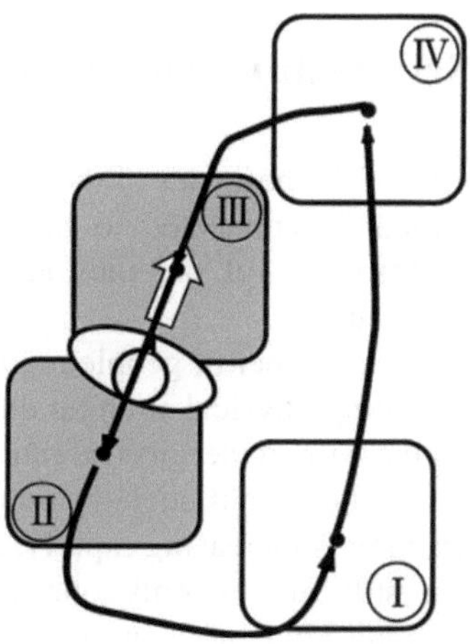

Fig. 8.20 Circulation of movable tiles in unidirectional mod

Cross-circulation (Fig. 8.21): This mode is adopted for directions of ±30–60°. The tiles used to create a new front surface move around to the left/right front (Path-1) or the left/right sides (Path-2) of the tiles involved in pulling back.

When a user of the CirculaFloor changes walking direction, the control program calculates the nearest phase of each tile using a template-matching technique corresponding to the new direction. Then the tiles are informed of the shortest path to their destinations.

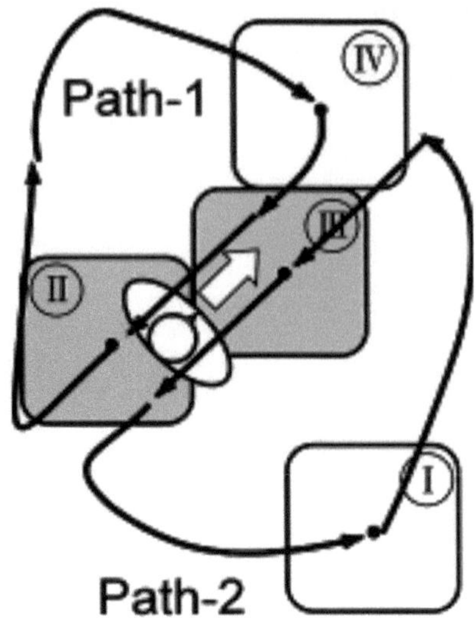

Fig. 8.21 Circulation of movable tiles in cross mode

8.5 Gait Rehabilitation Using a Locomotion Interface

One of the best uses of the GaitMaster is for walking rehabilitation. If the foot of a patient is connected to the motion platform, it can assist with walking. High performance of the motion platform to trace the foot is not required for this application.

The number of people requiring gait rehabilitation is increasing yearly owing to declining physical strength due to aging or being bedridden long-term, and also to an increase in the survival rates in the case of cerebral apoplexy, cerebral infarction, etc. In Japan, although the number of physical therapists who provide rehabilitation training is increasing rapidly, a large number of facilities that provide such training are still run by only one physical therapist. As a result, many patients stop training after the acute period during which their functions are restored to some extent and resume training for a maintenance phase in a condition called a plateau, where the functional recovery curve levels off.

We developed a simplified GaitMaster for rehabilitation [29]. It moves each foot on a motion platform with two DOF (back-and-forth and up-and-down), thus allowing repeated walking cycles. It is also easy to attach and detach, and it moderately restrains the body (Fig. 8.22). Given the range of movement of the human joints, the device is designed to move only the feet, leaving the user in control of movements of the joints in the legs, hips, and other parts of the body. In so doing, we have achieved an acceptable trade-off between the amount of exercise and moderate restraint provided. We also designed a rehabilitation program of training three times a week for about 20 min each time using this system. In this program, patients are given a goal: to achieve a speed of about 1.5 times that

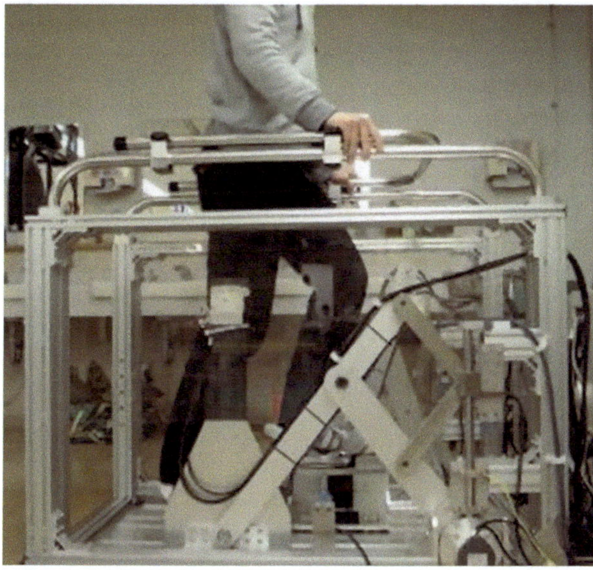

Fig. 8.22 Simplified GaitMaster for average increased walking velocity from walking rehabilitation

which they accomplished prior to the training in a 10-m walk. In moving towards this goal, the physical therapist considers the patient's condition each day to decide what training can be safely executed. Intermediate goals are set in the following way: strides are gradually increased to the target of normal strides for the relevant age group, and then walking speeds are gradually increased to the target values.

We confirmed improvement in the subjects' ability to walk. Some of the results are presented below. A total of 10 subjects took part in the rehabilitation program over a 6-month period, roughly divided into an "intervention period" and a "non-intervention period," which both included 4 weeks each for pre-evaluation, intervention/non-intervention of the system, and post-evaluation. Walking velocity over a 10-m distance was measured. Variations in walking velocities for weeks 5–12 were calculated against the baseline (BL) of the average walking velocities in the pre-evaluation period comprising weeks 1–4. Figure 8.23 gives the calculated average differences in the walking velocities of all the subjects and the average maximum 10-m walking velocities during the BL period and the maximum walking velocities for each week. Verification of the weekly values by a one-way layout repeated measurement variance analysis revealed significant variations from the BL values in the intervention period using the locomotion interface. On the other hand, no significant difference was found in the non-intervention period. We consider from these findings that the walking velocities of the subjects (plateau patients) were increased through use of this system. In the intervention period, walking velocities did not decrease from the 9th week onwards. This means that the effects of intervention by the system proved to be sustainable.

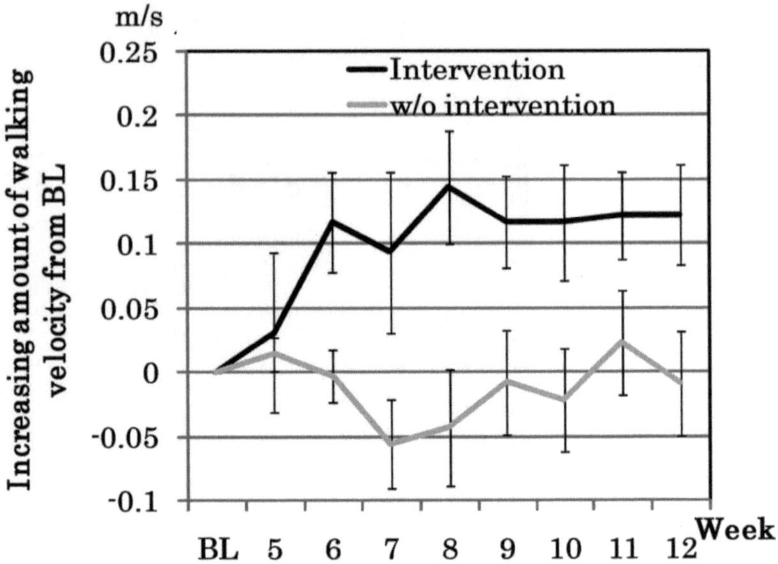

Fig. 8.23 Average increased walking velocity from the baseline (BL) period

8.6 Conclusion and Future Work

This chapter described some of the main topics with respect to haptic interfaces. A number of methods have been proposed to implement haptic interfaces. Future work in this research field will address the following two issues.

8.6.1 Safety Issues

Safety is an important problem in haptic interfaces. Inadequate control of the actuators may injure the user. The exoskeleton and tool-handling force displays have control problems in their contact surface for virtual objects. Vibration or unwanted forces can be generated and passed back to the user, which is sometimes dangerous. One of the major advantages of FEELEX is its safety. A user of FEELEX does not need to wear any special equipment while the interaction is taking place. Moreover, the contact surface of the FEELEX is physically generated, so it does not suffer from any control problems.

A locomotion interface has many important safety issues. Since these systems typically support the full body weight of the user, inadequate control can cause major injury to the user. Specialized hardware to keep the walker safe must be developed.

8.6.2 Psychology in Haptics

There have been many findings regarding haptic sensation. Most of these are related to skin sensations, and research activities that include muscle sensations are very few in number. Among these, Lederman and Klatzky's work is closely related to the design of the force display (Lederman and Klatzky 1987). Their latest work involves spatially distributed forces (Lederman and Klatzky 1999). They performed an experiment involving palpation. The subjects were asked to find a steel ball placed underneath a foam-rubber cover. The results showed that steel balls smaller than 8 mm in diameter decreased the success rate. This finding supports our specification for the FEELEX 2 in which the distance between rods is 8 mm. This kind of psychological study will assist in future development of haptic interfaces.

Haptics is indispensable for human interaction in the real world. Nevertheless, it is not commonly used in the field of human–computer interaction. Although there are several commercially available haptic interfaces, these are expensive and are limited in their functions. Image displays have been around for over 100 years. Today, image displays, such as TVs or movie projectors, are used in everyday life. On the other hand, haptic interfaces only have a 10-year history. There are still many obstacles to overcome before haptic interfaces can be incorporated in everyday use. However, haptic interfaces are seen as the new frontier of media technology and will certainly contribute to human life.

References

1. Iwata H (1990) Artificial reality with force-feedback: development of desktop virtual space with compact master manipulator. ACM SIGGRAPH Comput Graph 24(4)
2. Burdea G, Zhuang J, Roskos E, Silver D, Langlana L (1992) A portable dextrous master with force feedback., Presence 1(1)
3. Iwata H (1993) Pen-based Haptic virtual environment. In Proceedings of IEEE VRAIS'93
4. Iwata H (1994) Desktop force display. In: SIGGRAPH 94 Visual Proceedings
5. Massie T, Salisbury K (1994) The PHANToM haptic interface: a device for probing virtual objects. In: ASME Winter Annual Meeting, DSC-Vol. 55–1
6. Tachi S et al (1994) A construction method of virtual haptic space. In: Proceedings of ICAT'94
7. McNeely W (1993) Robotic graphics: a new approach to force feedback for virtual reality. In: Proceedings of IEEE VRAIS'93
8. Hirota K, Hirose M (1996) Simulation and presentation of curved surface in virtual reality environment through surface display. In: Proceedings of IEEE VRAIS'96
9. Murakami T, Nakajima N (1994) Direct and intuitive input device for 3D shape deformation. In: ACM CHI 1994, Conference on human factors in computing systems, pp 465–470
10. Sinclair M (1997) The haptic lens. In: SIGGRAPH 97 visual proceedings, p 179
11. Iwata H, Fujii T (1996) Virtual Perambulator: a novel interface device for locomotion in virtual environment. In: Proceedings of IEEE 1996 virtual reality annual international symposium, pp 60–65
12. Iwata H (1990) Artificial reality for walking about large scale virtual space. Hum Interface News Rep 5(1):49–52 (in Japanese)

13. Brooks FP Jr (1986) A dynamic graphics system for simulating virtual buildings. In: Proceedings of the 1986 workshop on interactive 3D graphics, Chapel Hill, NC. ACM, New York, pp 9–21
14. Noma H, Sugihara T, Miyasato (2000) Development of ground surface simulator for Tel-E-Merge system. In: Proceedings of IEEE virtual reality 2000, pp 217–224
15. Christensen R, Hollerbach JM, Xu Y, Meek S (1998) Inertial force feedback for a locomotion interface. In: Proceedings ASME Dynamic Systems and Control Division, DSC-Vol 64, pp 119–126
16. Darken R, Cockayne W, Carmein D (1997) The omni-directional treadmill: a locomotion device for virtual worlds. In: Proceedings of UIST'97
17. Poston R et al (1997) A whole body kinematic display for virtual reality applications. In: Proceedings of the IEEE international conference on robotics and automation, pp 3006–3011
18. Pratt DR et al (1994) Insertion of an articulated human into a networked virtual environment. In: Proceedings of the 1994 AI, simulation, and planning in high autonomy systems conference, pp 7–9
19. Slater M et al (1994) Steps and ladders in virtual reality. In: Virtual reality technology, World Scientific Publication, pp 45–54
20. Kontarinis DA, Howe RD (1995) Tactile display of vibratory information in teleoperation and virtual environment. Presence 4(4):387–402
21. Minsky M, Lederman SJ (1997) Simulated haptic textures: roughness. In: Symposium on haptic interfaces for virtual environment and teleoperator systems, Proceedings of the ASME Dynamic Systems and Control Division, DSC-Vol 58
22. Moy G, Wagner C, Fearing RS (2000) A compliant tactile display for teletaction. In: IEEE international conference on robotics and automation, April
23. Kawai Y, Tomita F (2000) A support system for the visually impaired to recognize three-dimensional objects. Technol Disabil 12(1):13–20
24. Burdea GC (1996) Force and touch feedback for virtual reality. Wiley, New York
25. Asanuma N, Yokoyama N, Shinoda H (1999) A method of selective stimulation to epidermal skin receptors for realistic touch feedback. In: Proceedings of IEEE virtual reality'99, pp 274–281
26. Kajimoto H, Kawakami N, Maeda T, Tachi S (1999) Tactile feeling display using functional electrical stimulation. In: Proceedings of ICAT'99, pp 107–114
27. Iwata H (1999) Walking about virtual space on an infinite floor. In: Proceedings of IEEE virtual reality'99, pp 236–293
28. Iwata H, Yoshida Y (1999) Path reproduction tests using a Torus Treadmill. Presence 8 (6):587–597
29. Yano H, Masuda T, Nakajima Y, Tanaka N, Tamefusa S, Saitou H, Iwata H (2008) Development of a gait rehabilitation system with a spherical immersive projection display. J Robot Mech 12(6):836–845

Chapter 9
Introduction to Mediated Communication

Hideaki Kuzuoka

Abstract "Mediated communication" is the research area that studies technologies to mediate communication in order to overcome the limitations of time and distance. Mediated communication studies are often discussed in the area of Computer Supported Cooperative Work (CSCW). This section first introduces the basic and some important research topics in this area, then describes some studies of mediated communication systems.

Keywords Mediated communication • Computer supported cooperative work • Human-robot interaction • Awareness • Non-verbal communication

9.1 Introduction

People's everyday communications are limited by voice and gestures that cannot reach over the distance, communication behaviors do not persist over time, and so on. To ameliorate such limitations, there is Mediated communication [1] which can act as a medium for whatever technology is in use. Two of the most common types are Computer-Mediated Communication (CMC) and Video-Mediated Communication (VMC). These types of studies are conducted in the research field of Computer-Supported Cooperative Work (CSCW).

The first half of this paper is an overview of CSCW and its important concepts. The second half is an introduction to Mediated Communication research that has been conducted by the authors.

H. Kuzuoka (✉)
Graduate School of Systems and Information Engineering, University of Tsukuba, Tsukuba, Japan
e-mail: kuzuoka@acm.org

Y. Sankai et al. (eds.), *Cybernics: Fusion of human, machine and information systems*,
DOI 10.1007/978-4-431-54159-2_9, © Springer Japan 2014

9.2 Overview of CSCW

CSCW refers to the general idea of using computers to support cooperative work, and the research field that is attempting to bring this concept to fruition. The research field of CSCW is not simply characterized by the technological aspects of its research goal such as system development, but also by the goal of understanding how people work cooperatively, what sorts of functions are needed to support such systems, and how such systems can change the cooperative work patterns of people. Therefore, the field of CSCW was begun by researchers from such fields as engineering, recognition science, psychology, sociology, management science, etc., who met and discussed methods for conducting actual cooperative research. However, because it is not easy to understand people as a group, it is said that people would be understood and systems gradually improved by repeatedly (1) testing and observing cooperative work, (2) conducting analyses and evaluations, and (3) creating and improving trial systems (Fig. 9.1) [2].

CSCW research is often categorized according to its temporal and spatial features. Temporal features include a synchronized type in which there is interaction in real-time, and a non-synchronized type in which information that it to be shared or exchanged is first stored on a computer. Spatial features include a face-to-face type in which participants share the same space, and the dispersed type in which they are geographically separated from one another. In addition, CSCW can also be categorized by combining the time axis with the space axis, as shown in Table 9.1.

In groupware for the face-to-face synchronized type, there are electronic meeting rooms. It uses computers to support face-to-face meetings so that the freedom of face-to-face communication will not be lost, and requires that cooperative work beyond face-to-face be enabled by computers. Typical of the dispersed, synchronized types of groupware are remote communication systems that utilize voice and video communications. In this type of research, the transmission of non-verbal information in face-to-face is an important topic for supporting remote communications. Various studies have been conducted to reveal the mechanism

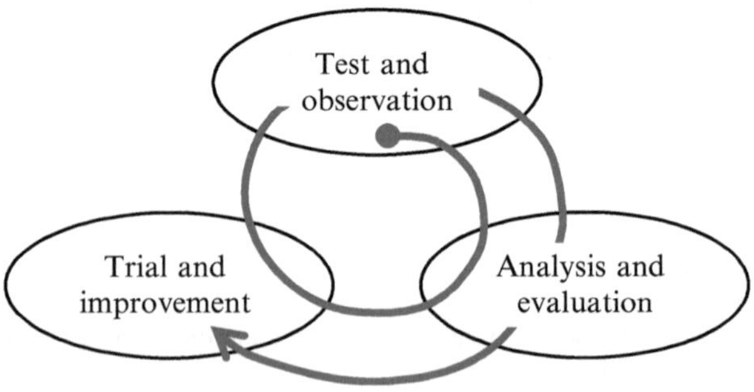

Fig. 9.1 Process of developing through repeated cooperative work

Table 9.1 Classifications of groupware by time and space

		Time	
		Synchronized	Non-synchronized
Space	Face-to-face	Electronic meeting system Single display groupware	Group memory
	Dispersed	Tele-conferencing system	Workflow system Social networking service Cooperative filtering

of human cooperation using sociological methods for analyzing mutual actions. Typical of dispersed, non-synchronized groupware are workflow systems. In this type of research, information used in cooperative work, analysis of the workflow, etc., must be analyzed and turned into a model that the computer can handle. However, the way that the system deals with frequently occurring exceptions is an important topic for achieving flexibility.

What is normally considered face-to-face non-synchronized type of cooperative work does not actually exist, but systems that can enable the exchange of various types of know-how through databases are categorized. For example, even working in the same office, people do not know what types of things their co-workers know. If such a database is available at such a time, then knowledge can easily be shared.

9.3 Research Fields of Mediated Communication

This section introduces specific research fields involved with mediated communication.

9.3.1 Electronic Meeting System

This is a system that is designed to support face-to-face meetings held in meeting rooms. Most systems like this involve placing a computer display in front of each participant, as well as setting up a large display that can be seen by everyone. All displays are set up so that they show the same thing, and if one of the participants writes something on the materials, then it is shown in the material of all of the other displays as well. The acronym for this system in which all participants share the same screen is WYSIWIS (pronounced "whizzy-whiz"), which is short for "What You See Is What I See". It is an important concept of CSCW [3].

9.3.2 Single Display Groupware

Single Display Groupware (SDG) is an application in which multiple users share one display to do cooperative work. Unlike cases where presentation videos are projected onto a screen so that they can be seen by all participants, SDG is equipped with an interface that allows parallel interaction among multiple participants.

Displays are largely divided into two types: one which has a vertical display screen like the kind used in presentations, and one where the screen is placed flat on a desk or table. There are many cases where either type can be used in meeting where there are just a few participants, but the first question of researchers is what type of input interface to develop. Myers et al. [4] proposed that multiple PDAs (personal digital assistants) be connected to a personal computer. By manipulating the user interface on the PDA screen, the application software displayed on the screen can be used simultaneously by multiple participants. With Dietz et al.'s DiamondTouch [5], beneath the screen on the desk/table, there are numerous tiny embedded antennas that emit signals that differ depending on their location. When a participant touches his or her screen with a fingertip, the fingertip receives a signal, and the signal is transmitted to a receptor that is attached to that participant's chair. Even if multiple participants touch the shared screen at the same time, each receptor can independently identify the location of the fingertip, so the system enables multiple participants to simultaneously process interactions with their fingers.

9.3.3 Teleconferencing System

This is a system that is designed to support meetings held at disparate locations using voice, video image, and computer communications. It is important to share materials at meetings, and various types of supporting groupware tailored to the type of supporting work have been developed. Already, there are many types of support software for general ordinary meetings on the market, which enable participants to freely write or draw using a pen or mouse. In architecture and production industries, there are prototype systems being developed that can allow the sharing of design sheets, blueprints, etc., and display them in 3D, and allow users, through virtual reality technology, to grasp objects in question directly with their hands and change their shape.

With that, in person-to-person communication it is well-known that eye contact plays an important role in turn taking and so on. Therefore, it is important to know who is looking at whom. However, in normal teleconferencing systems, it is not easy to reproduce proper eye contact. As a result, several different systems have been proposed to support this type of function [6–8].

It has been pointed out that communication in the production industry, at medical facilities, etc., places more emphasis not on face-to-face, but rather on the task at hand and corresponding gestures [9]. Therefore, in order to remotely support such types of work, video communication requires not the ability to have head-and-shoulder views of the participants in the discussion, but rather the object (s) in question.

9.3.4 Workflow System

As the name implies, "workflow" refers to the typical flow of work. For example, various documents such as vouchers or payment slips are usually sent in a certain arrangement in a certain order to sections or individuals. The groupware supporting such flows with computers is so-called workflow system, which can improve the efficiency of work without mistakes. There is great demand for workflow systems, and the number of products for business is increasing. However, making it easy to customize this system for individual companies, and enabling flexible response to exceptions, are becoming important topics of research.

9.3.5 Community Support

The development and popularization of technology that utilizes the Internet as a bulletin board has led to flourishing research that aims to support communication among a large but indefinite number of people who have something in common. This field is often called Community Support or Social Computing.

Social Networking Service (SNS) is a service that creates networks of people having a friendly relationship and can be said to be an important application for Community Support. For example, looking at the information of some user, the friends of that user can be seen at a glance. Next, looking at the friends' information, even more friends are displayed such that a network of participants with a friendly relationship can be displayed. Participants can exchange e-mails with each other, publicly show their diaries or journals, or can join a community with others who share their hobby. Typical examples of such service are Facebook and Twitter. While these sites are not the only ones to emerge as a result of groupware research, in CSCW they are often the target of analyses of the behaviors of people in online communities.

In the recommendation system, which is an important technology for supporting communities, a person's likely hobby(s) are predicted and recommended based on information about that person's favorites. For example, at Amazon, which is famous for online sales, information about a customer's books, etc., that they have bought, or own, or price information about books, etc., is compared with other users' data and used to recommend books, etc., that the customer might be interested in.

The technology for predicting a user's favorites by accumulating information about many users' favorites is called collaborative filtering. Research on collaborative filtering methods is being conducted not only for books, but also for a wide range of interests such as music and movies.

For such systems, important research topics include what sort of information users should enter, how can user information be acquired indirectly from the user's activities, how to figure out how to use such information, and how to recommend information that can be of benefit to the user (for example, see [10]).

9.4 Important Concepts

This section introduces some important concepts of mediated communication.

9.4.1 Awareness, Work Rhythms

Casual interaction is known to be important for members of a certain group to work together smoothly. For example, when suddenly coming up with an idea, or meeting someone by chance in the hallway, etc., unplanned meetings, informal conversation, etc., may be initiated [11]. What is playing a major role in such interaction is "informal awareness". For example, when performing work in the same room, it can somehow become apparent who is nearby, and what other people are trying to do [12]. However, in groups where the members are geographically dispersed, no awareness information is acquired, and casual interaction declines [11]. As a result, CSCW research has developed systems for supporting informal awareness, casual interaction, etc., in dispersed environments. For example, there is a method of taking periodic video snapshots of office staff and posting them on computers for viewing [13], a method for using icons to display actual images of members [14], and a method of using the movements of dolls, etc., on a desk to show actual images, state of activities, etc., of remote work partners [15].

The above research can be said to methods for indicating the current state of members. By collecting awareness information, Begole et al. identified certain rhythms seen of people at work and suggested that the members of the group shared these rhythms [16]. For example, the times that working people leave for work, eat lunch and return home are concentrated in a roughly regular time period. If such work rhythms are shared, it becomes possible to predict when and where members might meet, and communication can be made more efficient. Therefore, by collecting long-term data about the computer use time, online calendar, and the state of sending and receiving e-mail of each member used a computer, Begole et al. indicated that they could identify work rhythms.

Communication does not proceed merely by responding to occasional mutual actions, it also proceeds by constantly anticipating mutual actions. This is one factor involved in the smooth progress of team-based work. It will be important for future groupware to support such anticipations.

9.4.2 Body Movements

According to Ekman, body movements can be classified as emblems, illustrations, affect displays, regulators, and body manipulations [17].

Emblems are movements that are used to intentionally convey messages, and are used as substitutes for certain words and phrases. For example, movements of the neck to convey "yes" and "no", flashing the "V" sign to signify victory, or putting a finger to one's lips to signify "be quiet". Sometimes emblems are used by themselves, and sometimes they are also used together with spoken words. Furthermore, the timing of the use of emblems is also related to cutting off a conversation, and inflection at the end of a word. However, except for special cases where, for example, words cannot be used because of excessive noises, there are almost no cases of using multiple emblems in succession, and most are used by themselves. Because the vocabulary of such emblems is acquired through learning in each culture in the same way as language, there are almost no actions that are used to convey the same message in all cultures.

Illustrations are used in regard to the contents, flow, etc., of utterances and to emphasize and complement them. For example, when searching for the next word, speakers might wave their arm in the air, or imitate motions of people or animals, or draw the shape of something in the air, or point out the object in question, or make motions to depict a spatial relationship, among other things. Sometimes it is difficult to distinguish between emblems and illustrations, but in brief, emblems are used in place of conversation, while illustrations are actions that are only used during conversations. Therefore, persons of the same cultural sphere can understand the meaning of emblems merely by looking at them. In contrast, illustrations cannot be clearly understood if there are no words that are spoken with them.

Expressed emotions are facial expressions, gestures, etc., that signify emotional states, responses, etc., of individuals. However, in nearly all cases they depend on expressions, and are divided into such categories as happiness, sadness, fear, loathing, anger, and surprise. Affect displays appear without intention to try to convey a message, but as with British, Japanese, etc., it is possible to stifle them in academic, social, and other environments.

Regulators show understanding of what a conversation partner has said, and control the right to speak in a conversation. Thus, they are actions that facilitate the flow of the conversation. For example, nods indicates that showing an understanding as well as an interest in what another person is saying helps to maintain the conversation. When offering the "floor" to someone, momentary eye contact is made with that person, with a question asked with the end inflected. Actions such as adjusting glasses, or covering part of the mouth with the hand, are regulators that convey uneasiness.

Body manipulations (which are sometimes classified as "adapters" that include a wider array of body movements) are actions in which part of the body is used to get another person to do something. For example, this includes using things in a way that is contrary to the original purpose, like actions such as scratching one's head or licking one's lips, playing with a pencil, and so on. Unlike emblems, body manipulations are normally done subconsciously, and there is almost no regulation of the position that is used during a conversation. However, there are many instances in which such actions convey to others messages of unreliability or not being able to calm down.

9.4.3 Gaze

Although line of sight is often called "eye contact", that strongly implies that people are actually looking at each other's eyes. Therefore, in academia this is often referred to as "mutual gaze". By using this term, the person(s) being looked at can include others, not just a person who is involved in the conversation.

According to research conducted up to now, the functions of eyes during a conversation are divided into five categories: (1) turn taking, (2) mutual monitoring, (3) showing intentions, (4) expressing feelings, and (5) expressing inter-human relations. For example, when starting a conversation, the participants may gaze steadily at each other, or a speaker may look at other people's responses when he/she has finished speaking, or one person may be offering another person the right to speak by looking at him or her. This becomes material for judging the degree to which others are paying attention in order to monitor the level at which conversation partners show interest, understanding, etc. Furthermore, when point out something that a person wants others to see, it is possible to determine whether or not others are looking at the object in question.

9.4.4 Interpersonal Distance

The distance that one maintains with others is closely related to communication. According to Hall, who advocated proxemics, interpersonal distance can be classified into four categories: (1) intimate distance, which is up to 46 cm away from the other person, (2) personal distance, which is up to about 1.22 m away from the other person, (3) social distance, which is up to 3.66 m away, and (4) public distance, which is farther than 3.66 m [18].

Intimate distance is often observed in relationships such as those between lovers or between parent and child. In such cases, they are visually too close to each other, so voice is the main means of communication. Personal distance is a distance within which people can shake hands. In such cases, people can have a conversation at a medium volume while they clearly see each other's expressions. At that distance, it is possible to discuss such things as individual interests. At the social distance, it is no longer possible to see details in others' faces, but it is possible to have a conversation at a normal volume. Meetings with a small number of participants may correspond to social distance. In public distance, it is no longer possible to see

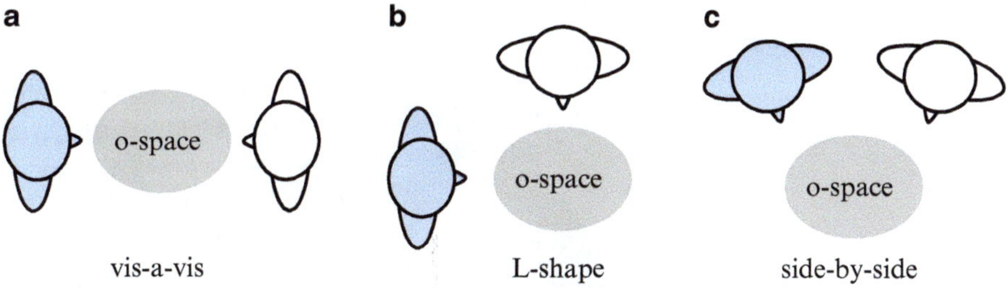

Fig. 9.2 Considered F-formation

details of conversation partners' faces, bodies, etc., but many people can see each other at the same time, and the volume of voices in the conversation starts to become louder. At more than 9 m away, it is necessary to shout or to increase volume with a megaphone or microphone, and people start to use numerous gestures. Such distance is used in formal speaking such as lectures and speeches.

9.4.5 F-Formation and Body Torque

When two or more people gather, they are likely to create and maintain an o-space, i.e., a space that all participants can look and speak into, and where they can handle objects of shared interest. The F-formation is a spatial formation of people that creates an o-space. In the case of two participants, typical F-formation arrangements are vis-a-vis, L-shape, and side-by-side (Fig. 9.2). When there are more than three participants, a circular formation is typically formed.

McNeill categorized F-formation into two types: social and instrumental [19]. A social F-formation consists only of people and is the same as Kendon's original definition. On the other hand, an instrumental F-formation includes a physical object as an element and participants normally gaze at that object in the space. Figure 9.3 is a typical example of an instrumental F-formation that can be seenduring a guided tour of a museum. In this example, the elements (i.e., the tour guide, visitors, and statue) are in a circular formation and all participants can gaze at the statue.

Kendon maintained that the orientation of the lower portion of the body is dominant in forming an o-space, compared to the effect of the upper body segments such as the head or upper part of the body below the neck (hereafter, called the "upper body"). On the basis of this assertion, Schegloff proposed the concept of "body torque" which means "*different or diverging orientations of the body segments above and below two major points of articulation–the waist and the neck*" [20]. According to Schegloff, the orientation of the lower part of the body relates to "dominant involvement" of the person, and the orientation of the shoulders and face relates to "subordinate involvement" [21].

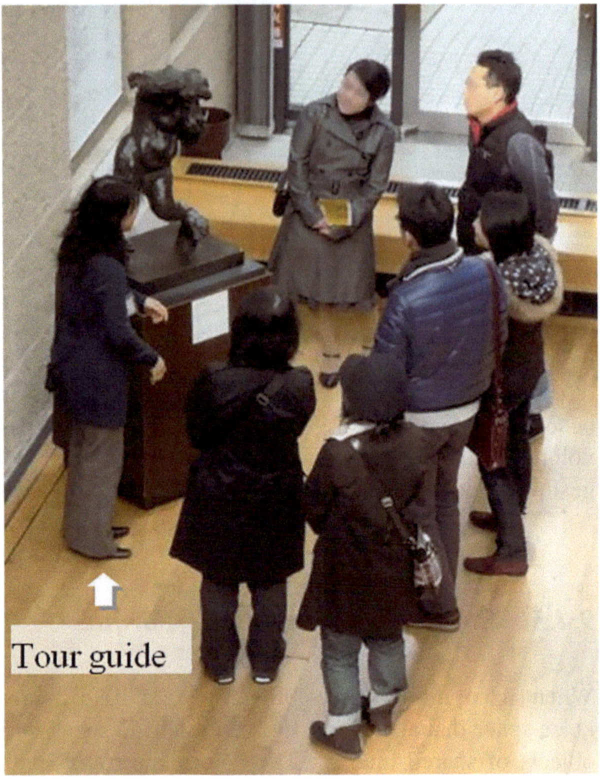

Fig. 9.3 Example of instrumental F-formation

9.4.6 Anisotropism in Video Mediated Communication

As a result of observing the affordance of remote communications systems, Gaver pointed out that non-verbal expressions of participants who were in one space (for example, eye contact) could not be correctly conveyed to participants in another space through such media as television cameras and monitors [22]. He called this phenomenon "anisotropism" of space connected by media. What is of particular concern in such cases is that the speaker presumes that his/her body actions may be recognized accurately by the interlocutors [23].

For example, during a teleconference, something being pointed to in a remote location shown through a display might be referred to as "that". However, the thing being pointed to is only shown in two-dimensional form on the participants' displays, and in their environments, they cannot correctly understand the object of the discussion. However, the person doing the pointing does not really notice that. Such a thing in simple conversation might not pose a problem, but in scenarios such as providing remote instruction in how to repair machinery, it might present a big problem.

9.5 Examples of Robot Mediated Communication

9.5.1 *SharedView: Supporting Remote Instruction of Physical Tasks*

SharedView is a system for an instructor in a remote location to provide instructions to workers in how to maintain, assemble, etc., equipment [24]. As shown in Fig. 9.4, because workers attach a small camera to their heads and the video images are sent to the instructor, the instructor can essentially see exactly what the workers are seeing. Using this display and hand gestures in front of it, the instructor can give instructions. Furthermore, since this display and hand gestures are captured again with the camera and shown on a small display attached to the head of the workers, the workers can see the gestures of the instructor that are superimposed over what they themselves looking at. In this way, the workers can receive instruction for work using hand gestures in a way that seems like they are facing the instructor. This technique can be applied not only for remote machinery maintenance but also to provide remote instruction for emergency procedures.

9.5.2 *GestureCam: A Robotic Camera with Remote Pointing Capability*

GestureCam is a small manipulator-type robot that is equipped with a laser pointer and camera (Fig. 9.5) [25]. By using this as a surrogate for an instructor who is in a remote location, this equipment can convey images at the instructor's line of sight and enable remote-controlled operations. When the instructor moves a manipulator (master) that has the same structure as the GestureCam, the GestureCam is controlled so that it takes the same attitude as the master. In this way, the instructor can freely look around the space where the worker is. The worker can see what the instructor is looking at by following the movement of the GestureCam.

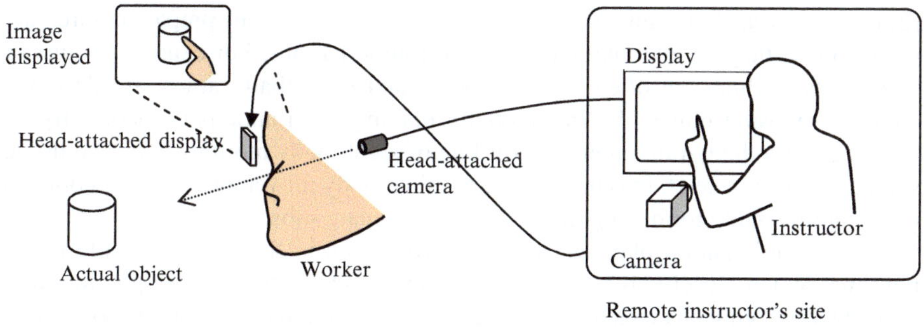

Fig. 9.4 Overview of the SharedView system

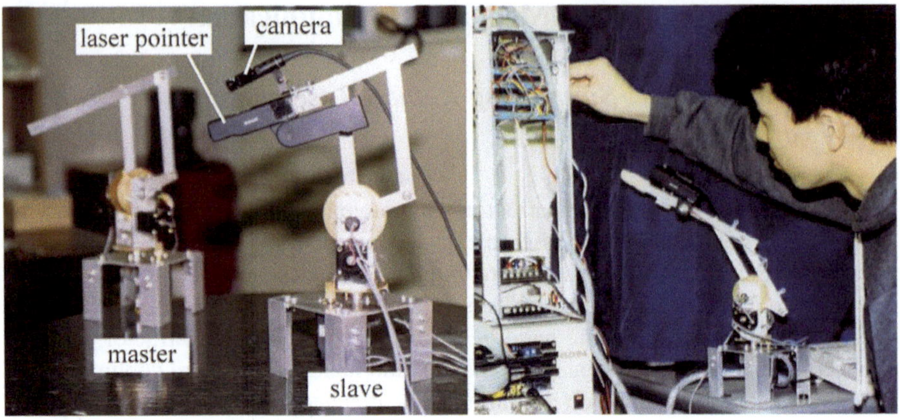

Fig. 9.5 GestureCam master and slave (*left*), and a view of instruction being given with GestureCam (*right*)

Because the laser pointer that is installed on the GestureCam is fixed in place in the same direction as the camera, the area being irradiated by the laser can also be remotely controlled by manipulating the posture of the GestureCam. In this way, the instructor can point out an object on the worker's side from a remote location.

GestureCam has enabled gaze awareness and gestures (limited to fingers) for objects arranged in three-dimensional space, which was not possible with conventional teleconferencing systems.

GestureCam is increasing both the accuracy and efficiency of work instruction given from a distance [26].

9.5.3 GestureMan-3: Supporting Predictability by Robot's Head Orientation

By observing the various utterances and physical movements made by people during conversations, it is possible to anticipate what interlocutors will attempt to do [27]. Humans can "tune into the same wavelength" because they prepare beforehand the response they should take based on their anticipations. For example, feints or "fake outs", which are often used in soccer and basketball games, are designed confuse opposing players by intentionally making them anticipate incorrectly by showing them the wrong intentions for line of sight, body motions, etc., and doing something else instead. In other words, physical body movements have become an important resource for having interlocutors anticipate subsequent moves.

In fact, anticipation plays an important role even in the case of simple finger pointing. When closely observing the harmonious movements of people, interlocutors, by observing changes in line of sight, head orientation, etc., before something is pointed out, turn their line of sight to that direction, showing that they are

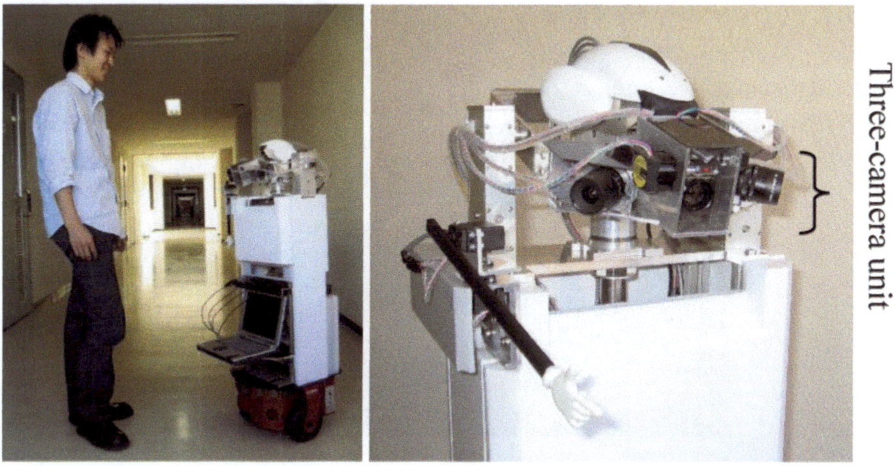

Fig. 9.6 GstureMan-3: Entire body (*left*) and enlargement of the head (*right*)

preparing for the gestures that should come next. In this way, the objects indicated by an interlocutor can be immediately recognized, and the next action can be undertaken.

With that, when there is a remote conversation using a remote-controlled robot, head movements that enable such anticipations are rarely expressed by the robot. In most cases, the robot's head is manipulated using a joystick, GUI on a computer screen, etc. For example, when a robot is mounted with a wide-angle camera, the manipulator can observe the wide-angle images on the monitor, so it is not necessary to change the direction of the camera by intentionally manipulating the robot's head. In contrast, when the camera's field of view is narrow, it is difficult to search for objects outside the line of sight, and there many instances when the robot's head has to be moved excessively, or, conversely, hardly moved at all.

GestureMan-3 is a robot that was developed to resolve these issues. There is no camera mounted on the robot's head; rather, there are three cameras laid out horizontally in a fan-shaped alignment on the robot's body (Fig. 9.6). There are three displays in front of the remote manipulator, and the images from the robot's camera are displayed widely from left to right (Fig. 9.7).

Therefore, in order to observe things from the robot's side, the manipulator can move his/her head laterally. The movements of manipulator's head are measured with a three-dimensional sensor, and the movements of robot's head are controlled so that they are synchronized with the manipulator's head movements. The robot's head is a simple directional indicator that helps the remote manipulator make interlocutors notice the direction the robot is looking at in the space.

This set-up makes it possible for changes in anticipated head intention to be expressed well through the robot, and it has become possible for harmonized movements to be made between remote locations. For example, Fig. 9.8 shows a scene where a remote manipulator is consulting about the arrangement of furniture

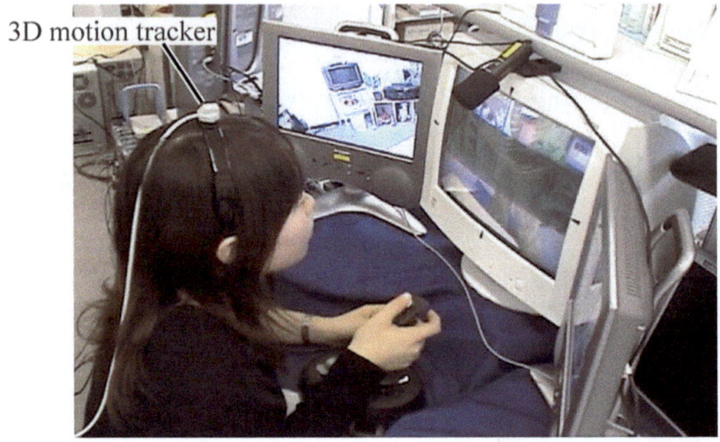

Fig. 9.7 User interface for remote manipulators

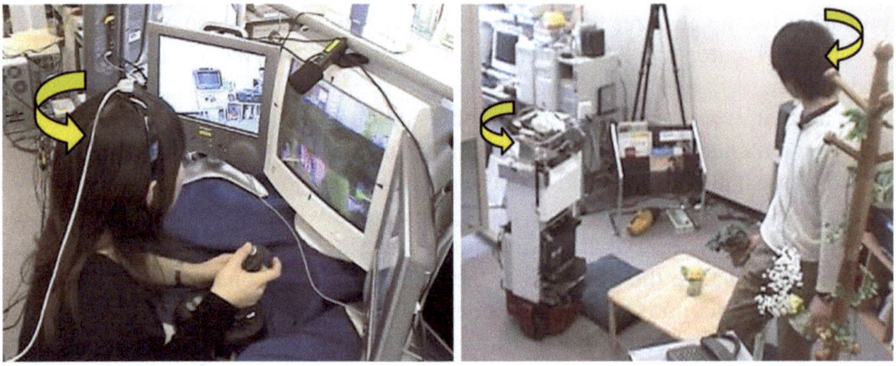

Fig. 9.8 An example of mutual orientation

in a house with a worker who is interacting with a robot. In this scene, the remote manipulator is searching for a place to put a potted plant. Immediately after the manipulator turns toward the left, the worker notices the movements of the robot's neck, and turns to look in the same direction. Integrated movement between the manipulator and the robot's head provides for harmonious physical movements of the worker and the manipulator through the robot. Many scenes can be seen where workers' direct indicative expression of "there" is easily understood.

In contrast, there are many examples seen of when the movements of the robot's head are not in concert with the manipulator, and the workers cannot find the places, objects, etc., that the remote manipulator is trying to indicate [28].

In order to support such anticipatory movements, it is important to design a user interface in which the remote manipulator can unconsciously induce anticipatory movements. For example, in the case of the GestureMan-3 interface, a wide, lateral view of the layout of the remote place is displayed, which enables the remote manipulator to generate natural left-right head movements. It is important that this movement be detected by a sensor, which can convert it into appropriate movements of the robot that can be exhibited without delay.

9.5.4 GestureMan-4: Reconfiguring Spatial Formation Arrangement by a Robot's Body Orientation

Museums are plagued by a shortage of tour guides. If a robot can automatically guide visitors, then this problem can be ameliorated. In order for the visitors to simultaneously see the exhibits and hear the guide's explanation, it is important for the guide and visitors to have an appropriate spatial arrangement, as shown in Fig. 9.3. Therefore, inducing visitors to form an appropriate spatial arrangement is considered to be one of the most important functions of a robot. As one means for accomplishing this, we decided to utilize the concepts of F-formation.

When the robot was explaining about exhibits at the museum, there were cases where we wanted visitors to focus their line of sight to the exhibit without changing their standing positions, while at other times, as shown in Fig. 9.3, we wanted to get them to move closer to the exhibit. In the case of the latter, if the robot's entire body was turned toward an exhibit, we could anticipate that the visitors would move toward the exhibit, based on knowledge about F-formation and body torque. On the other hand, when we wanted visitors to only go by their line of sight, we thought it was OK to only rotate the upper half of the robot's body to turn its line of sight toward the exhibit.

Therefore, the authors developed a robot with a degree of freedom to turn its neck, waist, and lower body (Fig. 9.9), and conducted an experiment to examine how the bodies of test subjects moved in accordance with the way that the robot's body was turned. Figure 9.10 shows a view of the experiment. Initially, the robot and human test subjects formed a vis-à-vis F-formation (Fig. 9.10 left), but when the robot's entire body was rotated clockwise toward an exhibit, the human subjects also moved toward the exhibit, forming an L-shaped arrangement (Fig. 9.10 right). On the other hand, when only the part of the robot from the waist up, or only its neck, was turned toward an exhibit, the probability that the human subjects would move was low [29]. Utilizing information obtained from this research, we are currently developing TalkTorque-2, which is a robot that can naturally express waist torque (Fig. 9.11).

Whiles these studies are not about mediated communication but rather concern autonomous robots, we can see that it would be desirable to have humans who are controlling robots from remote locations to have the robots able to express body torque, even in cases of remote communication through robots.

Fig. 9.9 GestureMan-4

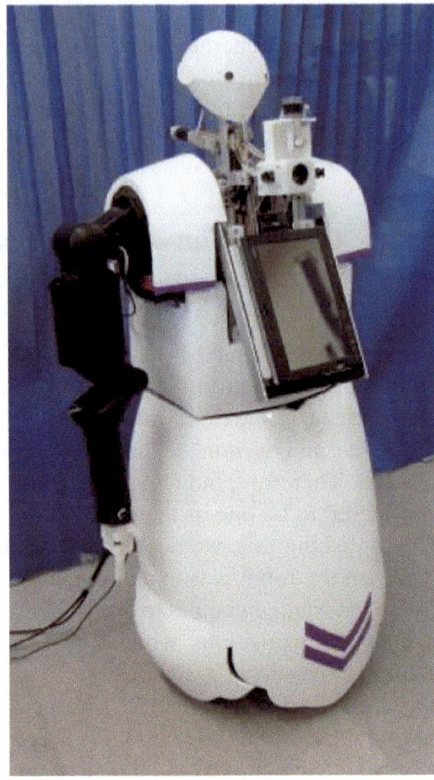

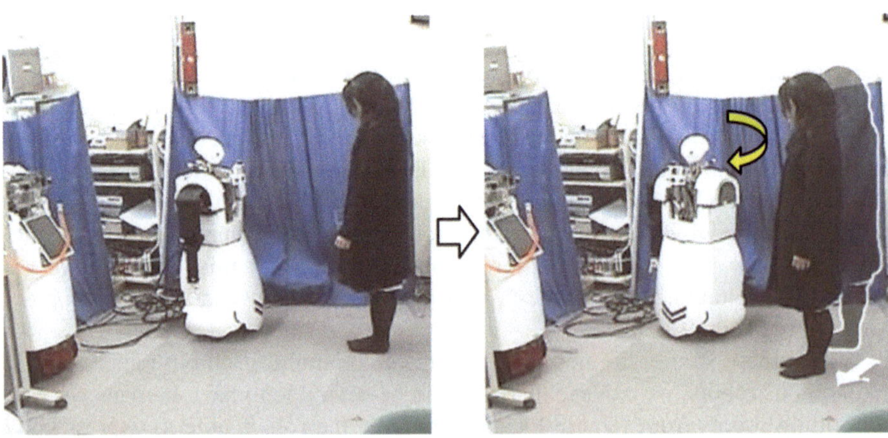

Fig. 9.10 Scenes from an experiment using GestureMan-4

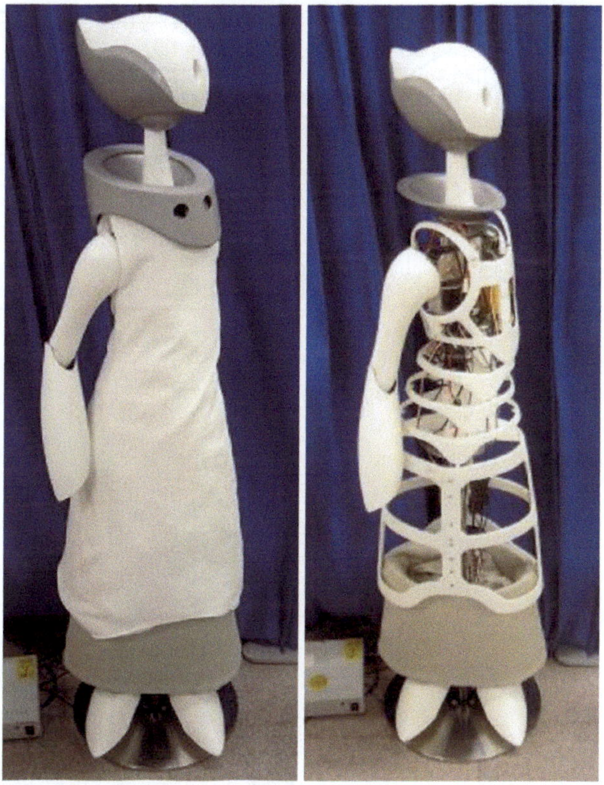

Fig. 9.11 External appearance (*left*) and inner structure (*right*) of TalkTorque-2

9.6 An Example of Video Mediated Communication System

Agora is a system that is designed to allow four participants dispersed in two different locations to have a meeting as if they were all sitting around one table [30]. An overview of the system is shown in Fig. 9.12, while Fig. 9.13 shows how the system looks when it is in use. The Agora system is comprised of a desk and 60-in. screens arranged in an L-shape around the desk. Video images of the upper bodies of the interlocutors in remote locations are projected from the back onto the L-shaped screens. In order to maintain eye contact, facial images of the interlocutors are taken with cameras that are attached at a height that is roughly eye-level. Because small, flat cameras are used, they do not get in the way.

Physical objects, hand gestures, etc., can be shared between remote locations using a technology that is similar to Double DigitalDesk [31]. In other words, a projector-camera pair are set up on each desk. The camera captures the way things look on the desktop and sends the image to the remote location, where the projector

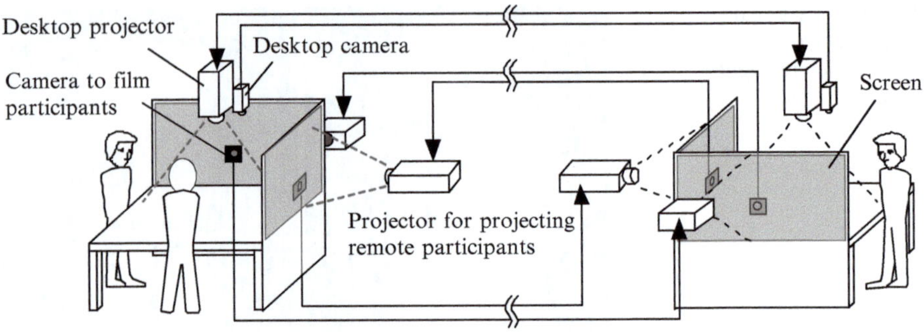

Fig. 9.12 Overview of Agora system

Fig. 9.13 Agora system in use

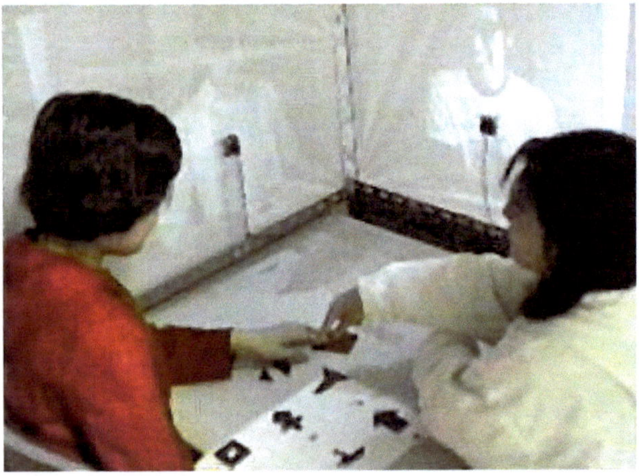

takes the desktop images sent from the remote location and projects them onto the local desk. In this way, there is a sequence of hand gestures seen on the desktop, and video images of the upper bodies of interlocutors can be seen, so it is easy to discern who is making hand gestures.

Agora has the following features in terms of physicality of actions:

- Use of gestures: All participants can use gestures for physical objects they have in common.
- Physical arrangement: Although they are fixed in place, the physical arrangements around the desk can be reproduced.
- Orientation: Orientations toward other participants, shared physical objects, etc., can be reproduced, even at remote locations.
- Mutual observation: The gestures, line of sight, body orientation and shared physical objects can be observed correctly and naturally to a certain extent.

- Sequentiality: Because actual images are directly transmitted, time lag caused by the system is minimized. As a result, various simultaneous, parallel interactions can be observed in as close to actual time as possible.

The reason why these have become possible is that since the screen and camera are arranged in three dimensions, the positional relation between torsos of the participants, their hands on the table, physical objects, etc., as well as the positional relationship of the participants themselves, can be reproduced, enabling people to do natural things they normally do and make mutual observations of these things.

9.7 An Example of Awareness Support System

Up to now, this paper has introduced research about broadband lines required for voice and video image communication. In contrast, this section will introduce an attempt to support daily awareness using a narrower band.

There are many instances where domestic and overseas branches of a company create project teams that straddle various branches. Digital but Physical Surrogates is a system that is designed to members of such teams that must be in diverse locations to sense each other's existence and freely converse with one another [30]. When a sensor installed in an office in a remote location detects movements by a member, a doll in another location moves, enabling members to sense the existence of other members (Fig. 9.14). When a member wants to engage in actual communication, they can activate the audio and video circuits by moving their face close to the video unit. If another member does not wish to receive the video circuit connection, all they have to do is put their surrogate doll on its side.

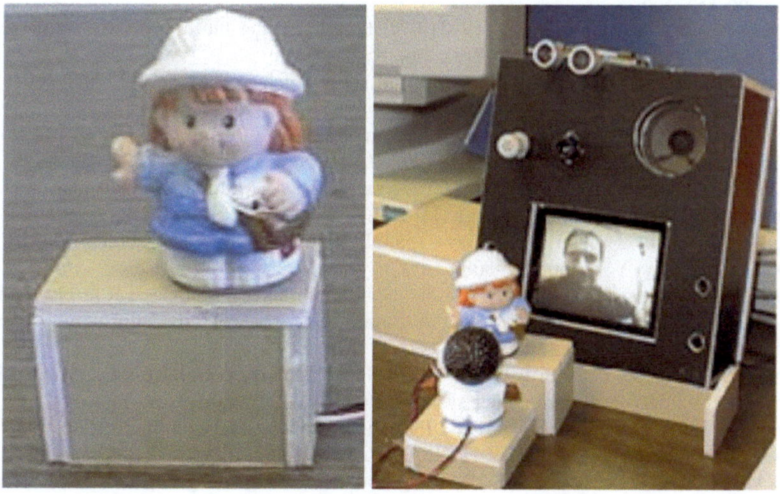

Fig. 9.14 An example of a surrogate (*left*) and surrogates in use (*right*)

9.8 Conclusion

This paper has presented an overview of mediated communication and examined specific examples of research. As was presented here, people's use of media is enabling communication that transcends the limits of time and space. Further, such communication systems are bringing major changes to people's social lives. Demand is leading to the creation of new systems that are even changing society itself, which in turn is leading to further new demands. This interactive cycle is turning at a rapid pace, and such changes are exceeding people's predictions. However, it is important that researchers have an attitude that attempts to understand the essence of human-to-human communication. It is also important to understand what types of communication are done when people are collocated, and how communication changes depending on the medium through which it occurs. The accumulation of knowledge and information about these topics will help us to develop even better communication systems.

References

1. Whittaker S (2003) Theories and methods in mediated communication. In: Graesser AC, Gernsbacher MA, Goldman SR (eds) The handbook of discourse processes. Erlbaum, New Jersey, pp 253–293
2. Tang JC, Minneman S (1991) Video whiteboard: video shadows to support remote collaboration. In: CHI 1991. ACM, New York, pp 315–322
3. Stefik M, Foster G, Bobrow D, Kahn K, Lanning S, Suchman L (1988) Beyond the chalkboard: computer support for collaboration and problem solving in meetings. In: Greif I (ed) - Computer-supported cooperative work: a book of readings. Morgan Kaufmann, Massachusetts, pp 335–366
4. Myers BA, Stiel H, Gargiulo R (1998) Collaboration using multiple PDAs connected to a PC. In: CSCW 1998. ACM, New York, pp 285–294
5. Dietz P, Leigh D (2001) Diamondtouch: a multi-user touch technology. In: UIST 2001. ACM, New York, pp 219–226
6. Ishii H, Kobayashi M (1992) ClearBoard: a seamless medium for shared drawing and conversation with eye contact. In: CHI 1992. ACM, New York, pp 52–532
7. Okada K, Maeda F, Ichikawaa Y, Matsushita Y (1994) Multiparty video conferencing at virtual social distance: MAJIC design. In: CSCW 1994. ACM, New York, pp 385–393
8. Nguyen D, Canny J (2005) MultiView: spatially faithful group video conferencing. In: CHI 2005. ACM, New York, pp 799–808
9. Nardi BA, Schwarz H, Kuchinsky A, Leichner R, Whittaker S, Sclabassi R (1995) Video-as-data: turning away from talking heads. In: Emmott SJ, Travis D (eds) Information superhighways. Academic Press, Duluth, pp 205–225
10. Bonhard P, Harries C, McCarthy J, Angela SM (2006) Accounting for taste: using profile similarity to improve recommender systems. In: CHI 2006. ACM, New York, pp 1057–1066
11. Kraut R, Egido C, Galegher J (1988) Patterns of contact and communication in scientific research collaboration. In: CSCW 1988. ACM, New York, pp 1–12
12. Cockburn A, Greenberg S (1993) Making contact: getting the group communicating with groupware. In: COCS 1993. ACM, New York, pp 31–41

13. Dourish P, Bly S (1992) Portholes: supporting awareness in a distributed work group. In: CHI 1992. ACM, New York, pp 541–547
14. Greenberg S (1996) Peepholes: low cost awareness of one's community. In: CHI 1996 companion. ACM, New York, pp 206–207
15. Kuzuoka H, Greenberg S (1999) Mediating awareness and communication through digital but physical surrogates. In: Extended abstracts of CHI 1999. ACM, New York, pp 11–12
16. Begole JB, Tang JC, Smith RB, Yankelovich N (2002) Work rhythms: analyzing visualizations of awareness histories of distributed groups. In: CSCW 2002. ACM, New York, pp 334–343
17. Raffler-Engel W (ed) (1983) Aspects of nonverbal communication. Swets & Zeitlinger, Lisse
18. Hall E (1966) The hidden dimension. Doubleday, New York
19. McNeill D (ed) (2005) Gesture, gaze, and ground, lecture notes in computer science. Springer, Berlin, pp 1–14
20. Schegloff EA (1998) Body torque. Soc Res 65(3):535–596
21. Goffman E (1963) Behavior in public places: notes on the social organization of gatherings. Free Press, New York
22. Gaver W (1992) The affordances of media spaces for collaboration. In: CSCW 1992. ACM, New York, pp 17–24
23. Heath C, Luff P (1991) Disembodied conduct: communication through video in a multi-media office environment. In: CHI 1991. ACM, New York, pp 99–103
24. Kuzuoka H (1992) Spatial workspace collaboration: a SharedView video support system for remote collaboration capability. In: CHI 1992. ACM, New York, pp 533–540
25. Kuzuoka H, Kosuge T, Tanaka M (1994) GestureCam: a video communication system for sympathetic remote collaboration. In: CSCW 1994. ACM, New York, pp 35–43
26. Kuzuoka H (1995) Can the GestureCam be a surrogate? In: ECSCW 1995. Kluwer, Dordrecht, pp 181–196
27. Auer P (2002) Projection in interaction and projection in grammar. InLiSt 33:1–39
28. Kuzuoka H, Kosaka J, Yamazaki K, Suga Y, Yamazaki A, Luff P, Heath C (2004) Mediating dual ecologies. In: CSCW 2004. ACM, New York, pp 477–486
29. Kuzuoka H, Suzuki Y, Yamashita J, Yamazaki K (2010) Reconfiguring spatial formation arrangement by Robot's Body Orientation. In: HRI 2010. IEEE, Piscataway, pp 285–292
30. Kuzuoka H, Yamashita J, Yamazaki K, Yamazaki A (1999) Agora: a remote collaboraiton system that enables mutual monitoring. In: Extended Abstracts of CHI 1999. ACM, New York, pp 190–191
31. Wellner P (1993) The DigitalDesk: supporting computer-based interaction with paper documents. In: Imagina 1993. Imagina and Centre National de la Cinematographie, Monte-Carlo, pp 110–119

[illegible]

Chapter 10
Robotics for Supporting Childhood Education

Fumihide Tanaka

Abstract This chapter describes an instance of Cybernics research for supporting human capabilities through the use of technologies. The main object here is childhood education. With increasing demand for a higher quality of childhood education, a new trend of using robotics technology to support childhood education is emerging. In conjunction with a discussion of robot ethics and social acceptance for robots, the new trend will be described.

Keywords Childhood education • Robotics • Human-robot interaction • Child-robot interaction • Robot ethics • Social acceptance • Childcare robot • Care-receiving robot • Learning support • Learning reinforcement • Developmental learning • Telerobotics • Telepresence robot • Tricycle-style interface • Distant communication • Distant education • Education support

10.1 Introduction

Early childhood education is an important global issue, with many different issues, and solutions for these issues occurring around the world. In Japan, the importance of early childhood education is receiving an unprecedented amount of attention, especially against the backdrop of declining birth rates. Moreover, as Japanese society has been gradually shifting from a high-growth stage to one of maturity, it is conceivable that, in addition to current value cores such as GDP and profit ratios, ethical and human considerations will gain more weight. In the context of such societal shifts, it is estimated that early childhood education will play an increasingly greater role.

F. Tanaka (✉)
Social ICT Research Center, Graduate School of Information Science and Technology, The University of Tokyo, Bunkyo-ku, Japan
e-mail: fumihide.tanaka@gmail.com

Y. Sankai et al. (eds.), *Cybernics: Fusion of human, machine and information systems*,
DOI 10.1007/978-4-431-54159-2_10,

This chapter describes some new technologies that support and expand early childhood education, recognizing it as an important social task. In the practical context of early education aimed at very young children, it is essential that children first become interested and enjoy the new technologies. Viewed from this perspective and as illustrated by several examples of field research presented in the following sections, recent robot technologies are attracting more attention as embodiments of technology. From these studies, it has become clear that robot technology strongly attracts a child's interest and that this can be used to good effect for applications in educational contexts. This chapter will describe support for early childhood education using robot technology and introduce the latest trends in global research.

10.2 Examples of Research on Using Robots in Actual Educational Contexts

This section introduces representative examples of research on robots in actual educational contexts.

The field experiment carried out by Kanda et al. [1] on the introduction of the communication robot Robovie in a primary school setting is an example of pioneer research in this field. A robot programmed to speak English was introduced in a primary school classroom, and the authors investigated the evolution of interactions between children and the robot, as well as the influence this had on the children's learning of English. The results showed that, although interaction between children and the robot was high in the first week but decreased in the second week, some data indicated that there was an effect of introducing the robot on the variation of the English language ability of some of the children.

Furthermore, in a follow-up experiment [2] carried out by the same authors over a 2-month period, several interesting ideas were tested, such as expressing new types of behavior and engaging in confidential discussions according to the cumulative number of interactions in order to achieve long-term interaction with the children. Additionally, the authors reported many findings regarding technical aspects such as the use of RFID tagging, which can serve as reference for future research.

Han et al. [3] also tested the effects of introducing an educational service robot on English-language learning for primary school students with a robot called IROBI, developed by the South Korean company Yujin Robotics. They carried out a three-pronged comparative experiment using conventional learning materials (books, audio tapes), e-learning materials via the computer screen, and IROBI. IROBI is designed to interact with the children using, among other functions, head expressions, conversation and the content-playing on an LCD in its chest area. The experiment has been carried out once (approx. 40 min) with 90 primary school students divided into three groups. The authors reported that IROBI proved most effective for all three items considered: concentration, interest and learning achievement.

Currently in South Korea, robot development (for example, the teacher robot EngKey, developed by KIST, the Korea Institute of Science and Technology) is being vigorously pursued as industry, government and academia work together to make up for the lack of English language teachers.

In all of the above examples, the subjects of educational support were children of primary school age and older, but experiments aimed at pre-school children have also been carried out. While pre-schoolers' language communication skills are less developed than those of primary school students, these experiments and observations carried out in the middle of the development stages provide insights for research that may be able to increase our understanding about human non-verbal communication skills and their development.

At the University of California, San Diego (USCD), there is an ongoing project aimed at supporting early education and furthering our understanding of human development and learning through the introduction of a robot in actual settings of early education such as nursery schools. Movellan et al. [4] have developed a robot called RUBI by inputting the knowledge gained from observations of actual education settings, beginning with observational studies conducted in nursery schools as described below. This research has indicated the potential robots such as RUBI have for promoting children's learning of yet-unknown languages [5].

Tanaka et al. [6] introduced a small human-like robot for approximately half a year in the above-mentioned nursery school at UCSD and conducted an observational study looking at the development of socialization between toddlers 2 years old and younger. It was shown using both quantitative and qualitative analytical methods that after several months of being with the children, the robot, which initially was treated as a foreign presence, had gradually come to be treated as a peer classmate. Moreover, based on these observations, the authors identified various conditions necessary for robots to attract a child's interest. Through the introduction of these conditions, advancements have been made in the development of robots, leading to more attractive (from the children's perspective) early educational support. As a concrete example of support, the same robot was made part of the morning dance routine in the nursery school (Fig. 10.1), making the daily activity program more fun and effective.

10.3 The Relevance of Robot Ethics

The topic of this chapter is deeply connected with the argument of so-called robot ethics. In a report by Sharkey [7] in the journal *Science*, the author called for special attention to be paid to the various ethical issues latently present in a series of childcare support robots. At that time, some of the robots developed to support childcare by the Japanese company NEC and the South Korean company Yujin

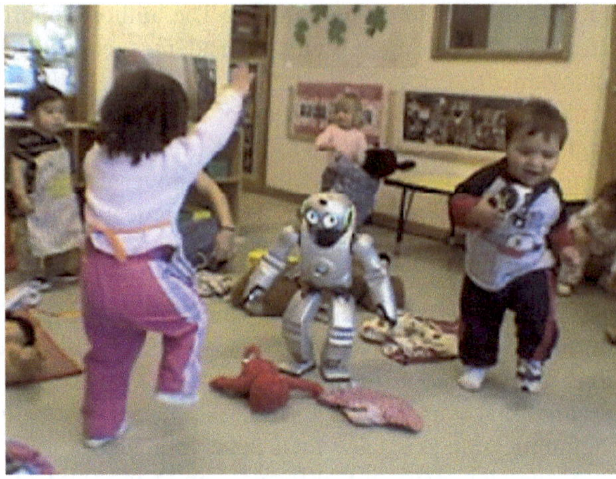

Fig. 10.1 Dance interaction between children and a robot (PNAS/ National Academy of Sciences, Copyright 2007)

Robotics (mentioned in the previous section) have started to be commercialized. Sharkey argued against such tendencies by stressing the need for caution as there are still many unknowns regarding the influence of continued interaction between robots and children on the latter's development. Additionally, the report also pointed out that these convenient technologies exert a secondary influence on the ambient environment, as there may be instances of completely relegating childcare to robots, of encouraging parents to neglect childcare duties, or of weakening the parent-child attachment that is indispensable for the child's emotional development.

The debate about such arguments continues in various media (for example, see an article at the special issue of *Interaction Studies* [8]). While these arguments have been criticized for being too extreme, robot developers nonetheless need to recognize that robot-children interactions involve not only physical impacts, but also effects on mental aspects, which are much harder to identify.

10.4 The Social Acceptance of Robot Technologies

In recent years, issues relating to how robot technologies are received by society and individuals (their social acceptance) have been gaining prominence in the field of Human-Robot Interaction (HRI). This theme is somewhat related to that of robot ethics mentioned in the previous section. Questions regarding robot ethics and their social acceptance have already been discussed in science-fiction literature for some time, but they have rarely been touched upon in the technically oriented academic field of robot engineering. Nevertheless, once we start to manipulate robots that interact with humans, and take into consideration the field research carried out in actual society, we must recognize that we cannot look lightly upon these issues.

More information regarding the research on social acceptance and cultural aspects in the HRI field is provided in the reference list [9].

Social acceptance is also an extremely important topic for this chapter, namely, robot technology applications in early childhood education. In the practical context of early education, interactions are not limited to researchers and developers, but also include interactions with ordinary people, such as teachers, parents, other children and so forth. As there are many different value systems among different people, occasionally there will be situations where great efforts will be required to gain the understanding of certain people. Nonetheless, as explained on the essential concepts of Cybernics, it is not enough for technologies to be developed; they also need to be accepted by people. Thus, one important requirement for the present research is to develop socially acceptable robot technologies.

10.5 Educational Support Using Care-Receiving Robots

In this section, we introduce the robot technology being developed by the authors for supporting early childhood education. We also describe how our awareness of aspects such as robot ethics and social acceptance, which were mentioned in the previous section, has contributed to the development of this technology.

As mentioned in Sect. 10.2, many of the early educational support robots were designed as substitutes for humans or parents, for the purpose of teaching or caring for children ("childcare robots"). Tanaka et al. [8, 10, 11], taking the opposite approach, have proposed the idea (Fig. 10.2) of making children teach or care for robots, thereby linking into the education of children. Because the robots discussed here receive care from children, they are called "care-receiving robots" (CRRs). In the following paragraphs we will expand on this concept.

First, the teachers or parents decide on the topic (e.g., how to greet others). Then, the teachers or parents guide the children on how to teach this topic to robots. For example, upon introducing a robot that cannot greet others in the classroom, they instruct the children to "teach the proper way of greeting" to the robot. Thereupon,

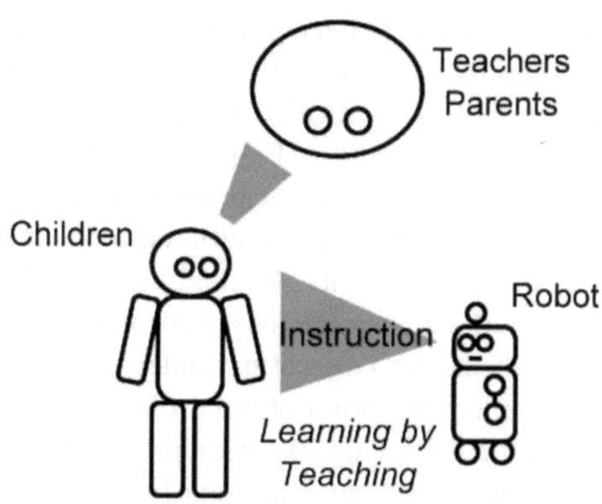

Fig. 10.2 Overview of educational support using a care-receiving robot

the children actively teach the robot the proper way of greeting and, consequently become familiarized themselves with how to greet others. The goal of this process is to increase the children's mastery of a particular topic as a result of giving instructions (learning by teaching).

This approach is based on the knowledge gained from the observational study conducted in the American nursery school mentioned in Sect. 10.2. During the observational study in the USCD affiliated nursery school, Tanaka et al. [6] discovered that the small human-like robot introduced in the classroom induced much more care-taking behaviors in the children than the other toys. The authors also found that these behaviors went on for longer periods of time when compared with other types of interactions occurring between the children and the robot. These findings suggested the possibility of this robot possessing characteristics that induced care-taking behaviors in the children, and the idea of care-receiving robots was born as an attempt to provide educational support by capitalizing on these characteristics.

Furthermore, the care-receiving robot induces the same kind of natural desire to care for others as that felt by children towards the dolls they are used to playing with, so we think that the ethical issues usually posed by childcare robots (as discussed in Sect. 10.3) are less prominent in this case. Today, the pros and cons of childcare robots are discussed at public symposiums mostly in Western countries where social acceptance of these technologies might be difficult. However, we think that this idea of the care-receiving robot proposed here will be more easily accepted by larger segments of society.

Continuing in this vein, Tanaka et al. [11] conducted verification experiments on care-receiving robots (CRR) in an actual setting. The verification process consisted of two stages: (1) ascertaining the feasibility of care-receiving robots, and (2) investigating the facilitating effects of "learning by teaching." The field experiment was carried out in Tsukuba City, in an actual learning setting at an English conversation classroom with children aged three to six. In this experiment, the CRR was a small human-like commercial robot called Nao, made by Aldebaran Robotics, that was remotely controlled from a separate room.

In the first experiment to ascertain feasibility, two types of CRR were introduced for comparison during lessons in which a total of 18 children participated. In the context of teacher-led lessons, the first Nao was remotely controlled to always act incorrectly (error rate 100 % condition) in the learning task, while the second Nao was remotely controlled to always act correctly (error rate 0 % condition). Basic vocabulary learning (English words for colors and shapes) similar to that used during normal lessons was selected as an example learning task. Using posters and cards, we prepared a scenario equivalent to that of a normal lesson. After completing the experiment, we analyzed the behavior based on video recordings. We observed a conspicuously high number of care-giving behaviors by the children towards the Nao operating under the "error rate 100 % condition," thus confirming the implementation potential (feasibility) of the CRR concept in this context.

In the following experiment to confirm the accelerative effects of "learning by teaching", we created a scenario whereby each of the 17 children joined the teacher and Nao in a three-person lesson for learning English verbs (approx. 30 min long). Since the purpose of this experiment was to test the learning effects in children, we first carried out a pre-test in an interview format, and then held a lesson during which participants identified four categories of previously unknown English words. The word cards used during this lesson were equivalent to those normally used in the classroom. An English verb was on each word card and a picture that showed the context in which that verb is used. The lesson was carried out as a game in which the teacher asked the child and Nao questions using the word cards. Whenever the teacher asked Nao (which was implemented as a CRR) for the meaning of a verb, Nao would invariably express a wrong behavior, so the teacher would then spoon-feed the correct behavior (direct teaching). For example, when using the word "brush", the teacher would make Nao pick up the toothbrush placed on the floor, then indicate the action of moving the brush from side to side in front of the mouth.

The teacher taught the participants in this experiment using the CRR for two randomly selected words out of the four word categories identified during the pre-test, while for the remaining two words the teacher used only the usual cards. After the lesson period, the participants in this experiment were free to play for 10 min alone with Nao ("free time"). After the "free time," a post-test was carried out using the same format as in the pre-test to investigate how many questions the children answered correctly by comparing them with the questions which could not be answered correctly at first. Additionally, another post-test using the same method was carried out 1 month after the experiment to investigate whether the participants in the experiment still remembered the words learned during the lesson.

The results of the experiment showed that the ratio of correct answers in the vocabulary post-test using the CRR was significantly higher than when the CRR was not used, confirming the accelerative effects of "learning by teaching" through the introduction of the CRR. Another interesting finding was that the ratio of post-test correct answers 1 month after the experiment was higher than the ratio of post-test correct answers on the day the experiment was carried out. According to interviews with the children's parents during the post-test 1 month later, after the experiment, many of the children, upon finding at home objects similar to those used during the experiment, were observed rehearsing the corresponding movements and confirming the proper way with their parents, even if Nao was not present on those occasions. These episodes hold great significance for the CRR concept. In brief, the essence of educational support using the CRR is to promote spontaneous learning for children by building on their natural desire to care for others, and these episodes indicate that it was precisely this phenomenon that was occurring.

Next, we carried out a detailed analysis of the teaching behavior displayed during the experiment by participants towards the CRR. We discovered that, besides the "direct teaching" method described above, children employed many methods of teaching, such as exemplifying the corresponding movement (gesturing) and offering verbal instructions about how to perform the movements (verbal teaching). We believe these results provide useful guidelines for designing a more effective CRR.

On the other hand, as a matter of critical self-examination, the CRR used during this experiment did not posses the capacity for developmental learning (even if taught, it quickly forgot and committed the same mistakes), so some of the children were clearly disappointed in this respect. The ideal CRR should possess the function of developmental learning. However, it is not yet clear what learning dynamics will be the most effective for children to teach the CRR, so we are carrying out further experiments with various learning dynamics.

10.6 Educational Environment Expansion by Telerobotics

In the previous sections we have outlined several examples of educational support using robot technologies. In this section we describe attempts to expand the educational environment using robot technologies and to connect this to educational support.

Currently, telerobotics is one of the most popular research topics in the field of robotics. In the past, one of humankind's dreams was to create an alter ego robot that could be remotely controlled to travel to distant lands and communicate with various people, and we have finally begun to glimpse the possibility of realizing such a dream in the not-too-distant future.

There is a long history of telerobotics in the field of robotics and originally the research proceeded in contexts such as work support where objects constituted the target searched for. However, in recent years, research targeting humans has made rapid progress in facilitating remote communication. The perspective of remotely controlling an alter ego robot has been broadened from the telexistence research pioneered by Tachi [12] to android research [13] in recent years. These technologies are developed to a very high degree, but at the same time they are extremely expensive. By contrast, there has recently been a trend led by Western venture companies (e.g. Willow Garage, VGO Communications, Inc., InTouch Health) to achieve remote communication using simple and cheap technologies, by having the mobile function performed by Skype on personal computers (sometimes referred to as telepresence technology). In the West, a change is occurring as this kind of technology is introduced in companies across Silicon Valley, in executive meetings, and in communication between doctors and patients in hospitals, among other venues.

As mentioned in the beginning section of this chapter, early education represents an important task in different societies, requiring us to never remain content with the status quo, but rather to continue making improvements. Experiments to improve education using telecommunication technologies are already being carried out in many areas. Furthermore, in the case of remote communication technology, the usage of Skype, etc., is starting to reach the practical stage.

In this context, experiments are being implemented to connect distant classrooms by using remotely controlled robots, with the goal of expanding various educational environments. Materials and methods have been improved in many

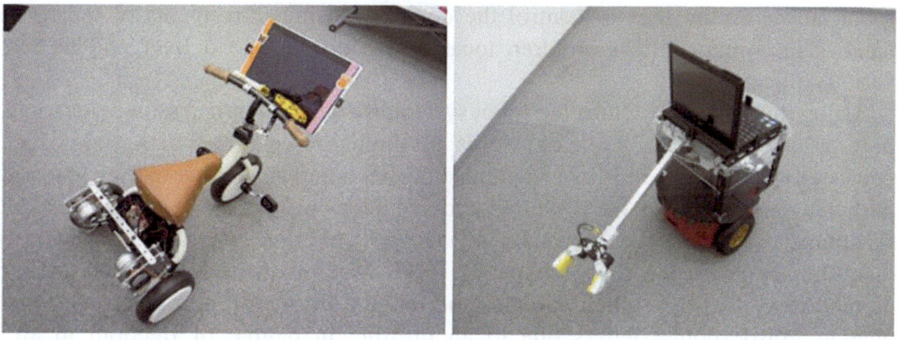

Fig. 10.3 Tricycle-style operating interface (*left*) and remotely controlled robot (*right*)

classrooms, but this technology extends the concept of space across classrooms, thus holding the potential to trigger a great breakthrough. The latest trends concerning such technologies will be introduced in this section.

In the case of the robot EngKey from KIST (introduced in Sect. 10.2), experiments have been initiated to hold English lessons by teachers residing in the Philippines or other English-speaking countries who remotely control the robot in the actual classrooms in South Korea in order to make up for the lack of English language teachers there. In present day South Korea, such national projects to support education proceed apace, while large-scale plans are being developed to introduce these technologies in many more classrooms in the future.

All of the remotely controlled robots that have been described so far are designed for adult operators; by contrast, the authors of this study are developing technologies with which the children themselves can remotely control the robots. In the following paragraphs we will describe our approach.

Tanaka et al. [14] have developed a tricycle-style interface (Fig. 10.3) that can be manipulated with ease even by children. Experiments using this interface have been initiated to achieve communication between children who are located in distant classrooms. In this context, we used the Internet to connect an English conversation classroom for children located in Tsukuba City with an international school located in Yokohama, then carried out a distant communication trial between Japanese children from Tsukuba and English native-speaker children from Yokohama.

A sensor (called a rotary encoder) that records the number of rotations has been installed on the rear wheels of the tricycle-style interface. By transferring data with the number of rotations for each wheel (left and right), the robot deployed in a distant place can be synchronized with back-and-forth and left-right movements. Additionally, a tablet PC is installed on top of the saddle, which allows us to observe the local conditions by communicating via Skype with the robot located at a distance. Conversely, the image of the operator is sent in real time to the robot, so the face of the operator is projected on the robot's side. Furthermore, a simple data glove containing flex sensors is installed inside a child-size cotton glove in the dominant hand of the operator; hand opening/closing data is sent to the remote robot, allowing the user to control the opening/closing movements of the robot hand. This system allows children located at a distance to deliver and receive various objects.

Using this remotely controlled robot system, we had children at remote locations play a lesson game of creating words in English. We prepared a task which consisted of creating words by arranging alphabet letters made of a spongy material with magnets attached on a whiteboard, while using the robot from a distant location. As a result, even normally shy Japanese children who find it difficult to talk directly with non-Japanese people could communicate using this system. Notably, in situations which revealed the robot's physical limits (e.g., not being able to grasp sponge letters due to an insufficient degree of freedom in arm movement), we observed instances of assistance (e.g., when the children on the robot side saw the robot struggling, they promptly tried to help), which, in turn, triggered mutual communication. The robot discussed in this section is remotely-controlled, so it is completely different from the human-like robots described in previous sections. Nevertheless, we find it fascinating that in this case as well, we could observe how a certain kind of robot "weakness" could exert a positive effect on human interactions.

10.7 Conclusions

In this chapter we have described the latest trends in robot technologies that support early childhood education. The discussion focused on two global trends: (1) directly supporting educational activities (lesson contents etc.) with robot technologies, and (2) expanding the educational environment by using robot technologies. At the same time, we stressed that besides technological development, considerations of ethics and social acceptance are also important, and introduced examples of research that support this view.

An interesting common factor that stood out from each of the examples described in Sects. 5 and 6 was the revelation that robot performance deficiencies can function as a "plus" in the context of human interaction. In the case of the CRR, we described an instance where a robot which was deliberately giving the wrong answers, was ultimately able to improve the learning abilities of human participants. In the case of the remote robot interface, we described an instance where the intended communication at a distance was induced on the basis of physical limits in the robot's performance.

We believe these observations can provide guidelines for new designs in the field of robotics. In brief, most robot development has been carried out within a value system that aims for higher performance in one way or another. However, we found that using a robot whose performance has been deliberately downgraded can also help to achieve a good HRI. Subsequently, this kind of robot "weakness" has become a new topic of design policy research.

The educational support described in this chapter provides examples and contains many elements of Cybernics and its new discoveries in human-support technologies. Here, the discussion on educational support focused on healthy people in an educational context, but even here, "human support" and "expansion" appeared as keywords. Furthermore, our attention was also drawn to issues of ethics and safety when new technologies are introduced into society. We want the reader to consider the overall landscape of the field of Cybernics by comparing these findings with different examples described in other chapters.

References

1. Kanda T, Hirano T, Eaton D, Ishiguro H (2004) Interactive robots as social partners and peer tutors for children: a field trial. Hum-Comput Interact 19(1–2):61–84
2. Kanda T, Sato R, Saiwaki N, Ishiguro H (2007) A two-month field trial in an elementary school for long-term human-robot interaction. IEEE Trans Robot 23(5):962–971
3. Han J, Jo M, Jones V, Jo JH (2008) Comparative study on the educational use of home robots for children. J Inf Process Syst 4(4):159–168
4. Movellan JR, Tanaka F, Fortenberry B, Aisaka K (2005) The RUBI/QRIO project: origins, principles, and first steps. In: Proceedings of 4th IEEE international conference on development and learning. IEEE Press, Osaka, Japan, pp 80–86
5. Movellan JR, Eckhardt M, Virnes M, Rodriguez A (2009) Sociable robot improves toddler vocabulary skills. In: Proceedings of the 4th ACM/IEEE international conference on human-robot interaction. ACM/IEEE, San Diego, USA, pp 307–308
6. Tanaka F, Cicourel A, Movellan JR (2007) Socialization between toddlers and robots at an early childhood education center. Proc Natl Acad Sci U S A 104(46):17954–17958
7. Sharkey NE (2008) The ethical frontiers of robotics. Science 322:1800–1801
8. Tanaka F, Kimura T (2010) Care-receiving robot as a tool of teachers in child education. Interact Stud 11(2):263–268
9. Nomura T, Suzuki T, Kanda T, Han J, Shin N, Burke J, Kato K (2008) What people assume about humanoid and animal-type robots: cross-cultural analysis between Japan, Korea, and the USA. Int J Hum Robot 5(1):25–46
10. Tanaka F, Kimura T (2009) The use of robots in early education: a scenario based on ethical consideration. In: Proceedings of the 18th IEEE international symposium on robot and human interactive communication. IEEE Press, Toyama, Japan, pp 558–560
11. Tanaka F, Matsuzoe S (2012) Care-receiving robot to promote children's learning by teaching: field experiments at a classroom for vocabulary learning. J Hum-Robot Interact 1:78–95
12. Tachi S (2003) Telecommunication, teleimmersion and telexistence. Ohmsha, Tokyo and IOS Press, Amsterdam
13. Ishiguro H (2006) Android science: conscious and subconscious recognition. Connect Sci 18 (4):319–332
14. Tanaka F, Takahashi T (2012) A tricycle-style teleoperational interface that remotely controls a robot for classroom children. In: Proceedings of the 7th ACM/IEEE international conference on human-robot interaction. ACM/IEEE, Boston, USA, pp 255–256

Chapter 11
Subjectivity-Kansei Computing

Takehisa Onisawa

Abstract The chapter first discusses subjective Kansei information, with features such as subjectivity, ambiguity, vagueness and situation dependence, with respect to the interaction between a human and a computer agent. Next, soft computing techniques including fuzzy theory, neural network models, and evolutionary computation are introduced to deal with subjective Kansei information. Finally, this chapter presents some study examples of Subjectivity-Kansei computing using soft computing techniques.

Keywords Kansei information • Cooperative agent • Human–agent interaction • Soft computing

11.1 Introduction

What is Kansei [1–5]? This technical term has a Japanese origin and no similar term is found in the English language. Daring to explain Kansei in English, Kansei is a human feeling that includes emotion, affectivity, impression, preference, subjectivity, and so on, and which is difficult to explain logically. In human face-to-face communication, not only verbal information, but also non-verbal information, such as voice pitch, facial expressions, and gestures, is used to ensure smooth communication. Kansei information is also used in human face-to-face communication. Changing the topic to human–system or human–agent interaction, interaction between a human and an agent can take many forms, for example, interaction in system fault diagnosis or medical diagnosis, interaction in route guidance, or giving advice to a human as a decision support system. The form of interactive design is also found in human–computer agent interaction. Through the interaction between

T. Onisawa (✉)
Faculty of Engineering, Information and Systems, University of Tsukuba, Tsukuba, Japan
e-mail: onisawa@iit.tsukuba.ac.jp

Y. Sankai et al. (eds.), *Cybernics: Fusion of human, machine and information systems*,
DOI 10.1007/978-4-431-54159-2_11, © Springer Japan 2014

a human and a system or computer agent, many different kinds of information are exchanged, e.g., numerical information, verbal information such as characters and symbolic characters, image information, intelligent information, and subjective Kansei information. In this chapter, we focus mainly on subjective Kansei information. Although hitherto subjective Kansei information has been ignored or eliminated from conventional information processing as noise because this kind of information cannot be dealt with objectively and logically, the importance of Kansei to the engineering field has recently been recognized because understanding human feelings and how these are affected is required for the construction of human-friendly systems and human–agent communication. In other words, it is necessary to analyze how a human feels about the design of an object or how a human is affected by, for example, musical works.

Before the main subject is discussed, we attempt to answer the following question: How is Subjectivity-Kansei related to Cybernics? The web page for Cybernics gives the following definition [6]:

> This project aims to create a new research field Cybernics. This is a new domain of frontier science that centers on cybernetics, mechatronics, and informatics, and integrates together human and robot. ... It is a complex interdisciplinary area in which robotics, brain science and neuroscience, information technology, ergonomics, KANSEI engineering, physiology, social science and even ethics are deeply intertwined.

These statements can be interpreted as follows. In the interaction between a human and a system or computer agent, when a human gives and receives items of information to and from a system or a computer agent, aspects of the human's evaluation, decisions, feelings, subjectivity and Kansei are included in the exchanged information and also in Cybernics. Thus, Subjectivity-Kansei is related to Cybernics and the concept of Subjectivity-Kansei is indeed integral to the field of Cybernics.

This chapter describes features of the information exchanged in the interaction between a human and a computer agent and explains some of the approaches to Subjectivity-Kansei information processing. Finally, some examples of Subjectivity-Kansei computing are presented.

11.2 Features of the Information Exchanged in Human–Computer Agent Interaction

When humans embark on creative activity such as music composition or the design of some object, e.g., a glass, they often require advice from other persons if they are unable to complete the task without assistance. This involves interaction between the person and the advisers. In Fig. 11.1, a human adviser is replaced by a computer agent as an adviser in the design of a glass. In this scenario, the role of the human is to request advice and evaluate the response, because even if a human cannot design a glass himself/herself, he/she does have an idea of the design image and can

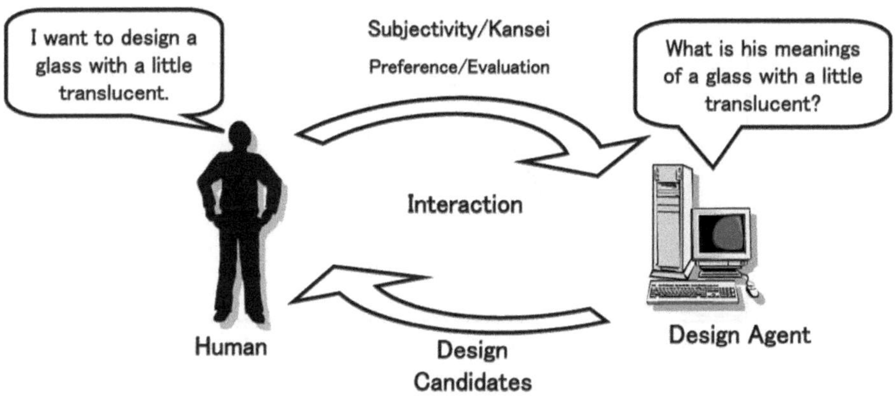

Fig. 11.1 Interaction between human and computer agent

evaluate whether design candidates are good. In this case, the design image of a glass is usually expressed by a sketch or in linguistic terms such as a *small short glass*, or *a slightly translucent glass*. Attached to such linguistic terms is the usual fuzziness that is dependent on individual human subjectivity, and thus, the meanings of the terms are dealt with as a type of Kansei information. The computer agent understands the meanings of the linguistic terms, ascertains the human's own interpretation through interaction, and presents design candidates that are tailored to the human's own taste. In this section, features of information such as subjectivity, ambiguity, vagueness, and situation dependence in the interaction are discussed [7–9].

11.2.1 Subjectivity

Objectivity is based on the standpoint that it is reasonable for all, and this is an important concept in conventional natural science. On the other hand, subjectivity is based on the standpoint that it is reasonable only for certain individuals or groups and does not consider whether it is reasonable for others. For example, a 175-cm-tall person recognizes a 185-cm-tall person as *tall*, whereas a 200-cm-tall person recognizes a 185-cm-tall person as *short*. Thus, should a 175-cm-tall person recognize a 180-cm-tall person as *tall*? This is a matter of subjective degree, and the answer is dependent on the actual individual doing the estimation. Furthermore, the estimation is not clear-cut in the sense that the boundary between *tall* and *not tall* is not clearly defined and incorporates an aspect of degree. Fuzzy sets [10] were proposed based on these concepts. Figure 11.2 shows an example of a fuzzy set for the label *tall* as defined by a 175-cm-tall person. Of course, a 200-cm-tall person may define a completely different fuzzy set for the label *tall*. It is necessary to consider human subjectivity in the interaction between a human and a computer

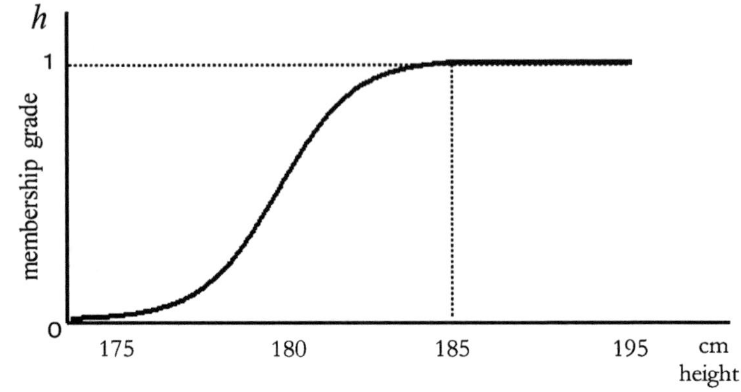

Fig. 11.2 Fuzzy set *tall*

agent since human subjectivity is included in information given and received during the interaction. Even in Kansei information processing, human subjectivity must be considered, since Kansei information is related to human subjectivity itself. Therefore, a system or a computer agent needs to be able to understand human subjectivity in the interaction between a human and a system or computer agent.

11.2.2 Ambiguity

The concept of objectivity is associated with that of uniqueness. On the other hand, the concept of subjectivity is associated with that of a diverse sense of values, which means, for example, that the interpretation of information is dependent on the person receiving the information or the situation in which the person is. A diverse sense of values that depends on subjectivity yields ambiguity, but it should be tolerated in the interaction between a human and a system or computer agent as shown in Fig. 11.1. Permitting a diverse sense of values implies permission of ambiguity. Only one sense of values yields uniqueness, and we can have only one objectively correct solution in a problem. On the other hand, a diverse sense of values allows various interpretations or different solutions of a problem. That is, we do not always have only one objectively correct solution or there is a possibility that we can have various types of solutions of a problem discussed in the interaction between a human and a computer agent if the solutions satisfy the human. Since human subjectivity, evaluation, and interpretation play central roles in the interaction between a human and a computer agent, ambiguity arising from a diverse sense of values must be permitted in the interaction. Therefore, a computer agent needs to understand human ambiguity, i.e., the diverse sense of values in the interaction between a human and a computer agent.

11.2.3 Vagueness

Since an objective system is designed to have a clear causal relation or a clear input–output relation, the system surely has a regular effect for a cause or a regular output for an input according to the relation. This idea leads to the concept of universality. On the other hand, a human does not necessarily have a regular input–output relation and may have several input–output relations incorporating his/her own peculiarities. Humans also seem to have incoherent input–output relations or inconsistent input–output relations depending on the circumstances. This vagueness arises from human subjectivity and ambiguity, i.e., a diverse sense of evaluation. Furthermore, this may be related to situation dependence, which is discussed in the next subsection. Therefore, a human sometimes arrives at a different decision or evaluation from the one he/she would have made on a previous day. It is important to permit this vagueness in the interaction between a human and a computer agent since human subjectivity, evaluation, and interpretation play central roles in the interaction.

11.2.4 Situation Dependence

It is assumed that an objective system has a regular input–output relation under some fixed condition. Therefore, the system has an output corresponding to an input and an input–output relation under the condition. This is the basic idea of conventional natural science. However, the information processing model of the interaction between a human and a computer agent as shown in Fig. 11.1 is not covered by this framework, since the framework does not permit subjectivity, ambiguity, or vagueness, and human subjectivity, evaluation and interpretation are dependent on the situation in which the human is. Not only the input, but also the situation in which the human is has an influence on the human's decision and/or evaluation. This means that the interaction between a human and a computer agent is surely situation-dependent.

11.3 Approaches to Information Processing in Human–Computer Agent Interaction

In the interaction between a human and a computer agent as shown in Fig. 11.1, the computer agent learns the human evaluation of the design candidates presented by the agent and the meaning of the evaluation through interaction with the human. The agent is then able to present acceptable solutions or design candidates in the sense that these solutions/design candidates are tailored to the human's own taste. In a conventional learning approach, certain evaluation functions are prepared and a solution is obtained in which the values of the evaluation functions are optimal. It is, however, difficult to define evaluation functions for humans, since information related to a human has features such as subjectivity, ambiguity, vagueness, and situation dependence, as mentioned in Sect. 11.2. Therefore, the computer agent in Fig. 11.1 needs to deal with these features of human information.

Soft computing [11, 12] techniques are considered one of the suitable approaches to information processing in the interaction between a human and a computer agent owing to the fact that the mechanisms of soft computing can handle the diverse features of human information. The idea of soft computing was proposed to deal with real-world information. In other words, soft computing tolerates inaccuracy of information by sacrificing information accuracy, since it is difficult to deal with real-world information in a way that seeks absolute correctness and strictness of information. Soft computing is also considered to be an all-encompassing technology for fuzzy theory, evolutionary computation including genetic algorithms, learning theory, and so on.

Nevertheless, soft computing has another side. As mentioned above, it is an all-encompassing technology including fuzzy theory, neural networks, evolutionary computation, and so on. Each methodology has its own advantages and disadvantages. For example, fuzzy theory is appropriate for knowledge representation in the form of words; that is, knowledge represented by fuzzy sets is understood easily. Fuzzy theory, however, is not appropriate for learning or optimization. On the other hand, a neural network model and evolutionary computation are appropriate for learning and optimization, but are not appropriate for knowledge representation. The idea behind soft computing is to replace the disadvantages of one methodology with the advantages of others.

11.3.1 Fuzzy Theory

There are many facets of vagueness, including incompleteness, randomness, imprecision, fuzziness, and actual vagueness. Fuzzy theory [13–15] deals with fuzziness, while probability theory deals with randomness, which is different from fuzziness. Randomness means uncertainty concerned with event occurrence; that is, randomness is uncertainty in forecasting whether an event will occur before the event does. This type of uncertainty goes away once the event occurs. For example, a weather reporter might say that the probability of rain the next day is 70 %. However, this type of uncertainty becomes clear the next day since it is then known whether there has been any rain. On the other hand, fuzziness in fuzzy theory is concerned with human subjectivity or the meaning of a linguistic term, e.g., a *tall* man or *low* temperature. What is the exact definition of a *tall* height or *low* temperature? These definitions differ from person to person.

Fuzzy theory includes fuzzy sets theory, fuzzy logic, and fuzzy measures and integrals. These concepts are introduced next.

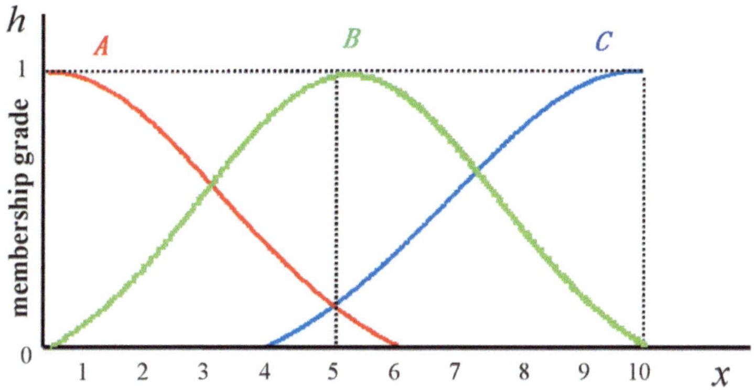

Fig. 11.3 Examples of fuzzy sets, *small numbers A*, *medium numbers B*, and *large numbers C*

Fuzzy Sets Theory A fuzzy set A is usually defined by a membership function h_A as in Eq. 11.1.

$$h_A(x) : X \rightarrow \quad [0, \ \ 1], \tag{11.1}$$

where X denotes the whole set and $x \in X$. For example, let X be the whole set of real numbers [0, 10], and let us consider a set of small numbers A, a set of medium numbers B, and a set of large numbers C in X. Figure 11.3 shows examples of these sets. In conventional set theory, an ordinary set $\widetilde{A}$, called a crisp set in this chapter to distinguish it from a fuzzy set and an ordinary set, is defined by a characteristic function $\chi_{\widetilde{A}}$ as in Eq. 11.2.

$$\chi_{\widetilde{A}}(x) : X \rightarrow \quad \{0, \ \ 1\}, \tag{11.2}$$

where X is the whole set and

$$\chi_{\widetilde{A}}(x) = \begin{cases} 1, & x \in \widetilde{A} \\ 0, & x \notin \widetilde{A} \end{cases}. \tag{11.3}$$

Figure 11.4 shows examples of set $\widetilde{A} = \{x | 0 \le x < 4, \ x \in X\}$, set $\widetilde{B} = \{x | 4 \le x < 7, x \in X\}$, set $\widetilde{C} = \{x | 7 \le x \le 10, \ x \in X\}$, and $X = \{x | 0 \le x \le 10, \ x \text{ is a real number}\}$. It can be seen from Eqs. 11.1 and 11.2 or from Figs. 11.3 and 11.4 that a crisp set is a special case of a fuzzy set.

Set Operations Although there are many definitions of the union, intersection and complement of fuzzy sets, these are usually defined as follows, based on Zadeh's definition [10].

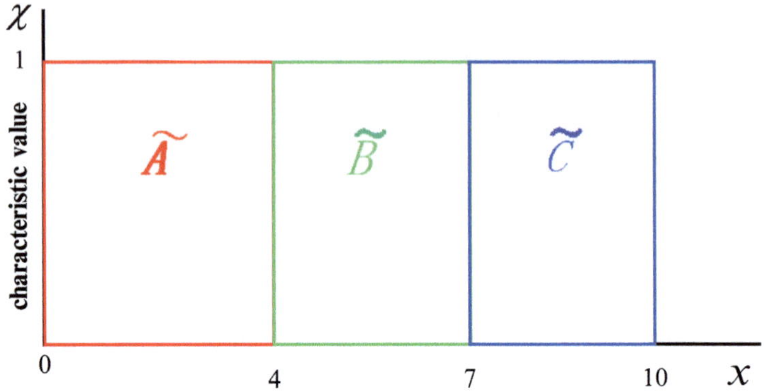

Fig. 11.4 Examples of crisp sets

Union of fuzzy sets is defined as

$$h_{A \cup B}(x) = h_A(x) \vee h_B(x), \tag{11.4}$$

where $\vee$ denotes the maximum.

Intersection of fuzzy sets is defined as

$$h_{A \cap B}(x) = h_A(x) \wedge h_B(x), \tag{11.5}$$

where $\wedge$ denotes the minimum.

Complement of a fuzzy set is defined as

$$h_{A^C} = 1 - h_A(x). \tag{11.6}$$

From these definitions it is evident that the inclusive middle law and inconsistency law do not necessarily hold in fuzzy sets.

$$h_{A \cup A^C}(x) = h_A(x) \vee \{1 - h_A(x)\} \neq 1, \quad h_{A \cap A^C}(x) = h_A(x) \wedge \{1 - h_A(x)\} \neq 0 \tag{11.7}$$

Figure 11.5 explains Eq. 11.7.

Extension Principle Let us consider a mapping *f* from set *X* to set *Y* by Eq. 11.8.

$$f\left(\widetilde{E}\right) = \left\{y \middle| y = f(x),\ x \in \widetilde{E},\ \ \widetilde{E} \subset X\right\}, \tag{11.8}$$

where *X* and *Y* are whole sets and $\widetilde{E}$ is a crisp set. Usually, $f\left(\widetilde{E}\right) \subset Y$. The concept of the mapping is extended to the mapping of a fuzzy set by the following definition called *an extension principle*.

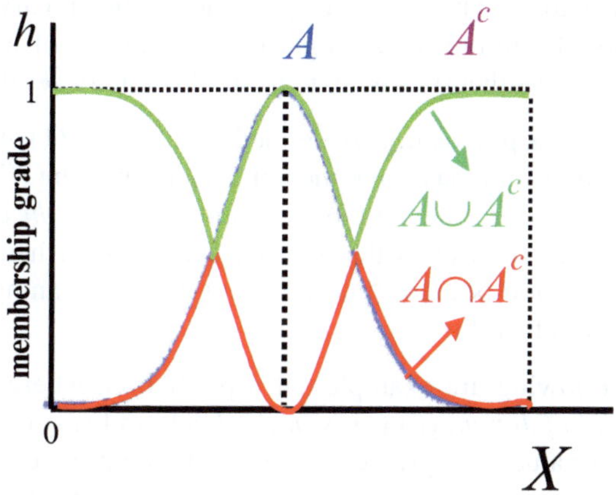

Fig. 11.5 $A \cup A^C$ and $A \cap A^c$

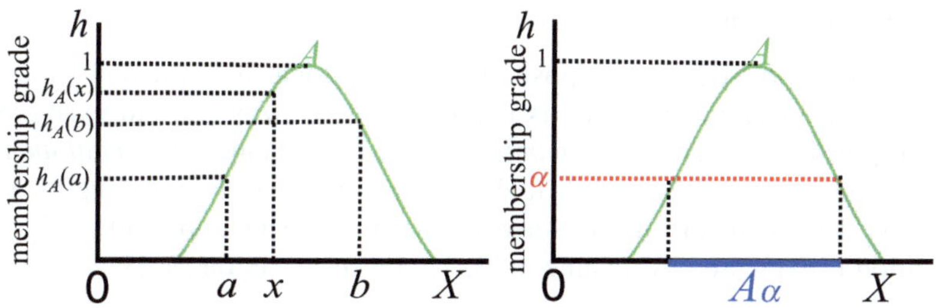

Fig. 11.6 Convex fuzzy set and α level set

$$h_{f(A)}(y) = \begin{cases} \sup\limits_{x \in f^{-1}(y)} h_A(x), & f^{-1}(y) \neq \phi \\ 0, & f^{-1}(y) = \phi \end{cases}, \tag{11.9}$$

where A is a fuzzy set of X.

Convex Fuzzy Set, Normal Fuzzy Set and α Level Fuzzy Set There are some specific definitions of a fuzzy set, a convex fuzzy set, a normal fuzzy set, and an α level set.

$$A \text{ is } a\ convex\ fuzzy\ set \Leftrightarrow \ for\ \forall a,\ \forall b \in X,\ \forall \tau \in [0,\ 1], \\ h_A(\tau a + (1-\tau)b) \geq h_A(a) \wedge h_A(b) \tag{11.10}$$

$$A \text{ is } a\ normal\ fuzzy\ set \Leftrightarrow \ \exists x \in X\ \ such\ that\ \ h_A(x) = 1, \tag{11.11}$$

$$A_\alpha \text{ is } an\,\alpha\ level\ set \Leftrightarrow A_\alpha = \{x | h_A(x) \geq \alpha,\ \ \alpha \in [0, 1]\}. \tag{11.12}$$

Figure 11.6 shows examples of these fuzzy sets.

Fuzzy Logic Fuzzy logic is based on fuzzy set theory, like binary logic is based on ordinary set theory. Therefore, fuzzy logic is an extension of binary logic in the same way that fuzzy sets theory is an extension of ordinary set theory.

Proposition In logic, a proposition is defined as follows. (1) A proposition is a statement. (2) A proposition has some meaning as a statement. (3) It is possible to evaluate the truth value of a statement. For example, *Tokyo is the capital of Japan* is a proposition of which the truth value is *true*. On the other hand, *a triangle is a circle* is not a proposition because this statement has no meaning and it is impossible to evaluate its truth value.

Prediction The following are examples of a prediction, where (x) is a variable: (i) (x) *is the capital of Japan*, (ii) (x) *is in the USA*, and (iii) (x) *is larger than 8*. Although the truth value of a prediction cannot be determined, if some value is substituted for (x) in a prediction, the prediction becomes a proposition and its truth value can be determined. For example, if (x) in prediction (i) has the value *Tokyo*, its truth value is *true*. On the other hand, if (x) in prediction (i) has the value *Tsukuba*, its truth value is *false*. The domain of (x), called the *universe of discourse*, must be defined beforehand.

Fuzzy Proposition A fuzzy proposition in fuzzy logic is expressed by a fuzzy statement, the meaning of which is expressed by a fuzzy set. An example of a fuzzy proposition is: *4 is a small number*, where the meaning of *a small number* is expressed by, e.g., A in Fig. 11.3. It should be noted that the meaning of *a small number* is dependent on the universe of discourse. The truth value of a fuzzy proposition is expressed by a value in [0, 1] or a fuzzy set on [0, 1].

Fuzzy Prediction A fuzzy prediction is expressed in the form: (x) *is* A, where (x) is a variable and A is a fuzzy set in the universe of discourse. The following are examples of a fuzzy prediction: (a) (x) *is a small number*, and (b) (x) *is young*.

Henceforth, a fuzzy proposition is written in the form, x *is* A, where x is not (x), but some noun, and A is a fuzzy set.

Modifier Let us consider the following fuzzy proposition with modifier m: x *is* mA. There are many types of modifiers, such as *very*, *more or less*, or *not*. When these modifiers are added to a fuzzy proposition, for example, *x is a small number*, the fuzzy proposition can be rewritten as follows: *x is a very small number*, *x is a more or less small number*, or *x is a not small number*. When a modifier is added to a fuzzy proposition, the meaning of the fuzzy statement is changed from $h_A(x)$ to $h_{mA}(x)$, where $h_A(x)$ and $h_{mA}(x)$ are the membership functions of fuzzy sets A and mA, respectively. Examples of the change in meaning of a fuzzy statement by means of a modifier are shown in Eq. 11.13.

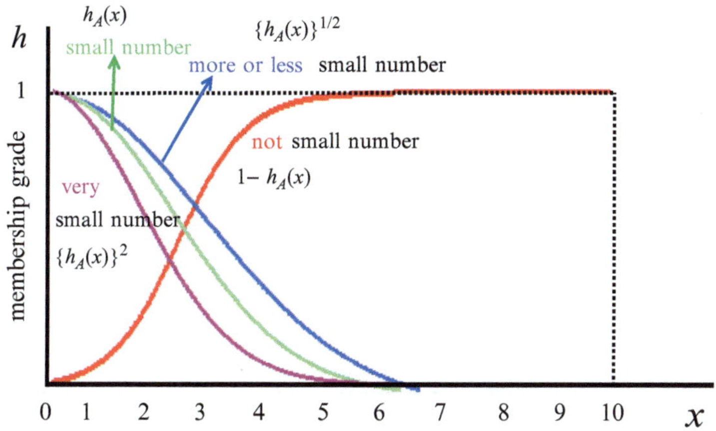

Fig. 11.7 Examples of modifiers

$$\begin{array}{l} x\,is\,A \;\Rightarrow\; x\ is\ very\ A \;:\; h_A(x) \;\Rightarrow\; \{h_A(x)\}^2 \\ x\,is\,A \;\Rightarrow\; x\ is\ more\ or\ less\ A \;:\; h_A(x) \;\Rightarrow\; \{h_A(x)\}^{1/2} \\ x\,is\,A \;\Rightarrow\; x\ is\ not\ A \;:\; h_A(x) \;\Rightarrow\; 1 - h_A(x). \end{array} \qquad (11.13)$$

Figure 11.7 illustrates these examples. Definitions of the change in meaning of a fuzzy statement by means of a modifier are not necessarily restricted to those in Eq. 11.13. For example, regarding modifier *very*, another definition can be considered as follows.

$$x\,is\,A \;\Rightarrow\; x\ is\ very\ A \;:\; h_A(x) \;\Rightarrow\; h_A(x-c), \qquad (11.14)$$

where c is the transformation value as shown in Fig. 11.8.

Composite Fuzzy Proposition Let us consider two simple fuzzy propositions, *x is A* and *x is B*. Using these propositions, the following three types of propositions are obtained.

$$\begin{array}{ll} x\ is\ A\ OR\ x\ is\ B, & A,B \subset X \\ x\ is\ A\ AND\ x\ is\ B, & A,B \subset X \\ If\ x\ is\ A\ \ Then\ y\ is\ B, & A \subset X, B \subset Y, \end{array} \qquad (11.15)$$

where *OR*, *AND*, and *If-Then* are logical connectives. These propositions are called composite fuzzy propositions. Moreover, the third proposition is called an implication, which is applied to fuzzy inference. The first and second propositions are rewritten simply as *x is A OR B*, and *x is A AND B*, respectively. As for the first and second propositions, although other types of composite fuzzy propositions shown in Eq. 11.16 can be considered, further discussion on these types of propositions are omitted in this chapter.

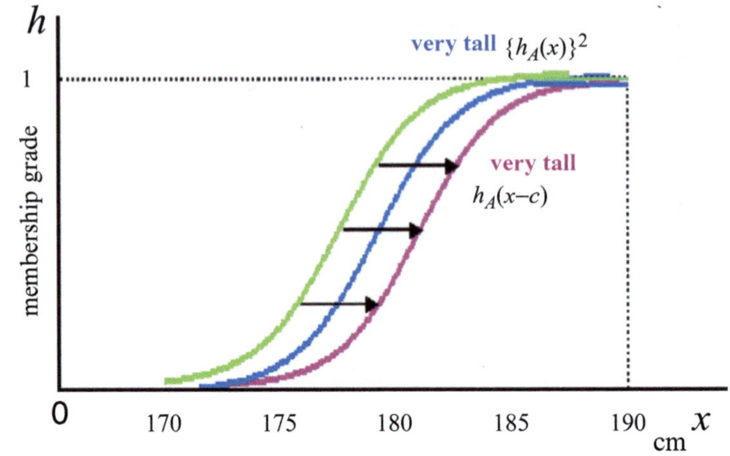

Fig. 11.8 Another definition of *very*

$$
\begin{array}{ll}
x \ is \ A \ OR \ y \ is \ B, & A \subset X, B \subset Y \\
x \ is \ A \ AND \ y \ is \ B, & A \subset X, B \subset Y.
\end{array}
\tag{11.16}
$$

Fuzzy Truth Value Let $Nv(P(a))$ be the truth value of proposition, P : *a is A*. The truth value in two-valued logic is either *true* or *false*; that is, $Nv(P(a)) \in \{0, \ 1\}$. On the other hand, the truth value in fuzzy logic is expressed by a numerical value in [0, 1]; that is, $Nv(P(a)) \in [0, \ 1]$. Usually, the truth value in fuzzy logic is defined by $Nv(P(a)) = h_A(a)$ based on the following idea, where $h_A(x)$ is the membership function of fuzzy set A. $Nv(P(a)) \rightarrow 1$ means that the truth value of P is more likely to be *true* in the sense of two-valued logic, while $Nv(P(a)) \rightarrow 0$ means that the truth value of P is more likely to be *false* in the sense of two-valued logic.

Let us consider the truth value of composite fuzzy propositions. And let us consider the two fuzzy propositions P_1 : *a is A* and P_2 : *a is B*, where A and B are fuzzy sets with their membership functions expressed by $h_A(x)$ and $h_B(x)$, respectively. The truth value of $P = P_1$ *OR* P_2 is defined as

$$
\begin{aligned}
Nv(P(a)) &= NV(P_1(a)) \vee Nv(P_2(a)) \\
&= h_A(a) \vee h_B(a).
\end{aligned}
\tag{11.17}
$$

The truth value of $P = P_1$ AND P_2 is defined by

$$
\begin{aligned}
Nv(P(a)) &= NV(P_1(a)) \wedge Nv(P_2(a)) \\
&= h_A(a) \wedge h_B(a).
\end{aligned}
\tag{11.18}
$$

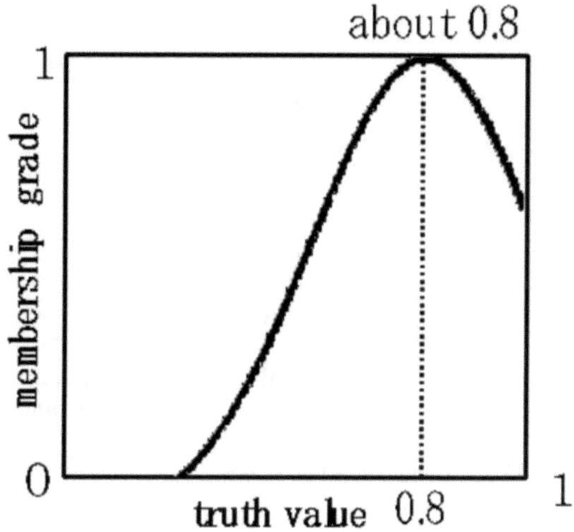

Fig. 11.9 Truth value *about 0.8*

The truth value of the fuzzy proposition with modifier m, $P : a \textit{ is } mA$, is defined as

$$Nv(P(a)) = h_{mA}(a). \tag{11.19}$$

The definition of the truth value of the fuzzy implication, $P = \textit{If } a \textit{ is } A \textit{ Then } b \textit{ is } B$, is not unique because there is some freedom in the truth value, with the exception of 0 and 1, when non-two-valued logic is introduced. Some of these are shown in Eq. 11.20, where $Nv(P(a,b))$ is the truth value of the fuzzy implication.

$$\begin{aligned} Nv(P(a,b)) &= \{1 - h_A(a) + h_B(b)\} \wedge 1 \\ Nv(P(a,b)) &= h_A(a) \wedge h_B(b) \\ Nv(P(a,b)) &= \{h_A(a) \wedge h_B(b)\} \vee \{1 - h_A(a)\}. \end{aligned} \tag{11.20}$$

Fuzzy Set as Truth Value Let the numerical truth value of fuzzy proposition, $P : a \textit{ is } A$, be 0.8, i.e., $Nv(P(a)) = 0.8$. The numerical truth value has some of following problems. Is it possible for a human to estimate the truth value of the fuzzy proposition as exactly 0.8? Or could 0.79 or 0.81 be accepted, instead of 0.8, as the truth value? Regarding the first question, it may be impossible to estimate exactly one numerical value as the truth value of a proposition. *About 0.8* or a linguistic term such as *more or less true* seems to be natural for a human as the evaluation of the truth value. This is also the answer to the second question. Therefore, a fuzzy set on [0, 1], e.g., *about 0.8*, is introduced as the truth value of a fuzzy proposition. Figure 11.9 shows an example of a fuzzy set expressing the truth value, *about 0.8*. Alternatively, the idea of a linguistic truth value is also introduced as the truth value of a fuzzy proposition. Figure 11.10 shows the linguistic truth values expressed by normal and convex fuzzy sets on [0, 1], where *completely true* means *true* in two-valued logic and *completely false* means *false* in two-valued logic.

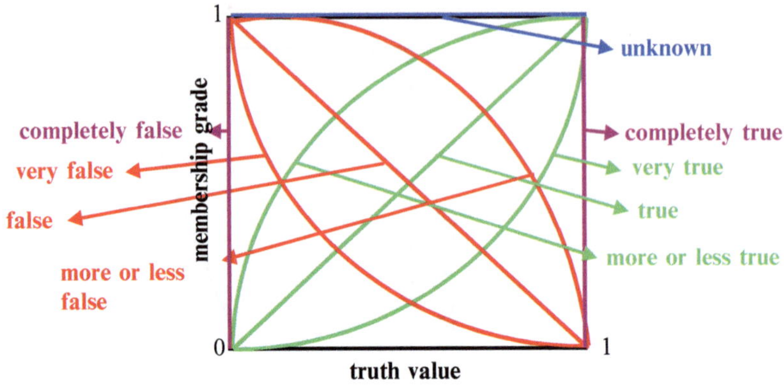

Fig. 11.10 Linguistic truth values

Truth Qualification Let us consider a fuzzy proposition and a fuzzy proposition with a linguistic truth value τ, P : a *is* A and P' : a *is* A *is* τ, respectively. The meaning of proposition P is qualified by the linguistic truth value τ. Given proposition, a *is* A, and linguistic truth value τ, truth qualification means obtaining statement a *is* A', such that the following two statements are equivalent in the sense of their meaning, that is, expressed by Eqs. 11.21 and 11.22.

$$a \ is \ A \ is \ \tau \ \approx \ a \ is \ A'. \tag{11.21}$$

$$h_{A'}(x) = h_\tau(h_A(x)). \tag{11.22}$$

where $h_A(x)$, $h_{A'}(x)$, and $h_\tau(v)$ are membership functions of fuzzy sets A, A' and τ, respectively, and $v \in [0,1]$. Equation 11.23 gives some examples of truth qualification.

$$\begin{aligned} &a \ is \ A \ is \ true \ \approx \ a \ is \ A \\ &a \ is \ A \ is \ very \ true \ \approx \ a \ is \ very \ A \\ &a \ is \ A \ is \ false \ \approx \ a \ is \ not \ A. \end{aligned} \tag{11.23}$$

Converse of Truth Qualification Given propositions, a *is* A and a *is* A', the converse of truth qualification means obtaining a linguistic truth value τ expressed by Eq. 11.24.

$$h_\tau(v) = \mathop{Sup}_{x \in h_A^{-1}(v)} h_{A'}(x). \tag{11.24}$$

Equation 11.25 gives examples of the converse of truth qualification.

$$\begin{aligned} &when \ h_{A'}(x) = h_A(x), && \tau = true \\ &when \ h_{A'}(x) = \{h_A(x)\}^2, && \tau = very \ true \\ &when \ h_{A'}(x) = 1 - h_A(x), && \tau = flase. \end{aligned} \tag{11.25}$$

Table 11.1 Truth value table for inference in two-valued logic

$/A/$	$/B/$	$/A \rightarrow B/$
T	T	T
T	F	F
F	T	T
F	F	T

T true, *F* false

Fuzzy Inference In two-valued logic, inference is performed based on the truth value table shown in Table 11.1, where symbols $/A/$, $/B/$, and $/A \rightarrow B/$ denote the truth values of propositions, *a is A*, *b is B*, and *If a is A Then b is B*, respectively, where sets A and B are ordinary sets. It must be noted that inference using information $/A \rightarrow B/{=}F$ is illogical. Therefore, the following four cases are considered for inference, based on Table 11.1.

1. Given $/A/{=}T$, what is the value of $/B/$? In this case, $/B/{=}T$ is inferred by Table 11.1. That is, it is possible to infer $/B/$.
2. Given $/A/{=}F$, what is the value of $/B/$? In this case it is not clear whether $/B/{=}T$ or $/B/{=}F$. Therefore, it is impossible to infer $/B/$.
3. Given $/B/{=}T$, what is the value of $/A/$? In this case it is not clear whether $/A/{=}T$ or $/A/{=}F$; that is, it is impossible to infer $/A/$.
4. Given $/B/{=}F$, what is the value of $/A/$? From Table 11.1, $/A/{=}F$ is inferred.

In two-valued logic the first type of inference is called *modus ponens* and the fourth type of inference is called *modus tollens*, expressed by Eq. 11.26.

$$\begin{aligned} &\frac{A \quad A \rightarrow B}{B}, \quad \text{modus ponens} \\ &\frac{B^C \quad A \rightarrow B}{A^C}, \quad \text{modus tollens.} \end{aligned} \tag{11.26}$$

Inference in two-valued logic is not applicable to the inference that a human usually does because if fact A is not the same as A in the implication $A \rightarrow B$, it is impossible to perform inference in two-valued logic, whereas a human usually performs the inference even if fact A' is a little different from A in the implication $A \rightarrow B$. Reasoning in fuzzy logic, called fuzzy inference, is expressed by Eq. 11.27.

$$\begin{aligned} &\frac{A' \quad A \rightarrow B}{B'}, \quad \text{fuzzy modus ponens} \\ &\frac{(B')^C \quad A \rightarrow B}{(A')^C}, \quad \text{fuzzy modus tollens.} \end{aligned} \tag{11.27}$$

Fuzzy modus ponens means that given implication $A \rightarrow B$ and fact A', similar to the if-part in implication $A \rightarrow B$, which means that A' is a little different from A in

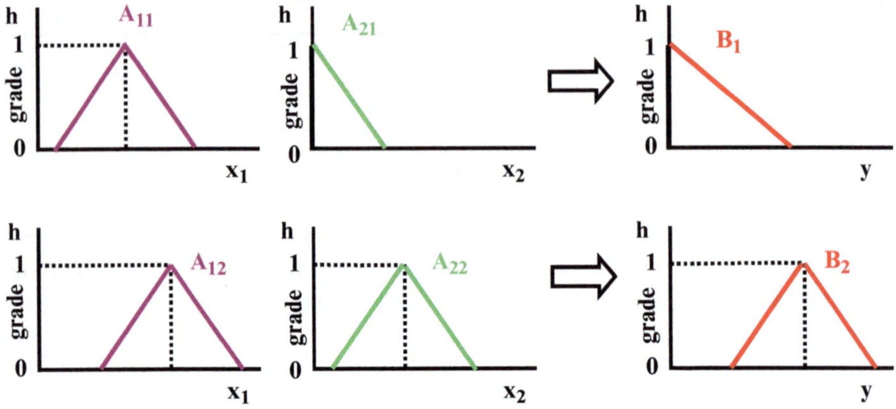

Fig. 11.11 Knowledge expression using fuzzy sets

the implication $A \rightarrow B$, fuzzy modus ponens infers some proposition B' similar to B in the implication $A \rightarrow B$, which means that B' is a little different from B. Fuzzy modus tollens means that given implication $A \rightarrow B$ and a fact, i.e., the negation of B' similar to the then-part in implication $A \rightarrow B$, which means that B' is a little different from B in the implication $A \rightarrow B$, fuzzy modus tollens infers negation of some proposition A' similar to A in implication $A \rightarrow B$, which means that A' is a little different from A in the implication $A \rightarrow B$. Next, we explain fuzzy modus ponens, which is expressed as Eq. 11.28.

$$h_{B'}(y) = \sup_x \{h_{A'}(x) \wedge h_{A \rightarrow B}(x, y)\}, \tag{11.28}$$

where $h_{A \rightarrow B}(x,y)$ shows the membership function of fuzzy implication with many definitions as mentioned above. For example,

$$\begin{aligned} h_{A \rightarrow B}(x, y)) &= \{1 - h_A(x) + h_B(y)\} \wedge 1 \\ h_{A \rightarrow B}(x, y)) &= h_A(x) \wedge h_B(y) \\ h_{A \rightarrow B}(x, y)) &= \{h_A(x) \wedge h_B(y)\} \vee \{1 - h_A(x)\}. \end{aligned} \tag{11.29}$$

Simplified Inference Method The inference method is explained using a simple example. Let us assume that we have the knowledge expressed by Eq. 11.30, which is expressed using fuzzy sets as illustrated in Fig. 11.11. The expression of knowledge is applicable to the expression of a fuzzy system's input–output relation as shown in Fig. 11.12. Furthermore, let us assume that information on x_1 and x_2 is given as $x_1 = x_{10}$ and $x_2 = x_{20}$. This means that the fuzzy system in Fig. 11.12 has inputs $x_1 = x_{10}$ and $x_2 = x_{20}$.

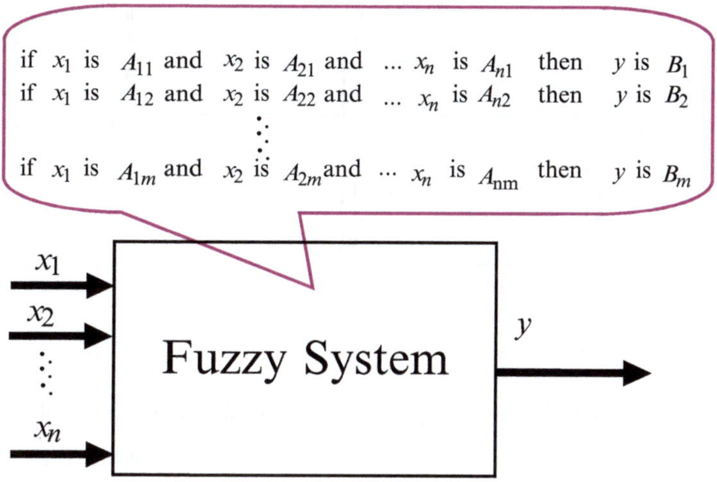

Fig. 11.12 Fuzzy system

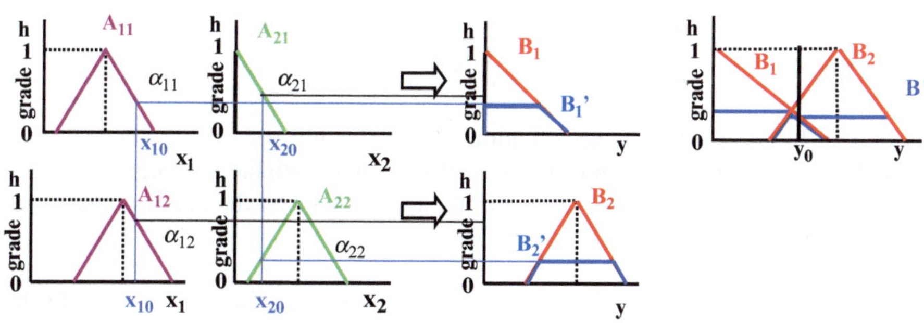

Fig. 11.13 Fuzzy inference procedures I

$$\begin{aligned} &\textit{If } x_1 \textit{ is } \mathrm{A}_{11} \textit{ and } x_2 \textit{ is } \mathrm{A}_{21} \textit{ Then } y \textit{ is } B_1 \\ &\textit{If } x_1 \textit{ is } \mathrm{A}_{12} \textit{ and } x_2 \textit{ is } \mathrm{A}_{22} \textit{ Then } y \textit{ is } B_2. \end{aligned} \tag{11.30}$$

The inference procedures are illustrated in Fig. 11.13. The satisfaction degree α_{11}, of x_{10} for fuzzy set A_{11} is obtained as shown in Fig. 11.13. The satisfaction degree α_{21}, of x_{20} for fuzzy set A_{21} is obtained in the same way. The satisfaction degree of the if-part for the first knowledge item is obtained by the min operation, $\alpha_{11} \wedge \alpha_{21}$. In this example α_{11} is obtained. Fuzzy set $B_1^{'}$ corresponding to fuzzy set B_1 in the then-part of the first knowledge item is obtained by $\alpha_{11} \wedge h_{B_1}(y)$, where $h_{B_1}(y)$ is the membership function of fuzzy set B_1. In the same way, fuzzy set $B_2^{'}$ corresponding to fuzzy set B_2 in the then-part of the second knowledge item is obtained. The result of fuzzy inference B', is obtained by

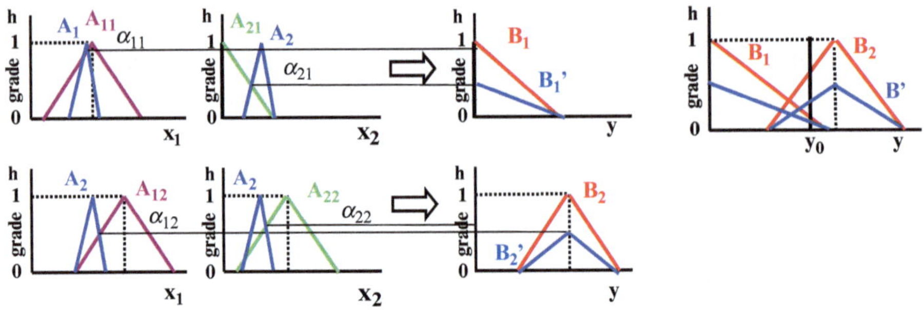

Fig. 11.14 Fuzzy inference procedures II

$h_{B_1'}(y) \vee h_{B_2'}(y)$, where $h_{B_1'}(y)$ and $h_{B_2'}(y)$ are membership functions of the fuzzy sets B_1' and B_2', respectively. The representative value y_0 is obtained by Eq. 11.31. This operation is called defuzzification.

$$y_0 = \frac{\int h_{B'}(y) y dy}{\int h_{B'}(y) dy}. \tag{11.31}$$

Figure 11.14 illustrates the situation where the information on x_1 and x_2 is expressed by fuzzy sets A_1 and A_2, respectively. The satisfaction degree of fuzzy set A_1 for A_{11} and that of fuzzy set A_2 for A_{21} are obtained by the max-min operation expressed in Eq. 11.32.

$$\alpha_{11} = \sup_x \{h_{A_{11}}(x) \wedge h_{A_1}(x)\} \quad \alpha_{21} = \sup_x \{h_{A_{21}}(x) \wedge h_{A_2}(x)\}. \tag{11.32}$$

In the same way, the satisfaction degree of fuzzy set A_1 for A_{12} and that of fuzzy set A_2 for A_{22} are obtained. B_1', B_2', and inference result B' are obtained in the same way as shown in Fig. 11.13.

Fuzzy inference is applicable to various fields of engineering, one of which is the system control field, i.e., fuzzy logic control. There are many complex systems whose behavior is difficult to express using differential equations. However, engineers typically do have some knowledge of these complex systems, and it is possible for them to express knowledge of the system behavior using certain linguistic rules in the form of if-then statements. As such, a fuzzy inference method can be applied to subsequent system modeling, system simulation, and system control.

Fuzzy Measures and Integrals What are measures? From a mathematical point of view, measures are numerical values given in order to measure something. For example, the length of a stick is expressed by a numerical value measured by a ruler or the weight of a person is expressed by a numerical value measured by a weighing device. Additivity is a basic property of measures. Let $m(A)$, $m(B)$, and $m(A \cup B)$ be the length of stick A, the length of stick B, and the length of the combined sticks A and B, respectively. Then, $m(A \cup B) = m(A) + m(B)$ is well known.

Equation 11.33 gives a mathematical definition of measures.

Let X and 2^X be a universal finite set and a power set of X, respectively. And let $A \subset X$ and $B \subset X$ be crisp sets. A set function $\rho : 2^X \to [0,1]$ satisfying the following properties is called a measure.

$$\begin{aligned} &(1)\ \rho(\phi) = 0 \\ &(2)\ \rho(X) = 1 \\ &(3)\ A \cap B = \phi \Rightarrow \rho(A \cup B) = \rho(A) + \rho(B), \end{aligned} \tag{11.33}$$

where ϕ is the empty set. The third property is essential to measures. The probability measure is one of the measures in mathematics.

When a human evaluates something, does the human always use measures satisfying additivity? If not, what does a relaxation of the property of additivity lead to?

Let us consider the situation in which a camera with a telephoto lens is sold by a vendor. Let $\$(A)$, $\$(B)$, and $\$(A \cup B)$ be the price of the camera, the price of the telephoto lens, and the price of the camera with the telephoto lens, respectively. In an ordinary camera shop a camera with a telephoto lens is sold at a price $\$(A \cup B) = \$(A) + \$(B)$, satisfying additivity. On the other hand, in a discount house a camera with a telephoto lens is sold at a price $\$(A \cup B) < \$(A) + \$(B)$. Customers have a feeling of profitability when buying a camera with a telephoto lens at this price. No one would buy a camera with a telephoto lens at a price $\$(A \cup B) > \$(A) + \$(B)$. It has been found that additivity plays an important role in pricing.

Fuzzy Measures Fuzzy measures are defined by Eq. 11.34.

Let X and 2^X be a universal finite set and a power set of X, respectively. And let $A \subset X$ and $B \subset X$ be crisp sets. A set function $g : 2^X \to [0,1]$ satisfying the following properties is called a fuzzy measure.

$$\begin{aligned} &(1)\ g(\phi) = 0 \\ &(2)\ g(X) = 1 \\ &(3)\ A \subset B \Rightarrow g(A) \le g(B), \end{aligned} \tag{11.34}$$

where ϕ is the empty set. The third property, *monotonicity*, is essential to fuzzy measures. Because of the monotonicity of fuzzy measures, and $A \cup B \supset A$, B and $A \cap B \subset A$, B, the following equation holds.

$$\begin{aligned} g(A \cup B) \ge g(A) \vee g(B) \\ g(A \cap B) \le g(A) \wedge g(B). \end{aligned} \tag{11.35}$$

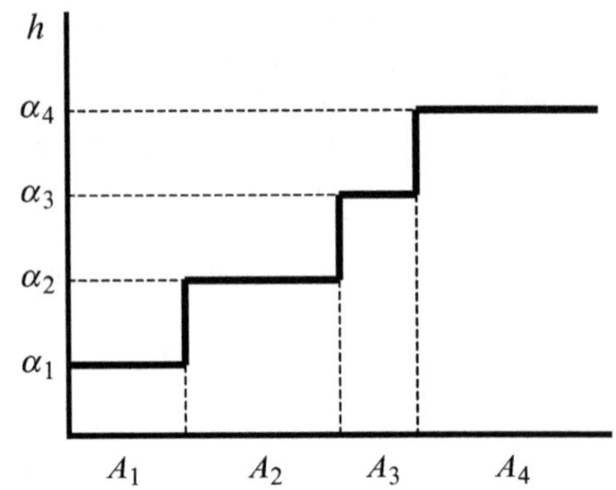

Fig. 11.15 Example of function h

Furthermore, under the condition $A \cap B = \phi$, one of the following three formulae holds.

$$\begin{aligned} g(A \cup B) &> g(A) + g(B) && : \text{super additivity} \\ g(A \cup B) &= g(A) + g(B) && : \text{additivity} \\ g(A \cup B) &< g(A) + g(B) && : \text{sub additivity.} \end{aligned} \tag{11.36}$$

From Eq. 11.36 it can be seen that fuzzy measures are an extension of conventional measures, i.e., Lebesgue measures, in the sense that fuzzy measures include additivity as a special case. Monotonicity is the relaxation of additivity.

Fuzzy Integrals Lebesgue integrals for Lebesgue measures, i.e., ordinary measures, are defined as follows. Let function $h : X \to [0,1]$ be defined by Eq. 11.37, where X is a universal set.

$$\begin{aligned} &h(x) = \sum_{i=1}^{n} \alpha_i \chi_{A_i}(x), \quad A = \bigcup_{i=1}^{n} A_i, \quad A_i \cap A_j = \phi, \quad i \neq j \\ &\chi_{A_i}(x) = \begin{cases} 1 : & x \in A_i \\ 0 : & x \notin A_i \end{cases}, \quad 0 \leq \alpha_1 \leq \alpha_2 \leq \ldots \leq \alpha_n. \end{aligned} \tag{11.37}$$

Figure 11.15 shows an example of function h, with $n = 4$. Lebesgue integrals of this simple function h are defined by the following formula:

$$\int_A h(x) d\rho(x) = \sum_{i=1}^{n} \alpha_i \rho(A_i) \tag{11.38}$$

where $\rho(A_i)$ is the Lebesgue measure of $A_i (i = 1, 2, \ldots, n)$. Lebesgue integrals denote the total sum of the area of this simple function as shown in Fig. 11.16.

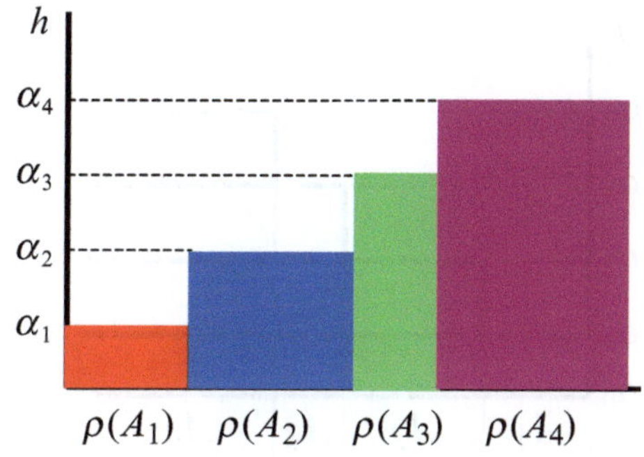

Fig. 11.16 Example of Lebesgue integrals

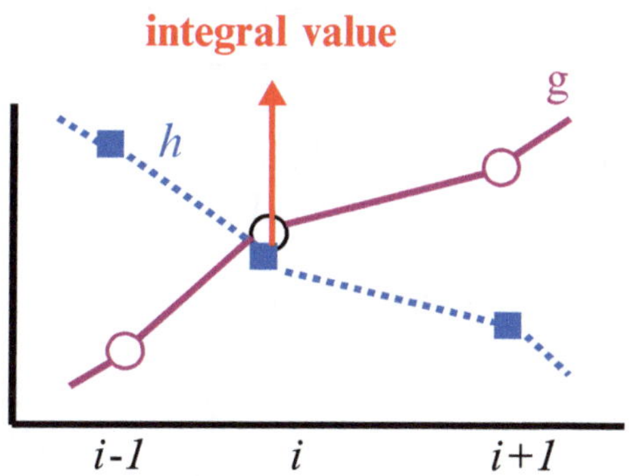

Fig. 11.17 Sugeno integrals

Two types of fuzzy integrals are introduced in this chapter. The first is Sugeno integrals and the other is Choquet integrals. Sugeno integrals of function $h : X \to [0,1]$ using fuzzy measure g are defined by Eq. 11.39.

$$\int h(x)\circ g(\bullet) = \max_{A\subset X}\left[\min_{x\in A}\{h(x)\wedge g(A)\}\right]. \tag{11.39}$$

If elements of universal set $X = \{x_1,x_2, \ldots,x_n\}$ are rearranged so that $h(x_1) \geq h(x_2) \geq \ldots \geq h(x_n)$, fuzzy integrals can be expressed by Eq. 11.40.

$$\int h(x)\circ g(\bullet) = \bigvee_{i=1}^{n}\{h(x_i)\wedge g(X_i)\}, \tag{11.40}$$

where $X_i = \{x_1,x_2, \ldots,x_i\}$. The integral value is obtained as shown in Fig. 11.17. As mentioned before, fuzzy measures are an extension of Lebesgue measures in the sense that they include additivity as a special case. Unfortunately, however, Sugeno integrals are not equal to Lebesgue integrals when the fuzzy measure satisfies additivity. Thus, Choquet integrals have been defined as another version of fuzzy integrals. Let function $h : X \to [0,1]$ be a simple function defined by

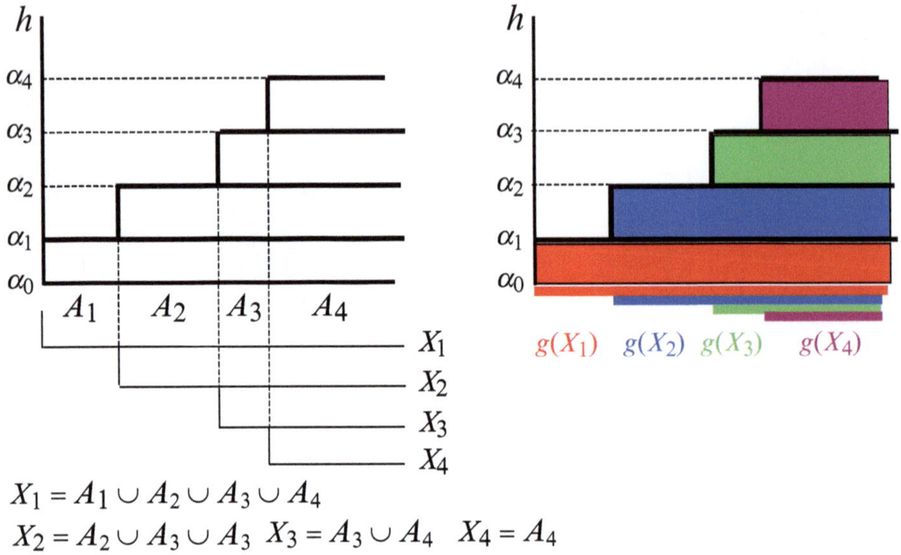

Fig. 11.18 Choquet integrals

$$
\begin{aligned}
h(x) &= \sum_{i=1}^{n}(\alpha_i - \alpha_{i-1})\chi_{X_i}(x), \\
\chi_{X_i}(x) &= \begin{cases} 1: & x \in X_i \\ 0: & x \notin X_i \end{cases}, \quad X_1 \supset X_2 \supset \ldots \supset X_n \\
0 &= \alpha_0 \le \alpha_1 \le \alpha_2 \le \ldots \le \alpha_n.
\end{aligned} \tag{11.41}
$$

Choquet integrals of function h using fuzzy measure g for the fuzzy integrals are defined by the following formula.

$$
(c)\int h(x)dg = \sum_{i=1}^{n}(\alpha_i - \alpha_{i-1})g(X_i). \tag{11.42}
$$

The total sum of the area of a simple function using Choquet integrals is shown in Fig. 11.18.

Choquet integrals are equal to Lebesgue integrals when the fuzzy measure satisfies additivity. This means that Choquet integrals as fuzzy integrals are an extension of Lebesgue integrals.

Applications Fuzzy measures and integrals are applied to a human evaluation model. Let us consider the situation in which a human evaluates some object using evaluation attributes as shown in Fig. 11.19. For example, let us consider the evaluation of rooms in apartment houses for the purpose of renting a room.

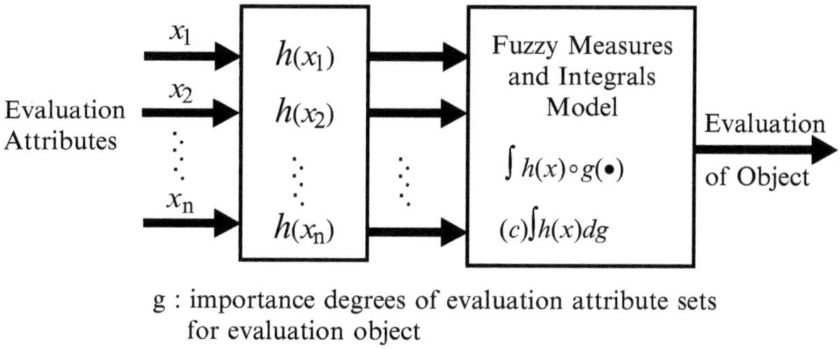

Fig. 11.19 Evaluation model using fuzzy measures and integrals

The following attributes are considered when renting a room: the rent, room size, distance from a station, year built, and so on. In this example, $h(x)$ denotes the evaluation value of each attribute for a given room, fuzzy measures show the degree of importance of attribute sets in the evaluation of rooms, and the fuzzy integral value denotes the evaluation value of a given room. The evaluation is performed in order to decide whether a given room should be rented.

Two types of problems are considered in applications of fuzzy measures and integrals. The first problem is the usual evaluation problem under the condition that fuzzy measures and evaluation of each attribute are given and that evaluation of each object is unknown. In the above example of evaluating rooms for the purpose of renting a room, this problem corresponds to the evaluation of a given room to decide whether to rent it. The fuzzy measures and integrals model is used for the evaluation of rooms during the room search. The second problem is the analysis of the human evaluation structure under the condition that evaluation of each attribute and evaluation of each object are given and that fuzzy measures are unknown. In the above example that considers the evaluation of rooms for rent, this problem corresponds to the analysis of the structure of a human's evaluation of the rooms. When a human evaluates rooms for rent, the analysis is performed based on those attributes to which the human has attached the greatest importance.

11.3.2 Neural Network Model

An artificial neural network model is an electrical analogy of the biological neural network connected by many biological nerve cells, called neurons [16–18]. A neuron has dendrites, an axon, and a synapse as shown in Fig. 11.20. A neuron receives signals from the synapses of neighboring neurons through dendrites, processes the received electrical pulses at the cell body, and transmits signals through an axon to a synapse as shown in Fig. 11.20. The electrical model of a typical biological neuron consists of a linear activator followed by a non-linear inhibiting function. Each synapse of a neuron has transmission efficiency and

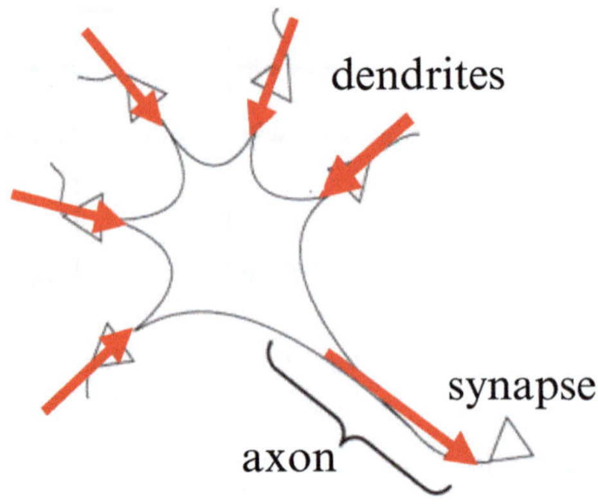

Fig. 11.20 Neuron

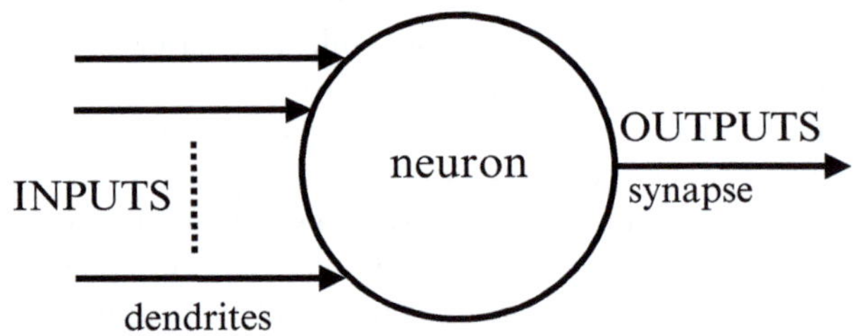

Fig. 11.21 Simplified neuron model

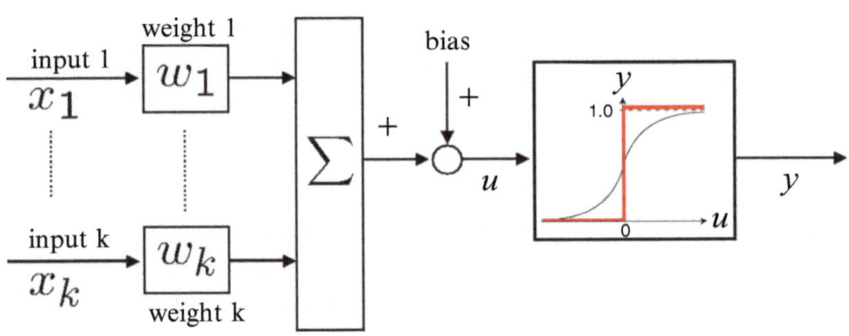

Fig. 11.22 Linear and non-linear parts of neuron model

outputs an exciting signal when the sum of the weighted input excitation exceeds some threshold value. Figure 11.21 depicts a model of a simplified neuron that is considered to be a multi input, single output system, while Fig. 11.22 shows part of the linear activation function yielding the sum of the weighted input signals and part of the non-linear inhibiting function comparing the sum with the threshold value. There are many types of artificial neural network models, including the multi-layered and mutually coupled neural network models. Figure 11.23 illustrates examples of these neural networks. A multi-layered neural network has three different layers: an input layer, an output layer and a middle layer, where the

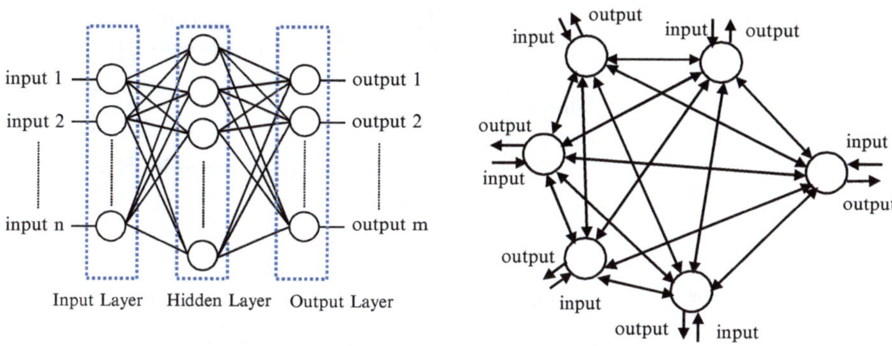

Fig. 11.23 Examples of neural network model

number of middle layers is either one or more than two and neurons in a layer are connected with neurons in another layer. On the other hand, in a mutually coupled neural network each neuron is connected with all other neurons.

For a learning problem in an artificial network model, the weights in the network undergo an adaptation cycle required to update the weights of the network until a state of equilibrium is reached, following which the weights no longer change. There are many kinds of learning methods for a neural network model, such as the Hebbian learning method, the competitive learning method, and the error back propagation learning method. A feed forward connection type neural network model is applied to pattern recognition, function approximation, and so on, while the mutually coupled neural networks model is applied to associative memory modeling optimization problems, and so on.

For more details refer to [16–18].

11.3.3 Evolutionary Computation

Evolutionary computation is a kind of searching algorithm based on biological evolution [18–20]. In this section, we focus specifically on the genetic algorithm (GA), which is one of the algorithms used to search for multi objective optimal solutions. GA was proposed by John Holland at the end of the 1960s based on Darwin's theory of evolution, i.e., the principle of Darwinism. Darwinism is based on the idea of natural selection and survival of the fittest, that is, only life adapting to its environment survives and evolves. As a result of the advancement in computing in the mid 1980s, many studies on GA have been carried out and GA has been applied to numerous fields.

A GA can find an optimal solution from many points of view in a wide solution space, making it appropriate for multi objective optimal solution problems. Furthermore, a GA also has a distinctive advantage in that if solutions are expressed and evaluated by some method, the GA can find an optimal solution without

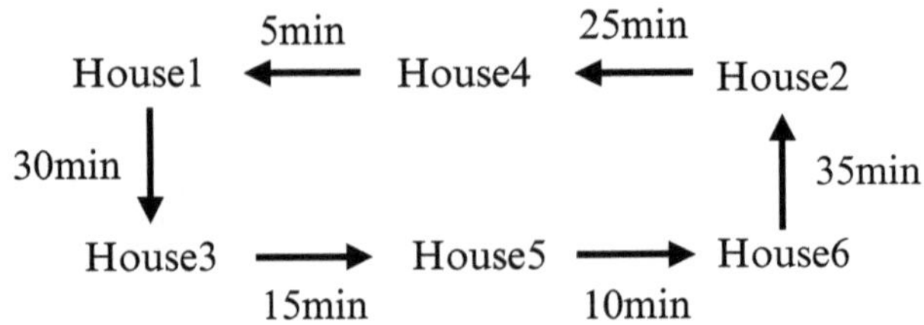

Fig. 11.24 Travelling salesman problem

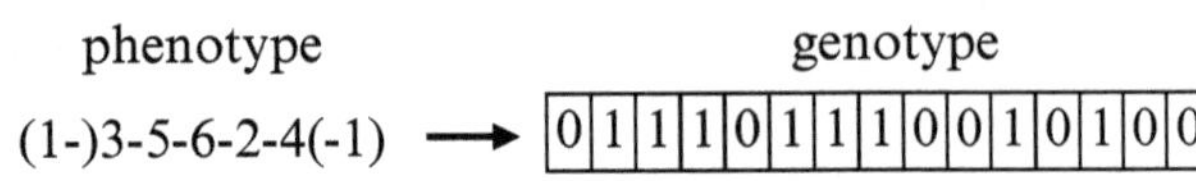

Fig. 11.25 Phenotype and genotype expressions

knowing the solving problem method or procedures. In terms of the expression of a solution, two expression methods are used. The first is the phenotype, i.e., the expression of a solution candidate in a real problem, while the other is the genotype expressing candidates of a solution as an individual in the GA. For example, let us consider the traveling salesman problem. A salesman starts at house 1, visits six other houses once each, and returns to house 1 in the shortest possible time, as shown in Fig. 11.24. The phenotype of a solution candidate expression is, e.g., 1-3-5-6-2-4-1. On the other hand, the genotype of the solution candidate expression is the expression in binary code. For example, the phenotype 1-3-5-6-2-4-1 is encoded as binary code, i.e., a chromosome, as shown in Fig. 11.25. As for the evaluation of a solution candidate, a fitness function is used, which is defined beforehand based on the objective of the given problem. In the traveling salesman problem, the fitness function is the time taken for traveling, e.g., 120 min for traveling 1-3-5-6-2-4-1.

Figure 11.26 depicts a flowchart of a GA. (1) In the first step, initial chromosomes are generated at random. In this step solution candidates of a real-world problem are encoded from a phenotype to a genotype, i.e., chromosomes, in the GA. (2) Each chromosome is evaluated as a solution candidate using a fitness function based on the given problem. In the traveling salesman problem, the time taken is calculated for each chromosome as its fitness value. (3) If an individual with a certain fitness value appears or if the GA operations have been repeated a fixed number of times, the GA procedures are stopped. Otherwise, the following GA operations are repeated. (4) Selection: the higher the fitness value individuals have, the more individuals will survive. The lower the fitness value individuals have, the more individuals will die. In this step various strategies are applied, such as roulette wheel selection, expected value selection, ranking selection, or tournament selection. This step is the implementation of the idea of natural selection. (5) Crossover: parts of chromosomes are replaced as shown in Fig. 11.27. There are many different crossover operations, such as one point crossover, many points crossover, and uniform crossover. (6) Mutation: parts of a chromosome are changed at random, as shown in Fig. 11.28. (7) Chromosomes for the next generation are generated using existing chromosomes and the abovementioned GA operations

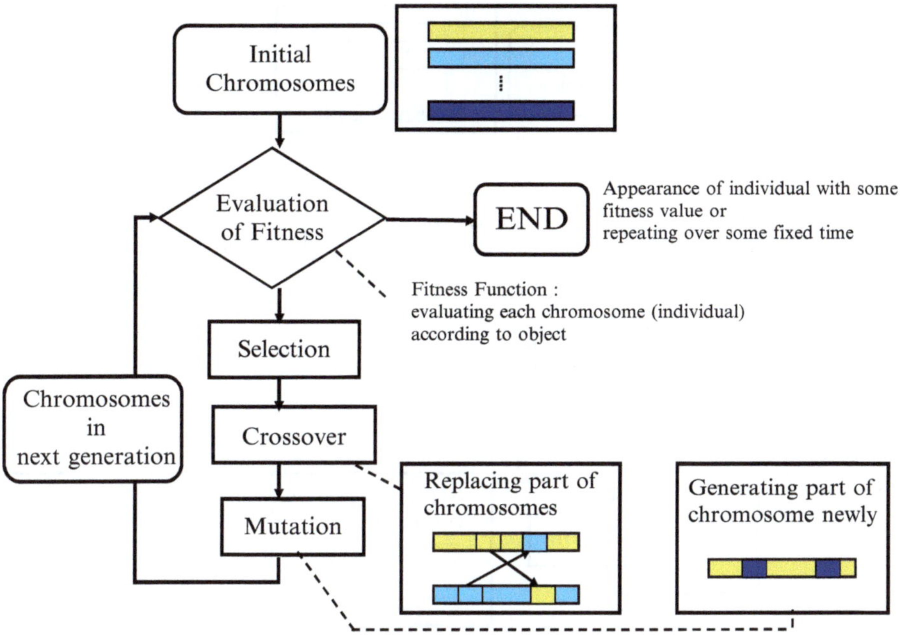

Fig. 11.26 Flowchart of GA

Fig. 11.27 Crossover

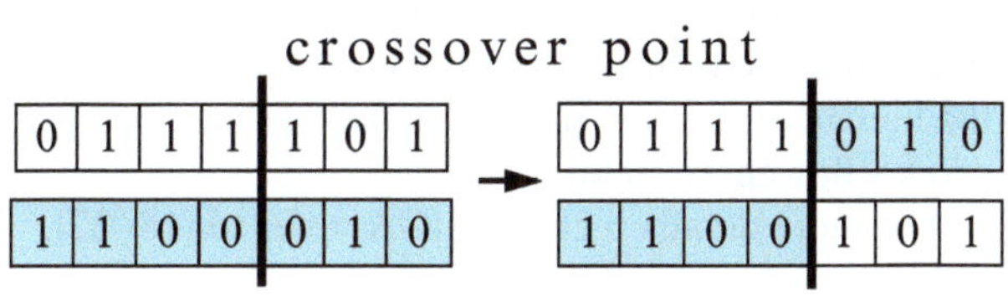

Fig. 11.28 Mutation

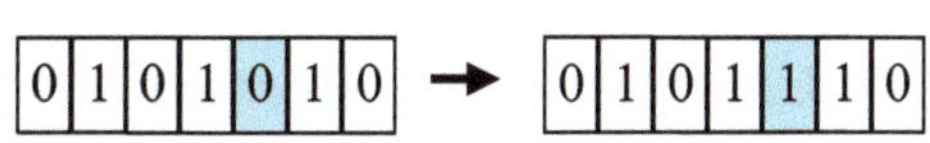

according to their fitness values. In this step various strategies, such as an elitist strategy, are applied. (8) Newly generated chromosomes are evaluated by the fitness function again, and procedures (3) through (8) are repeated.

In the above description of a GA, the question arises whether fitness functions can be defined for all problems. Let us consider the situation in which various pictures are to be evaluated from the viewpoint of a bright and lively picture. Can an objective fitness function be defined for the evaluation of brightness and liveliness? In real-world problems with complex problem structures or requiring evaluation of artworks related to human Kansei, it is usually difficult to define objective fitness functions. In such cases, however, humans can still evaluate solution candidates of the given problem, for example, evaluating pictures from the viewpoint of

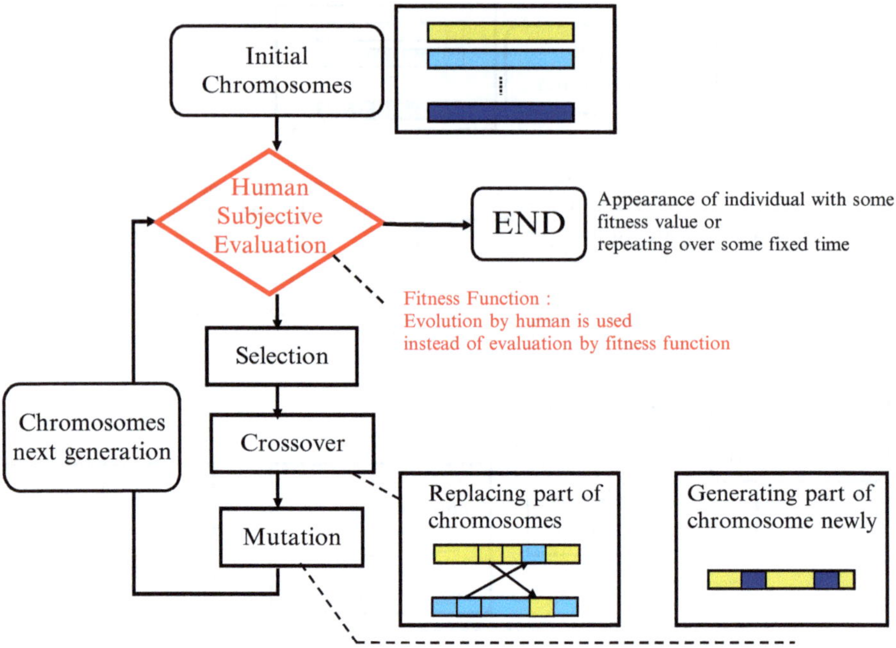

Fig. 11.29 Flowchart of IGA

brightness and liveliness. In order to deal with these problems, the concept of Interactive Genetic Algorithm (IGA) was proposed by Dawkins [21, 22]. In IGA, the human evaluation process is used instead of objective functions. Figure 11.29 gives a flowchart for an IGA.

For more details including IGA, refer to [18–22].

11.3.4 Case-Based Reasoning

Although case-based reasoning (CBR) [23, 24] is not necessarily included in soft computing technology, in this article, CBR is explained as one of the methods for Subjective-Kansei computing. CBR is a reasoning method based on experiential rules; that is, similar problems have similar solutions. Figure 11.30 presents an outline of CBR. (1) A given problem is analyzed and its features are extracted. (2) Cases that best fit the problem features are extracted from the case database. (3) These cases are applied to the given problem. If an extracted case has some features that do not fit the problem features, the case is modified. (4) If a case is evaluated to be a solution of the given problem, the case is saved as a success case. Cases that are evaluated not to be a solution are saved as failure cases so that the same failure is not repeated.

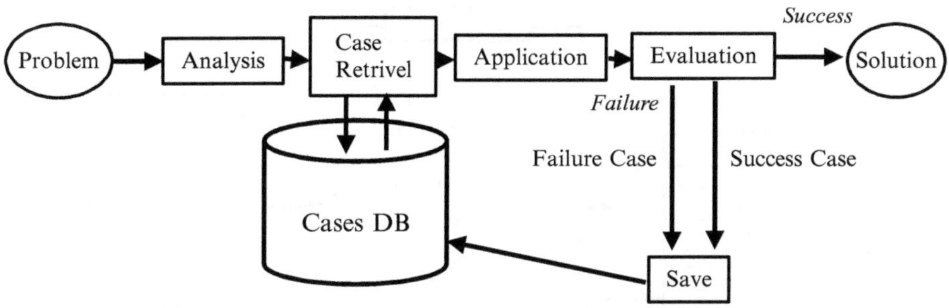

Fig. 11.30 Outline of CBR

CBR procedures can be explained by using the example of cooking miso soup. Let us assume that a user knows how to cook miso soup with tofu and cabbage and this is called Cook A's method. Now, this user tries to cook miso soup with tofu and wakame (a kind of seaweed), which is called Cook B's method. The process of cooking following Cook B's method is as follows. (1) The user recalls that Cook A's method is similar to that of Cook B. (2) This user modifies the cooking method of Cook A to correspond to that of Cook B; that is, one of the ingredients, cabbage, is changed to wakame. The cooking method is altered from cutting the cabbage and putting it into the miso soup to dunking wakame in water, cutting it, and then placing it in the miso soup. (3) The user applies the modified method to Cook B's method. (4) The user completes the cooking and eats miso soup with tofu and wakame.

CBR has been applied in medical diagnosis, fault diagnosis, trials, and so on. For more details, refer to [23, 24].

11.4 Application Examples

11.4.1 Caricature Drawing Using Words

Facial caricature drawings are usually created through image processing on a computer [25, 26]. However, this study has been carried out using words and a computer [27–29]. We introduce this study as an example of fuzzy theory applications.

A montage is usually constructed from a witness' testimony, and a facial sketch of a suspect is also drawn based on the information supplied by the witness. In this case, information from the witness is expressed using linguistic expressions. That is, impressions of a suspect's face and facial features are expressed in linguistic terms. A facial sketch artist interprets the meanings of the linguistic terms expressed by the eyewitness and draws the facial sketch. If the drawn sketch does

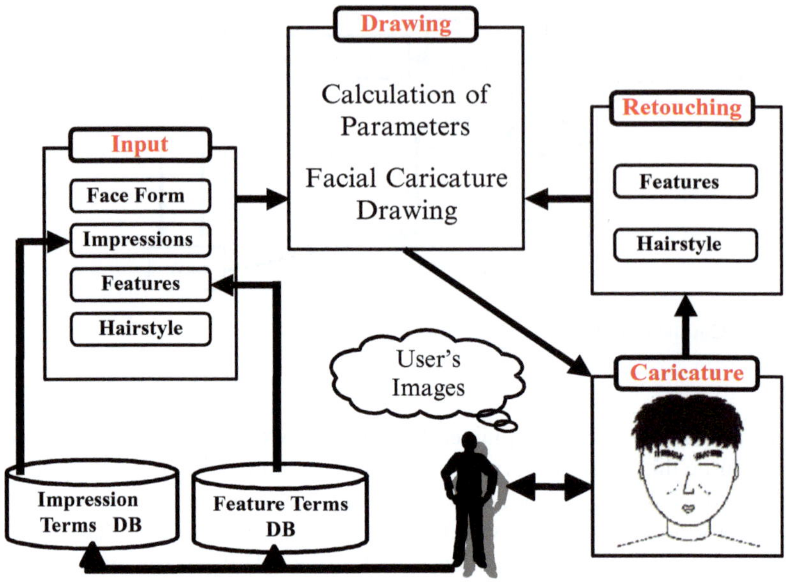

Fig. 11.31 Process of drawing facial caricatures

not match the witness' memory of the suspect's face and/or its facial features, the witness points out using words those parts of the sketch that need to be retouched, and the artist modifies the facial sketch based on the witness' comments. At the same time, the artist gains a better understanding of the meanings of the linguistic terms expressed by the eyewitness. In other words, the sketch artist draws the facial sketch of a suspect by learning from the eyewitness. Facial caricature drawing using words mimics the process of a facial sketch drawing based on the information of an eyewitness. Figure 11.31 shows the process of facial caricature drawing using words. The meanings of the input linguistic terms expressing impressions of the model's face, and its facial features are expressed by fuzzy sets. If the drawn facial caricature does not match the image of the model's face, the caricature is retouched according to words. The interaction between a human and a caricature drawing agent is performed in the feedback procedures shown in Fig. 11.31. The feedback denotes the evaluation of the drawn caricature as to whether images of the model's face are reflected in the caricature. Furthermore, the feedback procedures include a process of learning the meanings of linguistic terms expressing impressions and features of a model's face. When a model face caricature is drawn by several caricature artists, various types of caricatures are drawn, reflecting the different impressions and facial features of the model's face. This study considers subjectivity in facial caricature drawing. Figure 11.32 shows examples of facial caricature drawings.

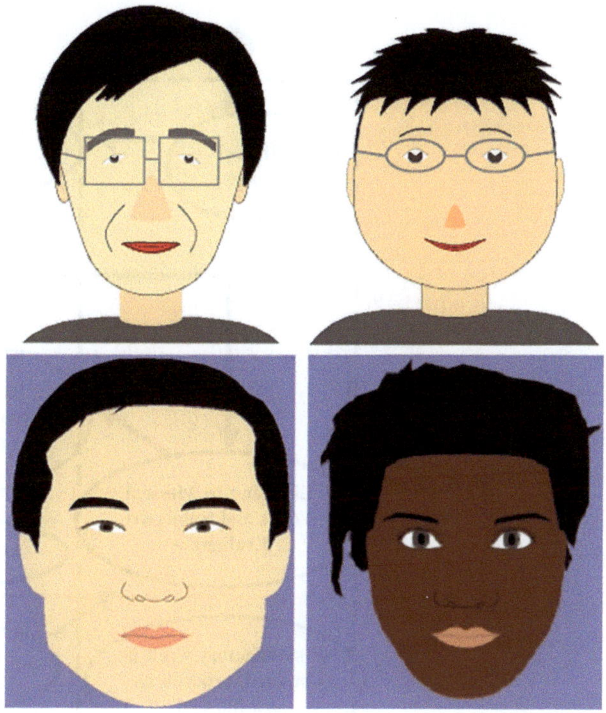

Fig. 11.32 Facial caricature examples

11.4.2 Music Composition Support

IGA has been applied to studies on music composition support or design support. This section mainly introduces a study on music composition support [30, 31]. Figure 11.33 shows the procedures for music composition. A user typically has his/her own mental image of a composed musical work. The music composition agent composes various musical works and presents these to the user. The human user listens to these musical works and evaluates them according to whether the presented musical works match his/her own image of the composed musical work. That is, the results of the GA operations are evaluated not by fitness functions, but by the human user himself/herself. The agent composes musical works again based on the user's evaluation. The procedures for music composition, presentation and evaluation are repeated until the user is satisfied with the presented musical work. Chromosomes expressing information on musical works are evolved according to the user's evaluation and finally contribute to a musical work matching the user's own image. The user's subjectivity and Kansei are reflected in the composed musical work. The music composition procedures of a human composer are similar to those of the interactive music composition agent, except that the human music composer is both the agent and user. A composer composes musical works, plays them, evaluates them and modifies them. These procedures are repeated until the

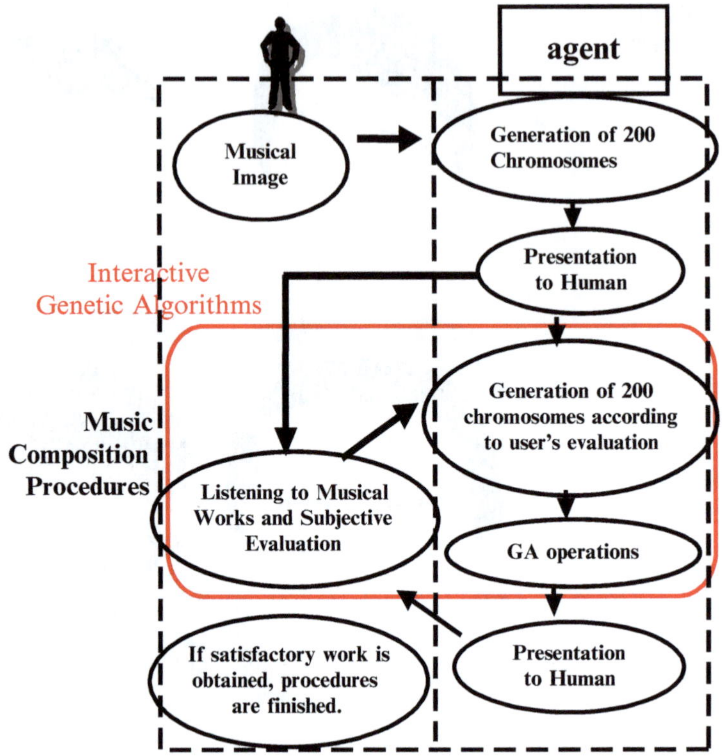

Fig. 11.33 Music composition procedures

composer is satisfied with the composed musical work. This study was extended to include operetta song generation based on impressions of a story scene using evolutionary computation, a neural network model, and Kansei information processing with the semantic differential method and co-occurrence of adjectives [32]. Figure 11.34 shows the operetta songs generated by this study, which reflect impressions of the story scenes represented by pictures (D), (B), (A), and (C) in this order. The procedures for clothes design and those for logotype design are similar to the ones shown in Fig. 11.33. Figure 11.35 shows examples of clothes design and logotype design obtained by these studies [33, 34].

11.4.3 Poker Game Partner Agent

A poker game is a type of game with imperfect information and bluffing, including slow play, as a strategy. Therefore, situation estimation and decision-making are usually difficult under the uncertainty of the poker game. This study considers the situation in which a human player makes a decision in cooperation with an

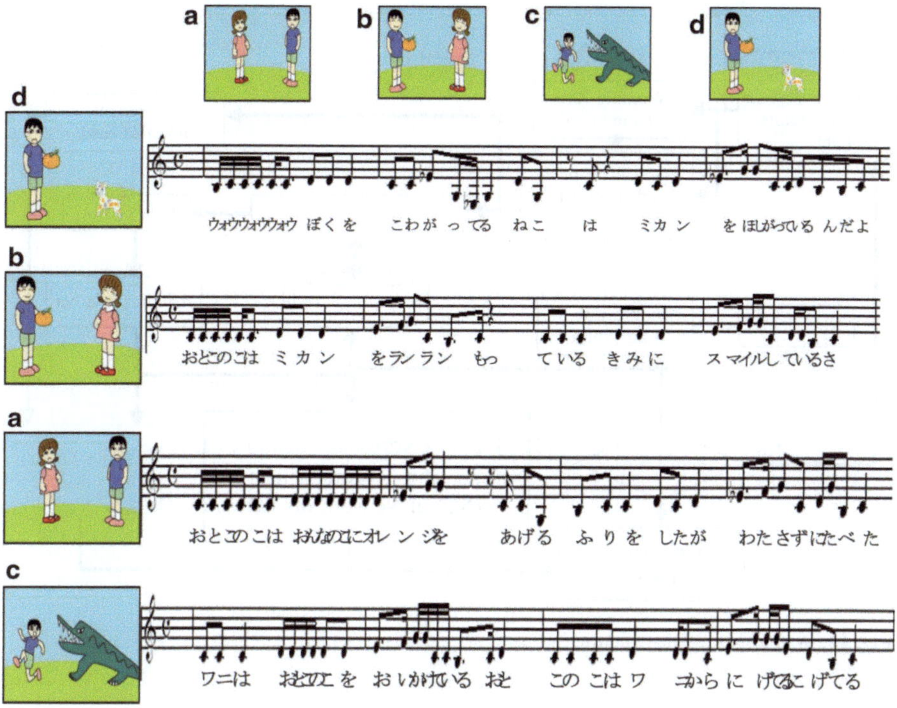

Fig. 11.34 Examples of composed operetta songs

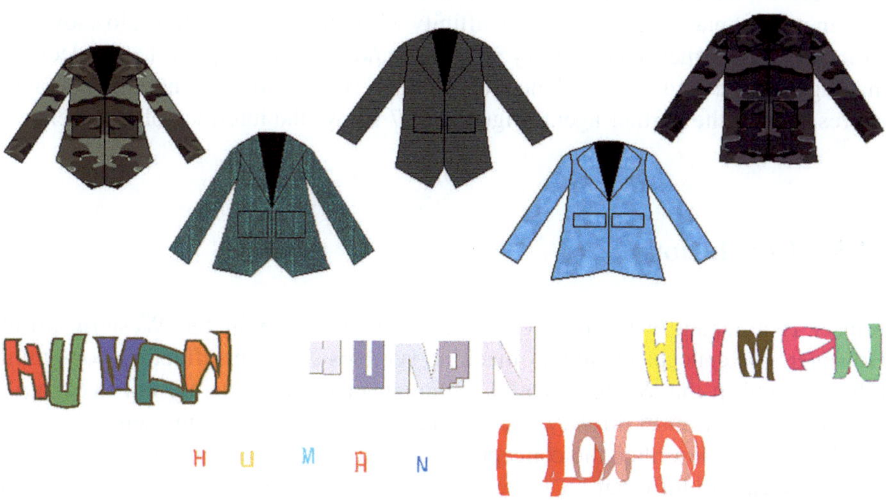

Fig. 11.35 Examples of clothes design and logotype design

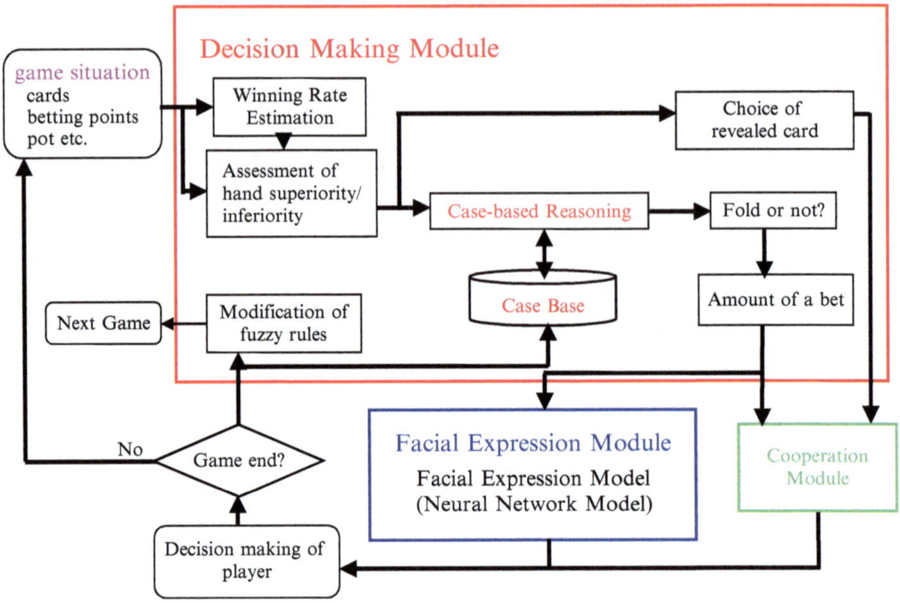

Fig. 11.36 Partner agent structure

agent [35–37]. As such, the agent is not merely a poker playing agent, but a partner agent that interacts with the human partner player on game strategy in a poker game. The partner agent presents not only linguistic expressions of game strategy or other advice, but also facial expressions according to the game situation so that the human partner player feels a sense of affinity with the agent. Figure 11.36 shows the structure of a partner agent. Fuzzy inference and CBR are applied to the decision making module and a neural network model is applied to generate the facial expressions of the partner agent. Figure 11.37 shows the interface of the agent.

11.5 Conclusions

Kansei is a Japanese term, and is difficult to translate in the Western world. However, the concept of human machine symbiosis [38] or affecting computing [39] is found in the Western world. Although these concepts are not necessarily associated with Kansei directly, they are related to Kansei in some sense.

This chapter described the concept of Subjectivity-Kansei computing for human subjective Kansei information processing in the interaction between a human and a computer agent. First, the features of human information such as subjectivity, ambiguity, vagueness, and situation dependence were introduced. These features

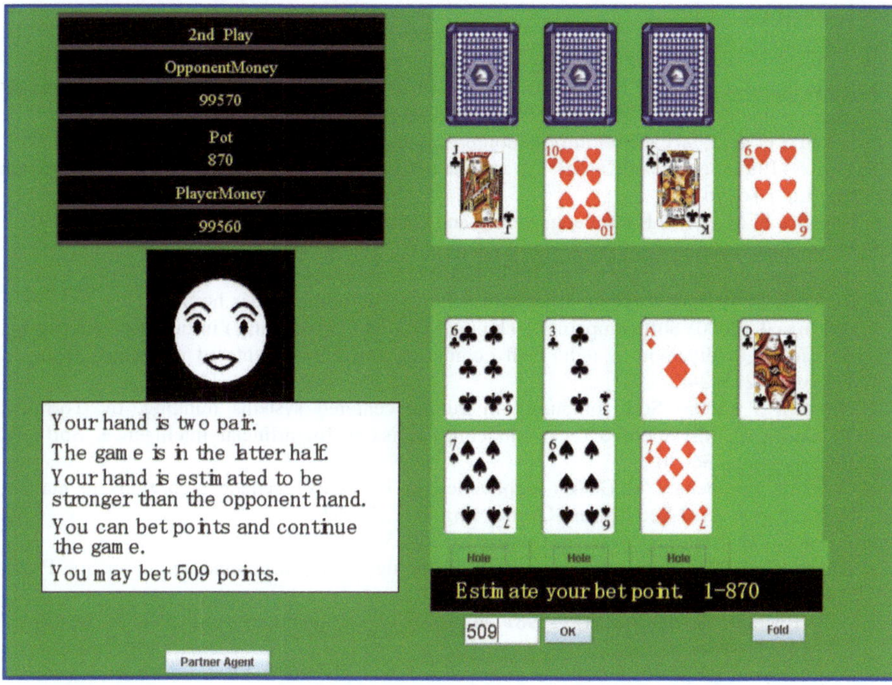
2nd Play
OpponentMoney
99570
Pot
870
PlayerMoney
99560
Your hand is two pair.
The game is in the latter half.
Your hand is estimated to be stronger than the opponent hand.
You can bet points and continue the game.
You may bet 509 points.
Hole
Hole
Hole
Estimate your bet point. 1-870
509
OK
Fold
Partner Agent

Fig. 11.37 Interface of agent

are quite opposite to the features of natural science, such as objectivity, uniqueness, universality, and reproducibility. Therefore, it is difficult to deal with Kansei information using a conventional approach requiring strictness or exactness of information. Next, other approaches for dealing with Kansei information were introduced, i.e., soft computing techniques comprising an all-encompassing technology including fuzzy theory, neural network models, and evolutionary computation. The techniques were designed to handle the features of human information and tolerate inaccuracy of information, albeit by sacrificing information accuracy. Finally, we introduced various study examples of Subjectivity-Kansei computing. The first considered sketch drawing using words and the application of fuzzy theory. The second was music composition support through the application of evolutionary computation, i.e., IGA. Finally, a poker game partner agent was introduced that incorporated fuzzy theory, neural networks, and CBR.

We sincerely hope that this chapter will contribute to ensuring that the importance of Subjectivity-Kansei computing in the interaction between a human and a computer agent gains the acknowledgement it deserves.

References

1. Japan Interdisciplinary Council (ed) (1993) Kansei and information processing–new possibility to computer science. Kyoritsu, Tokyo
2. Iguchi S et al (1994) Kansei information processing. Ohmusha, Tokyo
3. Tsuji S (1997) Science of Kansei – an approach to Kansei information processing. Saiensu-sha Co., Ltd., Tokyo
4. Nagamachi M (1997) Kansei engineering and comfort – preface. Int J Ind Eng 19(1):79–80
5. Japan Society for Fuzzy Theory and Systems (ed) (1998) Panel discussion: Kansei engineering. J Jpn Soc Fuzzy Theory Syst 10(3):426–444
6. Cybernics. http://www.cybernics.tsukuba.ac.jp/english/outline/index.html
7. Onisawa T (2000) Soft computing techniques in Kansei (emotional) information processing. In: Liu Z-Q, Miyamoto S (eds) Soft computing and human-centered machines. Springer, Tokyo, pp 215–248
8. Onisawa T (2005) Soft computing in human centered systems thinking. In: Torra V, Narukawa Y, Miyamoto S (eds) Modeling decisions for artificial intelligence. Springer, Heidelberg, pp 36–46
9. Onisawa T, Unehara M (2005) Application of interactive genetic algorithms to human-centered systems. J Soc Instrum Control Eng 44(1):50–57
10. Zadeh LA (1965) Fuzzy sets. Inf Control 8:338–353
11. Zadeh LA (1993) Applications of fuzzy technology and soft computing. J Jpn Soc Fuzzy Theory Syst 5:261–268
12. Li X, Ruan D, van der Wal AJ (1998) Discussion on soft computing at FLINS'96. Int J Intell Syst 13:287–300
13. Zimmermann HJ (1985) Fuzzy sets theory – and its applications. Kluwer-Nijhoff, Boston
14. Honda N, Ohsato A (1989) Introduction to fuzzy engineering. Kaibundo, Tokyo
15. Cox E (1998) The fuzzy systems handbook, 2nd edn. Academic Press, Cambridge, MA
16. Kosoko B (1992) Neural networks and fuzzy systems, a dynamical systems approach to machine intelligence. Prentice-Hall, Englewood Ciffs
17. Amari S (ed) (1993) New development of neural net. Saiensu-sha Co., Ltd., Tokyo
18. Konar A (2000) Artificial intelligence and soft computing, behavioral and cognitive modeling of the human brain. CRC Press, Boca Raton
19. Kitano H (ed) (1993) Genetic algorithm. Sangyo-Tosho, Tokyo
20. Fogel DB (1995) Evolutionary computation – toward a new philosophy of machine intelligence. IEEE Press, New York
21. Kitano H (ed) (2000) Genetic algorithm (4). Sangyo-Tosho, Tokyo
22. Takagi H (2001) Interactive evolutionary computation: fusion of the capabilities of EC optimization and human evaluation. Proc IEEE 89(9):1275–1296
23. Kolodner JL (1993) Case-based reasoning. Morgan Kaufmann, San Mateo
24. Nitta K (2005) Knowledge and inference. Saiensu-sha Co., Ltd., Tokyo
25. Hayashi J, Murakami K, Koshimizu H (1997) A method for automatic generation of caricature profile in PICASO system. Trans Inst Electron Inf Commun Eng D-II J80-D-II(8):2102–2109
26. Sato M, Saigo Y, Hashima K, Kasuga M (2003) An automatic facial caricature method for 2D realistic portraits using characteristic points. In: Journal of the 6th Asian design international conference, vol 1, E-40, Tsukuba
27. Onisawa T, Hirasawa Y (2004) Facial caricature drawing using subjective image of a face obtained by words. In: Proceedings of 2004 I.E. international conference on fuzzy systems, Budapest, p 1370
28. Benhidour H, Onisawa T (2008) Interactive face generation from verbal description using conceptual fuzzy sets. J Multimed 3(2):52–59
29. Benhidour H, Onisawa T (2010) Interactive learning of verbal descriptors meanings for face drawing system. J Adv Comput Intell Intell Inform 14(6):606–615

30. Unehara M, Onisawa T (2003) Music composition system with human evaluation as human centered system. Soft Comput 7(3):167–178, Springer
31. Unehara M, Onisawa T (2005) Music composition by interaction between human and computer. New Generat Comput 23(2):181–191, Ohmsha/Springer, Tokyo
32. Ishizuka K, Onisawa T (2010) Operetta songs generation system based on impressions of story scenes. In: Proceedings of joint 5th international conference on soft computing and intelligent systems and 11th international symposium on advanced intelligent systems, Okayama, pp 831–836
33. Ogata Y, Onisawa T (2008) Interactive clothes design support system, LNCS 4985, revised selected papers (the 14th international conference on neural information processing, WMC-2, 2007), Springer, Kitakyushu, pp 657–665
34. Yamamoto S, Onisawa T (2009) Interactive support system for logotype design based on user's feelings. In: Proceedings of the human interface symposium, Tokyo, pp 697–704
35. Ohsone K, Onisawa T (2008) Friendly partner system of poker game with facial expressions. In: Proceedings of 2008 I.E. symposium on computational intelligence and games, Perth, pp 95–102
36. Ohsone K, Onisawa T (2009) Cooperative partner agent of seven-card-stud poker. In: Proceedings of 2009 international fuzzy systems association world congress and 2009 European society for fuzzy logic and technology conference, Lisbon, pp 1595–1600
37. Osone K, Onisawa T (2011) Interactive learning agent of poker game. In: Proceedings of 12th international symposium on advanced intelligent systems, Suwon, pp 303–306
38. Gill KS (ed) (1996) Human machine symbiosis – the foundations of human-centred systems design. Springer, London
39. Picard RW (2000) Affective computing. The MIT Press, Cambridge, MA

Chapter 12
Human–Machine Coagency for Collaborative Control

Toshiyuki Inagaki

Abstract This chapter discusses some of the issues that are at the center of designing human–machine coagency where humans and smart machines collaborate and cooperate sensibly in a situation-adaptive manner. The first is the issue of authority and responsibility. It is argued that the machine may be given authority to improve safety and to alleviate possible damage to the human–machine system, even in a framework of human-centered automation. The second is the issue of the human operator's overtrust in and overreliance on automation, where it is argued that possibilities and types of overtrust and overreliance may vary depending on the characteristics of the automated system. The importance of the design of a human–machine interface and human–machine interactions is included in the discussion.

Keywords Human supervisory control • Function allocation • Human-centered automation • Authority and responsibility • Overtrust and overreliance • Levels of automation

12.1 Introduction

Many complex industrial processes are semi-autonomous, where computers control the processes based on directives given by human operators. The configuration of such human–machine systems is called *human supervisory control* [1]. Why are these processes semi-autonomous, rather than being fully automated? The most obvious reason is that we cannot foresee in the design phase all possible events that may occur during the expected lifetime of the processes. Thus, although designers have tried to replace human operators with machines for higher efficiency or

T. Inagaki (✉)
Graduate School of Systems and Information Engineering, University of Tsukuba, Tsukuba, Japan
e-mail: inagaki.toshiyuki.gb@u.tsukuba.ac.jp

Y. Sankai et al. (eds.), *Cybernics: Fusion of human, machine and information systems*,
DOI 10.1007/978-4-431-54159-2_12,

reliability, their attempts have not been entirely successful [2]. Actually, human operators have to be on-site to perform the task of "completing the system design," that is, adapting the system for situations that the designers did not anticipate [3].

It then becomes an important design decision to determine what humans should do and what machines should do. One design strategy is to allocate to machines every function that can be automated, and to allocate to operators the leftover functions for which no automation technologies are available. Another strategy is to find an allocation that ensures economic efficiency. Such design strategies are typical examples of *technology-centered automation* [4]. This may remind readers of Charlie Chaplin's *Modern Times*, which portrays a comic yet unpleasant world in which seemingly intelligent machines demand that humans obey or adapt to the machines.

Human-centered automation is what is needed to realize an environment in which humans and machines can work cooperatively in a more sound and comfortable manner [5]. However, in spite of the popularity of the term, it is still not clear what human-centered automation really means. In fact, there are several different meanings of human-centered automation, as pointed out by Sheridan [6]. He discusses the possible and even probable contradictions that may be found in the "definitions" of human-centered automation [6].

Human–machine systems are not yet free from problems, such as (a) loss of *situation awareness*, in which operators fail to grasp the process state exactly [7]; (b) *automation-induced surprises*, in which operators fail to understand what the computers are doing and why [8, 9], and finally (c) *complacency*, in which operators monitor processes less often than is required (or is optimal) [10, 11]. These problems tell us that human–machine interaction is not well designed even in modern processes created with highly advanced technologies.

This chapter discusses some of the issues that are at the center of designing human–machine coagency where humans and smart machines collaborate and cooperate sensibly in a situation-adaptive manner. One of the main topics in this chapter is the issue of authority and responsibility. It is argued that the machine may be given authority to improve safety and to alleviate possible damage to the human–machine system, even in a framework of human-centered automation. The second is the issue of the human operator's overtrust in and overreliance on automation, where it is argued that the possibilities and types of overtrust and overreliance may vary depending on the characteristics of the automated system. The importance of the design of a human–machine interface and human–machine interactions is included in the discussion.

12.2 Human Supervisory Control

The classical definition of human supervisory control of complex systems emerged in the 1960s during research on teleoperated lunar vehicles and manipulators [12]. A problem to consider in 1967 was the long delay between the ordering of a remote

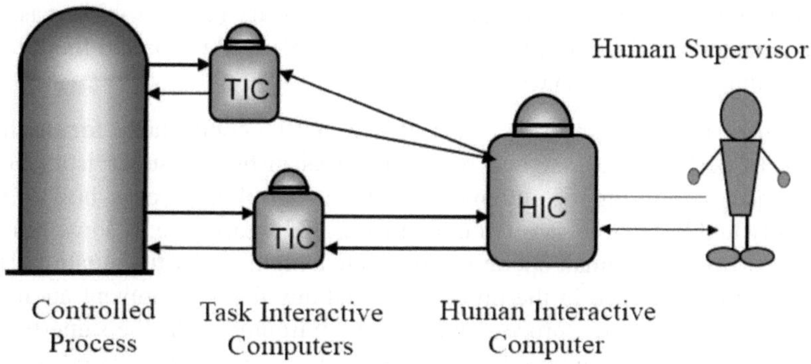

Fig. 12.1 Human supervisory control model

manipulator and the feedback from it. Instead, a supervisory control structure was proposed, where a remote computer would communicate with the manipulator, orchestrating intermediate events between orders (short-range goals) by remote closed-loop control. Back "on earth", the local computer handled the "supervisory loop", and the loop was closed by the operator. The local computer could also mimic predicted behavior of the manipulator feedback providing direct "quasi-feedback" [12].

There are many modern technical systems that are controlled by machine intelligence (or computers) under human supervision. Nuclear power plants, glass-cockpit aircraft, and computerized manufacturing systems are typical examples of such systems. These systems are neatly represented by a human supervisory control model [1].

The human supervisory control model distinguishes four units, as depicted in Fig. 12.1: (a) the human supervisor, (b) the human-interactive computer (HIC), (c) one or more task-interactive computers (TICs), and (d) the technical process to be controlled. The human supervisor decides what to do and issues commands to a HIC that has the capability to communicate with the human supervisor. The HIC understands high-level language to interpret directives given by the human supervisor, provides him/her with system state information in an integrated form, and issues decision aids or alert messages when appropriate. Upon receiving a supervisor's directive, the HIC issues the necessary commands to at least one TIC. The TIC then performs feedback control using its actuators and sensors.

Deciding what to do is one of the tasks that the human supervisor must perform. Sheridan [1] distinguished five phases of the human's supervisory control effort:

(i) Planning what needs to be done over some period of time and matching these requirements with available resources;
(ii) Teaching the computer what it needs to know to perform its assigned function for that time period;
(iii) Monitoring the automatic action to check that everything is proceeding as planned;

(iv) Intervening in the automatic action when necessary (such as in the case of an emergency situation or after completion of a planned task); and finally
(v) Learning from experience.

As can be imagined from (i) to (v), it may not be comfortable for the human operator to perform the assigned roles and tasks in human supervisory control. For instance, monitoring the automation and the controlled process, both of which are usually highly reliable, is often monotonous and wearisome. If something goes wrong, however, the human operator jumps into a highly stressful situation. He/she is requested to intervene in the process without any delay to prevent an anomaly from propagating into the process and/or the environment. At the same time, the human operator is not supposed to shut down a normal process based on a false alarm, which makes an intervention task very difficult and stressful.

12.3 Collaboration Failures Between Humans and Machines

Let us take, as an example, a highly automated aircraft. It is recognized that aviation automation has contributed to the improvement of aircraft safety. Nevertheless, aircraft incidents and accidents still occur. We realize that sometimes automation can result in incidents or accidents that were not possible in the "old days". Given below are a couple of examples.

(a) The automation (TIC) is strong enough to counteract effects caused by an anomaly occurring in the aircraft. However, the automation is sometimes *silent* [13]; it does not explicitly tell pilots how hard it is to control the aircraft. Pilots may thus often fail to recognize what is happening. An example of this is an in-flight upset incident in 1985, when a Boeing 747 aircraft dived 32,000 ft near San Francisco. The rightmost (#4) engine failed while flying at 41,000 ft on autopilot, and the aircraft began to suffer an undesirable yaw movement. The autopilot attempted to compensate the yaw movement by lowering the left wing; the rudder could not be used at the time. The pilots were busy focusing their attention on the decreasing airspeed. After some unsuccessful attempts to increase the airspeed, the captain finally decided to disconnect the autopilot so that he could fly the aircraft manually. Upon autopilot disconnection, the aircraft rolled to the right, nosed over, and dived steeply until the captain regained control of the aircraft at 9,500 ft. For further details of this incident, refer to ([5], p. 308), amongst others.
(b) The automation (HIC) may *surprise* pilots by doing what the pilots did not explicitly order. Suppose a pilot directed the HIC to do task A. The HIC may think that task B must be done simultaneously, and may perform both tasks without conveying its decision clearly to the pilot. The pilot would then be confused about the aircraft's behavior. They may say, "what is the autopilot

doing, and why is it doing that?" The crash of an Airbus A330 aircraft at Toulouse in 1994 is such an example. The accident occurred in a test flight to investigate the performance of the autopilot during an engine-out go-around. The pilot commanded the autopilot on at 6 s after takeoff. The goal of the autopilot was to climb to the 2,000 ft altitude that had already been set. The autopilot calculated at which point it had to activate the altitude acquisition transition mode (ALTSTAR) to achieve a smooth level-off. The calculation was done while both engines (the A330 is a two-engine aircraft) were operating perfectly and the aircraft was climbing very fast, at a vertical speed of 6,000 ft/min. Eight seconds after takeoff, the left engine was reduced to idle, to simulate an engine failure. At the same time, the autopilot activated the ALTSTAR mode, but the pilots did not realize the mode change. Under the simulated engine failure condition, the aircraft could climb at only 2,000 ft/min. To achieve the already calculated climb rate (6,000 ft/min), the autopilot continued pitching the aircraft up. Although the pilots realized that something was wrong, they could not understand what the autopilot was doing or why. Since there was no pitch limit in the ALTSTAR mode, the pitch angle reached 31.6°. At that stage, the captain disconnected the autopilot. It was, however, too late to regain control of the aircraft. For further details of this incident, see [14], amongst others.

12.4 Function Allocation

Suppose we need to design a human–machine system with specific missions or goals. We first have to identify functions that are needed to accomplish the goals. We then get to the stage of function allocation. *Function allocation* refers to the design decisions that determine which functions are to be performed by humans and which by machines. Various strategies for function allocation have already been proposed.

12.4.1 Traditional Strategies for Function Allocation

Rouse [15] classified traditional function allocation strategies into three types. The first category is termed *comparison allocation*. Strategies of this type compare the relative capabilities of humans versus machines for each function, and allocate the function to the most capable agent (either the human or the machine). The most famous MABA-MABA (what "men are better at" and what "machines are better at") list is possibly the one edited by Fitts [16], and reproduced in Table 12.1.

The second type is called *leftover allocation*. Strategies of this type allocate to machines any function that can be automated. Human operators are assigned the leftover functions for which no automation technologies are available.

The third type is *economic allocation*. Strategies of this type try to find an allocation that ensures economic efficiency. Even if some technology is available

Table 12.1 The fitts list

Humans appear to surpass present-day machines with respect to the following:
1. Ability to detect small amounts of visual or acoustic energy
2. Ability to perceive patterns of light or sound
3. Ability to improvise and use flexible procedures
4. Ability to store very large amounts of information for long periods and to recall relevant facts at the appropriate time
5. Ability to reason inductively
6. Ability to exercise judgment
Present-day (in the 1950s) machines appear to surpass humans with respect to the following:
1. Ability to respond quickly to control signals and to apply great forces smoothly and precisely
2. Ability to perform repetitive, routine tasks
3. Ability to store information briefly and then to erase it completely
4. Ability to reason deductively, including computational ability
5. Ability to handle highly complex operations, i.e., to do many different things at once

Taken from Fitts [16], Hancock and Scallen [17], and Price [18]

to automate a function, if the cost of automating the function is higher than that of hiring a human operator, the function is assigned to the operator.

Note here that the traditional strategies just described consider "who does what." Such design decisions yield function allocations that are *static*. In other words, once a function has been allocated to an agent, the agent is responsible for the function at all times.

12.4.2 Static Function Allocations Are Not Always Appropriate

Suppose design decisions are made using either the leftover or the economic allocation strategies. These strategies do not reflect any human characteristics or viewpoints, and the resulting function allocation may be puzzling for operators. An operator may ask, "Am I meant to be responsible for this function, or is the automation?" Also, there is no guarantee that the allocations provide the operators with job satisfaction.

The comparison allocation may be better for the operators than either the economic or leftover allocation. However, the comparison allocation is not free from criticism either. Price [18] and Sharit [19] claimed that the list by Fitts is overly generalized and non-quantitative. Sheridan [6] pointed out that, "in order to make use of the Fitts MABA-MABA list, one needs data that are context dependent, but these data are mostly unavailable" (p. 59). He argued, referring to the ideas of Jordan [66], that "the idea of comparing the human with the machine should be thrown out but the facts about what people do best and what machines do best should be retained," and "the main point of retaining the Fitts list is that people and machines are complementary" (p. 59). A *complementary strategy* can be seen in KOMPASS [20].

Even though operators are allocated only those functions in which people surpass machines, this superiority may not hold at all times and for every occasion. Operators may get tired after long hours of operation, or they may find it difficult to perform the functions under the given time constraints. This implies that "who does what" decisions are not sufficient; instead "who does what and when" considerations are needed for the success of function allocation, which means that function allocation must be dynamic.

12.4.3 Adaptive Function Allocation

Suppose that a human and a machine are to perform their assigned functions for some period of time. The operating environment may change as time goes by, or performance of the human may degrade gradually as a result of psychological or physiological reasons. If the total performance or safety is to be strictly maintained, it may be wise to reallocate functions between the human and the machine. A scheme that modifies function allocation dynamically depending on the situation is called *adaptive function allocation*. The automation that operates under an adaptive function allocation is called *adaptive automation* [21–27].

Adaptive function allocation makes use of selected criteria to determine whether, how, and when functions need to be reallocated. The criteria reflect various factors, such as changes in the operating environment, loads or demands on operators, and performance of operators (see, e.g., [22, 27]).

Note that an active agent for a function may change from time to time in an adaptive function allocation. In such a case, it is said that the authority (for controlling the function) is traded from one agent to another. In other words, *trading of authority* means that either the human or the computer is responsible for a function, and an active agent changes alternately from time to time [1, 27].

Who makes the decision on trading of authority? More precisely, who decides whether the control of a function must be handed over and to which agent? Must a human operator decide, or may the machine (or the computer) decide? The former type is called the *human-initiated trading of authority*, and the latter the *machine-initiated trading of authority*. Which strategy is to be adopted is a hard problem to solve, as will be discussed later.

12.5 Machine Support for Human Information Processing

Four stages can be distinguished in human information processing: (a) perception, (b) situation understanding, (c) action selection, and (d) action implementation. It is well known that humans can fail in a variety of ways at each stage of information processing. Machines are supposed to provide humans with support at each stage. Parasuraman et al. [28] claimed that "the four-stage model of human information processing has its equivalent in system functions that can be automated," and they described human–machine interactions by distinguishing the following four classes of functions: (1) information acquisition, (2) information analysis, (3) decision and action selection, and (4) action implementation.

In order to understand how machines can perform these four classes of functions, let us consider two examples in aviation.

Example 1 The *traffic alert and collision avoidance system* (TCAS) is a family of airborne devices designed to help pilots avoid mid-air collisions [29]. Its functionality includes the following:

1. Information acquisition: The TCAS transmits interrogations at 1,030 MHz that transponders on nearby aircraft respond to at 1,090 MHz. By decoding the replies, the position and altitude of the nearby aircraft can be ascertained.
2. Information analysis: Based on the range, altitude, and bearing of a nearby aircraft, the TCAS performs range and altitude tests to determine whether the aircraft is a threat.
3. Decision and action selection: When the nearby aircraft is declared a threat, the TCAS selects an avoidance maneuver (to climb or descend) that will provide adequate vertical miss distance from the threat. If the threat aircraft is equipped with TCAS, the avoidance maneuver will be coordinated with the threat aircraft.
4. Action implementation: The TCAS issues a resolution advisory (RA) to inform the pilot of the appropriate avoidance maneuver. However, the TCAS does not perform any avoidance maneuvers itself.

Example 2 The *enhanced ground proximity warning system* (EGPWS) is designed to help pilots avoid a ground collision [30]. The functionality of this system is described as follows:

1. Information acquisition: The EGPWS collects air data, radio altitude, barometric altitude, and airplane position through various other systems, including the Flight Management System, GPS, and the airplane air data system.
2. Information analysis: Having received the above data, the EGPWS determines a potential terrain conflict by using its self-contained worldwide airport and terrain databases. The EGPWS displays the terrain as dotted patterns with colors indicating the height of the terrain relative to the current airplane altitude.
3. Decision and action selection: The EGPWS continuously computes terrain clearance envelopes ahead of the airplane. If these envelopes conflict with data in the terrain database, the EGPWS sets off alerts.
4. Action implementation: The EGPWS issues a caution-level alert approximately 40–60 s before a potential terrain conflict, and sets off a warning-level alert approximately 20–30 s before a conflict. However, the EGPWS does not perform any conflict avoidance maneuvers itself.

It is clear from Examples 1 and 2 that it is not the machine (TCAS or EGPWS) but the human pilot who implements a collision avoidance maneuver. Why is the action implementation stage not fully automated in these examples? The answer lies partly in the principles of human-centered automation.

12.6 Human-Centered Automation

12.6.1 Principles of Human-Centered Automation

Human-centered automation is an approach to realize a work environment in which humans and machines collaborate cooperatively (see, e.g., [4–6, 31–33]). Of the various application domains, it is aviation for which human-centered automation has been defined in the most detail. Aviation has a long history of automation and has experienced both its benefits and costs (see, e.g., [5, 34]). The principles of human-centered automation, given in Table 12.2, have resulted from studies to resolve the costs of automation, such as the out-of-the-loop performance problem, loss of situation awareness, complacency or overtrust, and automation surprises (see, e.g., [4, 5, 8, 13, 35–38]).

12.6.2 Domain-Dependence of Human-Centered Automation

Human-centered automation can be domain-dependent and thus must be established properly for each transportation mode: e.g., "human-centered automation for automobiles" can be quite different from "human-centered automation for aviation systems" as defined in Table 12.2. Such domain-dependence may stem from the quality of human operators and time criticality [39].

Quality of Human Operators The quality of human operators varies depending on whether they are professional or non-professional. Professional operators, such as airline pilots, are trained thoroughly and continuously so that their knowledge and skills are great enough to use smart and sometimes complicated machines correctly. On the other hand, in cases of non-professional operators, such as private

Table 12.2 Principles of human-centered automation in aviation

The human bears the ultimate responsibility for the safety of an aviation system
Therefore:
* The human must be in command
* To command effectively, the human must be involved
* To be involved, the human must be informed
* Functions must be automated only if there is a good reason for doing so
* The human must be able to monitor the automated system
* Automated systems must, therefore, be predictable
* Automated systems must be able to monitor the human operator
* Each element of the system must have knowledge of the others' intent
* Automation must be designed to be simple to learn and operate

car drivers, it would not be sensible to assume that their levels of knowledge and skills are high. Their understanding of the machine functionality could be incomplete, or even incorrect.

Example 3 Adaptive cruise control (ACC) systems are designed to reduce the driver's workload by freeing him/her from frequent acceleration and deceleration. Sometimes, these systems may be differentiated into two classes: high-speed range ACC and low-speed range ACC. When there is a leading vehicle to follow, both ACC systems control the speed of their host vehicle so that the time gap to the target vehicle may be maintained. Suppose the sensor loses sight of the target vehicle; the high-speed range ACC remains in its active state. In the case of low-speed ACC, the behavior differs depending on the control logic design. Two designs are possible. One allows the ACC to stay in its active state, while the other puts it into a standby state. It is hard to tell which design is better. Loss of mode awareness or automation surprises can occur in both design types, but in different ways. Inagaki and Kunioka [40] conducted an experiment with a PC-based driving simulator where no information was displayed regarding the state of the ACC. Subjects were requested to carry out procedures of perception, decision-making, and action implementation based on their mental models. Even after training or experience with the ACC systems on the simulator, loss of mode awareness and automation surprises were observed, which reflect the overtrust in and distrust of automation, and inertness of mental models.

Time Criticality Time criticality differs appreciably depending on the transportation mode. Consider the following examples in which an automated warning system is available to the operator.

Example 4 When a nearby aircraft is declared a threat, the TCAS selects an avoidance maneuver (to climb or descend) and issues an RA to inform the pilot of the appropriate avoidance maneuver (see Example 1). The estimated time to the closest point of approach is 15–35 s. The pilots are thus meant to respond to the RA within 5 s.

Example 5 Nowadays, certain types of automobile are equipped with a *forward vehicle collision warning system*. This system detects a vehicle in the front and measures its speed and the distance to it using a distance radar (mostly, a laser radar or a millimeter-wave radar) sensor mounted on the vehicle. If there is a possibility of collision with the vehicle in front, the system sets off a collision warning. The estimated time to collision is at most a few seconds.

As can be seen in the above examples, if the collision warning were against another aircraft, there would be sufficient time for the pilot to grasp the situation, validate the given warning, and initiate a collision avoidance maneuver. In the case of the automobile, however, time criticality is extremely high, and the driver has only a small amount of time to avoid a collision, as explained in Example 5.

12.7 Two Questions on Human-Centered Automation

The principles of human-centered automation given in Table 12.2 seem to be convincing. However, there are two questions that may not be easy to answer, namely: (1) Does the statement that, "The human must be in command," have to hold at all times and for every occasion? (2) What should the machine do if it detects inappropriate behavior or performance while monitoring the human? Is the machine only allowed to give warnings? Or, is it allowed to act autonomously to resolve the detected problem?

12.7.1 Who is in Charge and in Command?

Humans may not always be able to cope with the given situation. Consider the following example.

Example 6 The ITARDA (Institute for Traffic Accident Research and Data Analysis) analyzed data of automobile collisions that occurred in Japan during the period 1993–2001. Among all the collisions of four-wheeled vehicles, they extracted 359 head-on or rear-end collisions for which microscopic data were available with respect to the following: vehicle speed and location at which the driver perceived the possible danger, vehicle speed immediately before the collision, and vehicle speed at the time of the collision. They found that 13.9 % of the drivers tried to avoid the collision by steering and braking, 42.6 % by braking alone, and 5.6 % by steering alone. Surprisingly, 37.9 % of the drivers neither changed the steering direction nor applied the brakes [41].

How can we design a system that assists the driver when a collision is imminent? Consider the following two types of *advanced emergency braking system* (AEBS).

Example 7 (AEBS of type 1) The radar sensor monitors the vehicle in the front. When the system determines, based on the distance and relative speeds of the vehicles, that a collision is to be anticipated, it issues a warning to the driver and retracts the seatbelts.

Example 8 (AEBS of type 2) When the system determines that a collision is to be anticipated, it issues a warning to the driver and retracts the seatbelts, as in the case of type 1. When the system determines that a collision is imminent and that the driver is late in responding to the situation, it retracts the seatbelts firmly and applies an automatic emergency brake.

The AEBS of type 1 enhances the driver's situation awareness (SA). If the driver applies the brakes quickly enough, no collision will occur. However, if the driver fails to respond to the situation, the system provides no active help, and therefore a collision would be inevitable. The AEBS of type 2 has two layers of assistance: enhancement of the driver's SA, and trading of authority from the human to the machine, when appropriate. Trading of authority occurs in this case to support action implementation when the driver fails to take action at the right time. The system applies the emergency brakes, not based on the driver's directive, but based on its own decision. Note that one of the principles in Table 12.2, "the human must be in command," is violated here. However, that does not necessarily mean that an AEBS of type 2 should not be allowed. On the contrary, Example 6 suggests the need for machine-initiated trading of authority in emergencies.

Professional operators may also fail to respond appropriately to the situation encountered, as shown in the following example.

Example 9 An analysis of *controlled flight into terrain* incidents of commercial jet airplanes during the period 1987–1996 found that 30 % of the accidents occurred when the traditional *ground proximity warning system* (GPWS) failed to detect terrain ahead, while 38 % were due to late warning of the GPWS or improper pilot response [30].

Problems of "no warning" or "late warning" may be resolved by introducing the EGPWS (see Example 2), which enhances the pilot's understanding of the height of the terrain relative to the aircraft altitude. The problem of "pilot's late response" may not be fully resolved by the EGPWS, since it is the human pilot who is responsible for a collision avoidance maneuver. However, there is a system in which the collision avoidance maneuver is initiated automatically. The automatic ground collision avoidance system (Auto-GCAS) for combat aircraft is such an example [42]. When a collision with the terrain is anticipated, the system gives a pull-up warning. If the pilot takes aggressive collision avoidance action, the system does not step in any further. If the pilot does not respond to the warning, the system takes over control from the pilot and executes an automatic collision avoidance maneuver. When no further threatening terrain is found, the system returns control back to the pilot. Thus, the Auto-GCAS determines when to intervene and when to return command of the aircraft back to the pilot.

Even in case of aircraft, a machine-initiated action implementation has been playing important roles in relieving the pilot's physical and/or mental load. One of classical example is the *mach-trim system*. When an aircraft flies at a high speed, it receives a pitch-up moment and thus the control column needs to be pushed forward to maintain the altitude. If airspeed becomes higher than a certain value, aircraft obtains a pitch-down moment and thus the control column must be pulled back, which caused difficulty in old days in maneuvering aircraft. Now the mach-trim system handles the problem without human intervention and creates positive stability for the aircraft.

Another example may be the *thrust asymmetric compensation* (TAC) system on the twin-engine Boeing 777. The TAC helps the pilot to cope with the yawing effect when an engine fails during the takeoff role. When the TAC senses that the thrust levels differ 10 % or more between the two engines, it initiates rudder control automatically so as to minimize the yaw and to make it possible for the pilot to center the control column.

More recent examples can be found in the A350. Airbus Corporation is trying to develop an automatic system that, upon a TCAS RA, initiates an appropriate maneuver to steer the aircraft away from a potential mid-air threat without input from the flight crew [43]. Airbus is also considering equipping the A350 with an automatic system that would provide a warning to the flight crew when unsafe cabin pressure is detected. If the crew does not cancel the warning or take positive control of the aircraft, the system performs an automatic side-step maneuver to the right of the designated airway to avoid conflict, and then puts the aircraft into a rapid descent at maximum operating speed [44]. These classical and new examples show that automatic action implementation based on the machine's decision is of value even in the aviation domain.

12.7.2 What if the Machine Finds that the Human's Action is Inappropriate?

A human's control action or directive to the machine may be classified into three categories: (1) a control action that needs to be carried out in a given situation; (2) a control action that is allowable in the situation and thus may either be done or not done; and (3) a control action that is inappropriate and thus must not be carried out in the situation. Assuming some sensing technology (or machine intelligence, provided by a computer), two states may be distinguished for each control action: (a) "detected," where the computer determines that the human is performing the control action, and (b) "undetected," in which the control action is not detected by the computer.

Figure 12.2 depicts all possible combinations of a control action and its state. Among these, case α shows the situation where the computer determines that the human operator is (too) late in performing or ordering a control action that must be carried out in the given situation. A typical example of case α in the automobile domain is that, in spite of rapid deceleration by the leading vehicle, a following driver does not apply the brakes owing to some distraction. Case β indicates a situation where the computer determines that the human operator has misunderstood the given circumstances and the control action that he/she is taking or has requested does not suit the situation. A typical example of case β is when a driver is about to change the steering direction to enter an adjacent lane without noticing that a faster vehicle is approaching from behind in that lane.

A question that must be asked for case α is whether the computer should be allowed to initiate without human intervention the control action (such as applying the brakes) that the human should have taken, or whether the computer is allowed only to set off a warning to urge the human to perform manually the control action that the situation requires. A question asked for case β is whether the computer should be allowed to prohibit the control action (such as altering the steering direction to make a lane change) that the human is trying to do, or whether the

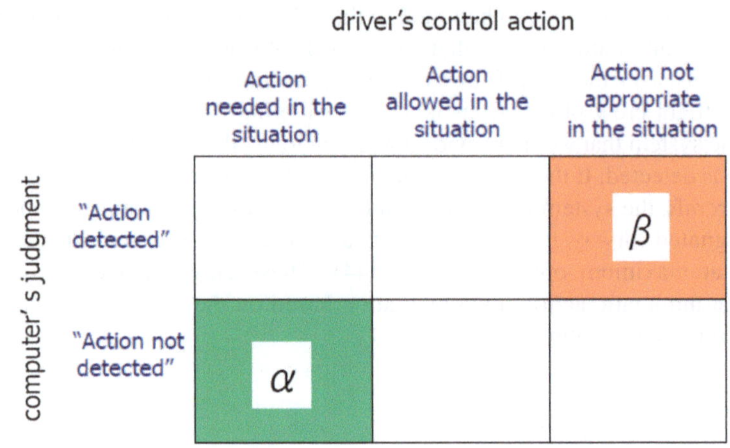

Fig. 12.2 Control actions in a given situation

computer is allowed only to set off a warning to tell the human that his/her action should be stopped immediately.

Suppose the computer always knows what control action is appropriate, besides just detecting (or not) whether a control action has been taken. Then it would be almost obvious that the computer should be allowed to initiate the control action that the human failed to perform in case α, and to prohibit the human's control action that does not suit the given circumstances in case β, considering the following facts: (1) humans do not always respect or respond to warnings, and (2) humans need a certain amount of time to interpret the warnings and thus a time delay is inevitable before effective actions can be taken. It is, however, too optimistic to assume that the computer never makes an error in judging whether the human's response to the situation is inappropriate. Inagaki and Sheridan [45] have analyzed in a probability theoretic manner the efficacy of the computer's support in both cases α and β, under a realistic setting that the computer's judgment may be wrong. They have proven that the computer should be allowed to act autonomously in certain situations via machine-initiated trading of authority based on its decision.

There are some studies that have analyzed the efficacy of the computer's support for cases α and β by conducting cognitive experiments [46–48]. The question posed in these studies was, "What type of support should be given to a car driver when it is determined, via some sensing and monitoring technologies, that the driver's situation awareness may not be appropriate to a given traffic condition?" For cases α and β in Fig. 12.2, two types of driver support were compared: (a) warning-type support in which an auditory warning is given to the driver to enhance SA, and (b) action-type support in which an autonomous safety control action is executed to avoid a collision. Although both types of driver support were effective, the investigators also observed some problems.

The warning-type driver support is fully compatible with human-centered automation, because the driver always retains final authority over the automation. Most drivers who participated in the experiments in [46–48] accepted the warning-type support for both cases α and β. However, the warning-type of driver support sometimes failed to prevent a collision when the driver did not respect the warning. A driver's typical and 'reasonable' disregard for a correct warning occurs when the warning is based on an object that is invisible to the driver. This fact suggests a limitation of a purely human-centered automation design in which the human remains the final authority at all times and for every occasion.

The machine-initiated action taken for case α may be straightforward, viz., merely implement the control action that the human failed to perform in a timely manner. For case β, machine-initiated control actions are classified into two groups: (a) *hard protection*, in which the human is not given authority to override the computer's corrective control action initiated based on its judgment that "the human's action does not suit the situation"; and (b) *soft protection*, in which the human is given authority to override the computer's corrective control action, even though the computer has determined that "the human's action does not suit the situation".

It is reported in [46, 48] that action-type support with hard protection characteristics sometimes failed to receive *acceptance* from drivers, although it was successful in collision prevention. The most prominent reason for this lack of acceptance is as a result of the hard protection characteristic in cases when there is a conflict of intention between the human and the computer. The soft protection type action support may also fail to prevent a collision from occurring, especially when the driver misinterprets why protective action has been triggered and for which object. It may not be sensible to blame the drivers even though they 'interpret' a given situation incorrectly, because they might have to interpret the situation based on limited information collected within a limited time period. An issue that arises is how to design a human–machine interface and interaction for cases when something is invisible to the driver, yet visible to the machine.

12.8 Overtrust and Overreliance

If machines are capable of correcting and preventing 'erroneous or inappropriate' behavior of the human operator, as discussed in Sect. 12.7, the human operator will trust and rely on the machines. Problems may occur if the human operator places too great a trust in or reliance on the machine without learning or knowing its limitations. This section presents a theoretical framework for describing and analyzing the human operator's overtrust in and overreliance on smart machines, and illustrates the framework with examples of assistance systems for car drivers [49].

12.8.1 Overtrust

Overtrust in an advanced driver assistance system (ADAS) is an incorrect diagnostic decision to conclude that the assistance system is trustworthy, when it actually is not. This section gives two axes for discussing overtrust in the assistance system. The first axis is the *dimension of trust* and the second the *chance of observations*.

Dimension of Trust The first axis describes in what way the driver can overrate trust. Lee and Moray [50] distinguished four dimensions of trust: (a) foundation, representing the fundamental assumption of natural and social order; (b) performance, resting on the expectation of consistent, stable, and desirable performance or behavior; (c) process, depending on an understanding of the underlying qualities or characteristics that govern behavior; and (d) purpose, resting on the underlying motives or intents. Three types of overtrust can be distinguished depending on which of the dimensions, (b) through (d), is overrated; the first dimension, (a), is usually met in the case of an ADAS.

Overrating dimension (b) can be explained by the following thought pattern of a driver: "The assistance system has been responding perfectly to all the events that I have encountered so far. Whatever event may occur, the system will take care of it appropriately." Improper evaluation of dimension (c) is seen in the case where a driver who has been using an assistance system without having read the user manual is thinking, "It would be quite alright even if I do not know the details of how the system functions." Overestimation of dimension (d) is illustrated by the case where a driver believes that "I do not understand why my assistance system is doing such a thing. However, it must be doing what it thinks is necessary and appropriate."

Chance of Observations The second axis for investigating overtrust describes how often the driver can see the assistance system functions. The chance of observations affects the ease with which a mental model of the assistance system is constructed. The possibility of a driver's overtrust can differ depending on whether the assistance system is for use in normal driving or in an emergency.

Consider the ACC as an example of an assistance system to reduce driver workload in normal driving. Based on the large number of opportunities to observe the ACC functioning repeatedly in daily use, it would be easy for the driver to construct a mental model of the ACC. If the driver has been satisfied by the 'intelligent' behavior of the ACC, it would be natural for him/her to place trust in the assistance system. However, the trust can sometimes be overtrust. Suppose the driver encounters a new traffic condition that is seemingly similar to a previous one, but is slightly different. By expecting that the ACC should be able to cope with the situation without any intervention by the driver, the driver could be overestimating the functionality of the ACC.

Next, consider the AEBS as an example of an assistance system activated only in an emergency to ensure the driver's safety. It would be rare for an ordinary driver to see the AEBS working, and he/she may not be able to construct a complete mental model of the system owing to the limited number of chances to experience the

AEBS working. Drivers may have been told (by the car dealer, for instance) that the AEBS would be activated automatically in an emergency. However, they may not be fully convinced because of the lack of opportunities to observe for themselves that the AEBS works correctly and consistently when necessary.

12.8.2 Overreliance

Overreliance on an ADAS is an incorrect action selection decision determining to rely on the assistance system by placing overtrust in it. Regarding overreliance on automated warning systems, there are relevant studies in the aviation domain (see, e.g., [36, 51–53]). Suppose that the automated warning system almost always alerts the human when an undesirable event occurs. Although it is possible for a given alert to be false, the human can be confident that there is no undesirable event as long as no alert is given. (A similar situation can occur in the automobile domain when the driver is provided with a communication-based alert from the road infrastructure to let the driver know of an approach or existence of cars on a crossroad behind some buildings). Meyer [52] used the term ‘reliance’ to express this response by the human. If the human assumed that the automated warning system would always give alerts when an undesirable event occurred, the human’s thinking would constitute overtrust in the warning system, and the resulting reliance on the warning system would be overreliance. The definition of overreliance on the ADAS, given at the beginning of this section, is a generalization of that of overreliance on warning systems in previous studies in the sense that the goal of the assistance system is not only to set off warnings but also to execute control actions.

Two axes are provided for overreliance on assistance systems. The first axis represents the *benefits expected* and the second the *time allowance for human intervention*.

Benefits Expected The first axis describes whether the driver can derive some benefit by relying on the assistance system. Suppose the driver assigns the ACC all the tasks for longitudinal control of the vehicle. This may enable the driver to find time to relax his/her muscles after stressful maneuvering, or to allocate cognitive resources to finding the correct route to the destination in complicated traffic conditions. In this way, relying on the assistance system sometimes yields extra benefit to the driver, when the system is used in normal driving.

The discussion can be quite different in the case of the AEBS. The AEBS is activated only in an emergency, and the time duration for the AEBS to fulfill its function is very short, say only a few seconds. It is thus not feasible for the driver to allocate the time and resources, saved by relying on the AEBS, to something else to derive extra benefit from only a few seconds. A similar argument may apply to other assistance systems designed for emergencies.

Time Allowance for Human Intervention The second axis, time allowance for human intervention, describes whether the driver can intervene in the assistance system's control if the driver determines that the system performance differs from what he/she expected. In the case of the ACC, it is not difficult for the driver to intervene to override the ACC if its performance is not satisfactory. However, in the case of the AEBS, it would be unrealistic to assume that the driver could intervene in the control by the AEBS if he/she decides that the AEBS's performance is not satisfactory, because the whole process of monitoring and evaluating the AEBS's performance as well as the decision and implementation of intervention must be done within a few seconds.

12.8.3 From Collision Damage Mitigation to Collision Avoidance

Based on the framework given in Sects. 12.8.1 and 12.8.2, the design guidelines for the AEBS were revised in 2011 by a task force of the Advanced Safety Vehicle (ASV) project, Ministry of Land, Infrastructure and Transport (MLIT), Japan.

If the host vehicle is approaching the leading vehicle relatively quickly, most AEBSs first tighten the seatbelt and add a warning to urge the driver to apply the brakes. If the AEBS determines that the driver is too late in braking, it applies the brake automatically based on its decision. However, in Japan the AEBS has been implemented as a *collision damage mitigation system*, instead of a *collision avoidance system*. Behind the design decision to 'downgrade' the AEBS, there has been concern among the regulatory authorities that "if an ADAS were to perform every safety control action automatically, the driver would become overly reliant on the assistance system, without paying attention to the traffic situations himself or herself."

Although the above 'concern' seems to be reasonable, there have been some discussions in the ASV project that more precise investigations are necessary so as not to lose opportunities for drivers (especially elderly drivers) to benefit from an assistance system that would back them up or even override them when appropriate. The MLIT set up a task force in December 2009 in the ASV project to investigate future directions for driver assistance in the light of (1) driver's overtrust in and overreliance on the ADAS, and (2) authority and responsibility between the driver and the automation.

The following argument was made by the ASV task force: "Since the AEBS is activated only in cases of emergency, it would be very rare for an ordinary driver to see how the system works (i.e., chance-of-observation axis). It is thus hard for the driver to construct a precise mental model of the AEBS, and may be hard for him/her to engender a sense of trust in the system (i.e., dimension-of-trust axis). However, it is known that people may place inappropriate trust (i.e., overtrust) without having any concrete evidence proving that the object is trustworthy.

Now, let us assume that the driver places overtrust in the assistance system. We have to ask whether the driver may rely on the system excessively (i.e., overreliance). In case of AEBS, even if the driver noticed that the system's behavior was not what was expected, no time may be left for the driver to intervene and correct it (i.e., time allowance for human intervention). In spite of that, does the driver rely on the AEBS and allocate his/her resource to something else at the risk of his/her life (i.e., benefits expected)? The answer would be negative."

The ASV task force approved the above argument and decided that the AEBS should be developed as a collision avoidance system, instead of a collision damage mitigation system. The task force investigated design requirements for such a collision avoidance AEBS so that it would not interfere with the driver's own actions (by ensuring that it applied the automatic brakes at the latest time possible), but would still effectively avoid a collision with an obstacle ahead. Human factor viewpoints played major roles in determining the design requirements for the timing of the AEBS to initiate automatic emergency braking and its deceleration rate. In fact, these were determined by analyzing drivers' braking behavior in normal and critical traffic conditions. Moreover, a couple of conventional requirements for the AEBS were abolished from the human factors viewpoints (e.g., to reduce mode confusion or automation surprise). Based on the conclusions of the ASV task force, the MLIT has been revising the design guidelines for the AEBS. The new guidelines will be announced to the public in 2012.

12.9 Combination of Agents with Limited Capabilities

Suppose we are trying to design an ADAS that *makes the invisible visible* by providing information or images of objects or events that the driver cannot see directly, gives an alert when the driver is late in responding to the situation, and provides control inputs to the host vehicle when necessary. It is not an easy task to implement an ADAS that can cooperate well with the human driver. Coagency between the driver and an ADAS would fail quite easily if the interface and interaction were not appropriate. Let us consider an ensemble of a human driver and an ADAS, where each of the agents has limited ability. Figure 12.3 illustrates the combinations of limited capabilities of the driver and the ADAS [54].

Region 1 depicts the situation where both agents can see the objects. However, an automation surprise can occur if what the driver sees is different from what the ADAS sees and if the driver fails to notice this. Figure 12.4 illustrates a situation where the driver was astonished by the ACC's acceleration; the driver had expected the ACC to slow down in response to the deceleration of the leading vehicle A that the ACC had been following thus far. This case represents an actual experience by the author. A probable cause of the acceleration by the ACC could be that the ACC detected vehicle B and switched the target vehicle from A to B. In the author's host vehicle, the instrument panel displayed an indication implying that the ACC was

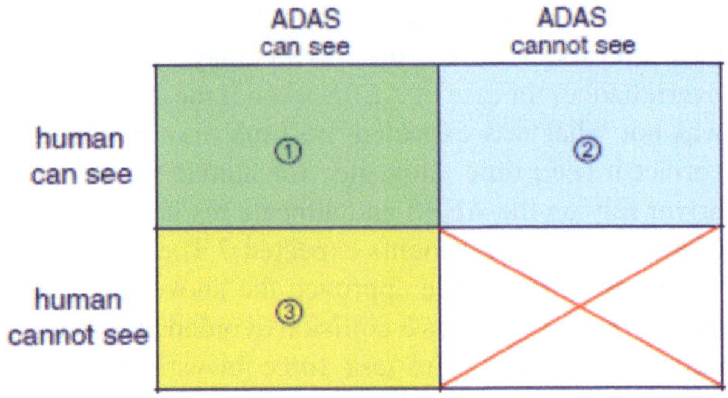

Fig. 12.3 Combination of agents with limited capabilities

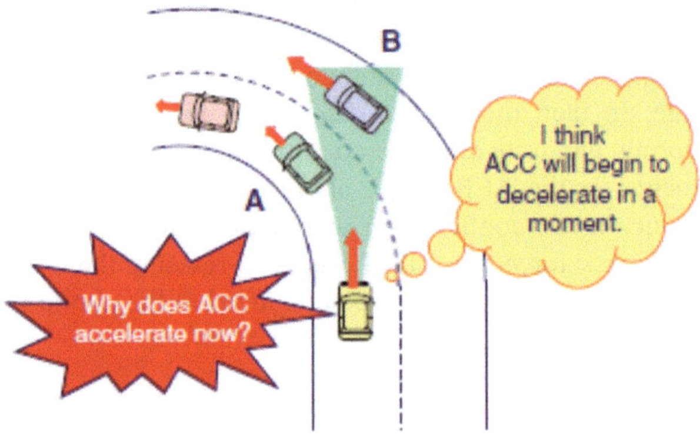

Fig. 12.4 What the driver see ≠ what the ADAS sees

following 'a target vehicle.' It did not explain which was the target vehicle or that the target vehicle had indeed changed.

Even when what the driver sees is exactly the same as what the ADAS sees, problems may occur if the way of thinking differs between the two agents. A typical case is illustrated in Fig. 12.5, where one agent tries to avoid a collision into an object by braking, while the other agent avoids this by changing the steering direction.

Region 2 depicts the situation where the ADAS cannot see the object that the driver sees. A typical case is shown in Fig. 12.6. While following vehicle A with the ACC, the driver noticed that vehicle B in the adjacent lane might be cutting in just ahead. The driver then expected the ACC to initiate deceleration shortly. However, the ACC did not decelerate. On the contrary, it accelerated. This case illustrates another of the author's actual experiences. The reason for the surprising behavior by the ACC is that the ACC did not sense vehicle B because it was outside the sensor range, and accelerated in response to the acceleration of vehicle A. No human interface is currently available to visualize a sensor's range, which means that there are no clues to help the driver recognize the extent of what the ACC can see.

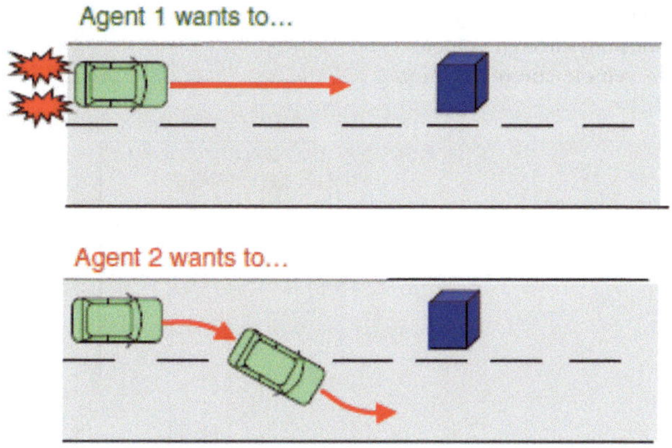

Fig. 12.5 Conflict of intentions

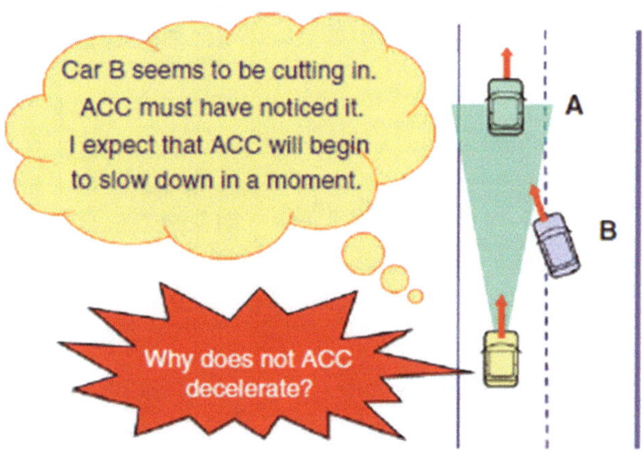

Fig. 12.6 Failure to recognize limit of capability

Region 3 represents the situation where the ADAS can see what the driver cannot see. The support offered to the driver by the ADAS aims to make the invisible visible. A typical case is depicted in Fig. 12.7, where the driver tries to find the right moment to enter a through street. It is hard for the driver to check whether cars are approaching from the right because the building on the corner blocks the driver's view to the right. The ADAS provides the driver with an alert message, "A car coming from right!" based on the information obtained through vehicle-to-vehicle or vehicle-to-infrastructure communication. If the human interface is poorly designed, it may not be easy for the driver to understand whether the alert was aimed at vehicle A or B in Fig. 12.8. If the alert is given too early and the driver has experienced a *false alert* before, he/she may suspect that the given alert is yet another false alert (Fig. 12.9).

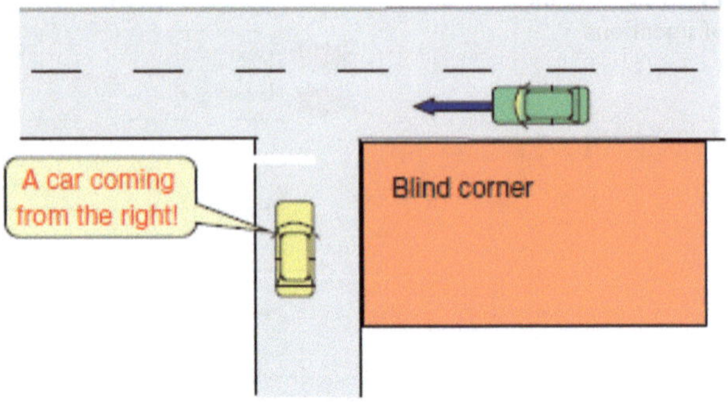

Fig. 12.7 Proximity warning through vehicle-to-vehicle communication

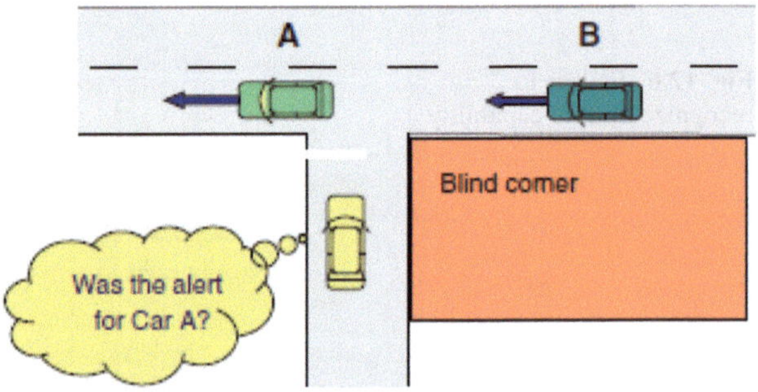

Fig. 12.8 Ambiguity caused by an imprecise interface

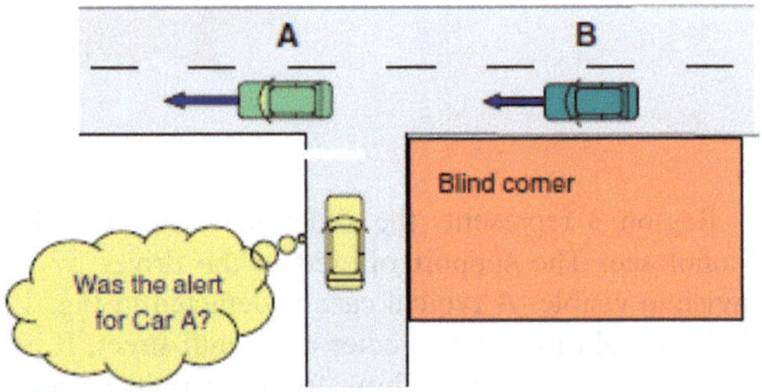

Fig. 12.9 Warning may be disregarded without any validation

The difficulties in the above cases stem from the fact that the driver cannot see the car (or cars) that the alert is attempting to highlight. No concrete evidence is available for the driver to validate the alert. All that the driver can do is either believe in the alert (i.e., wait at the intersection for a while) or ignore the alert (i.e., turn into the through road). This is an issue of *trust*; the driver's attitude toward the alert may be judged in hindsight as appropriate trust, overtrust, or distrust.

12.10 Viewpoints for Designing Human–Machine Coagency

Let us discuss how we should design the functionality to assist human operators appropriately and in a context-dependent manner. Discussions should consider two aspects: enhancement of situation awareness, and design of authority.

12.10.1 Enhancement of Situation Awareness

Human interface design is a central issue for enhancing situation awareness, avoiding automation surprises, and establishing appropriate trust in automation. The implemented human interface must enable the human to: (1) recognize the intention of the automation, (2) understand why the automation thinks what it does, (3) share the situation awareness with the automation, and (4) show the limits of the functional abilities of the automation.

Enhancement of situation awareness corresponds well with the human-centered automation concept, in which the *human locus of control* is claimed. However, as noted earlier, non-professional operators may not be able to cope with the given situation. Even professional operators may not respond to the situation appropriately; recall the mid-air crash on July 1, 2002, in which two TCAS-equipped aircraft collided over southern Germany [55, 56]. When a conflict developed between the two TCAS-equipped aircraft, the TCAS software determined which aircraft should climb and which should descend. One of the aircraft descended according to the TCAS resolution advisory. The other aircraft also descended, despite its TCAS instructing the pilot to climb, thus causing the mid-air collision. As described by Example 1 in Section 12.5, the TCAS is not given any authority to force a pilot to follow its resolution advisory.

12.10.2 Design of Authority

Human-computer interactions can be described in terms of the *level of automation* (LOA). Table 12.3 gives an expanded version, in which a new LOA appears between levels 6 and 7 in the original list by Sheridan [1]. The added level, called level 6.5, was first introduced in [57] to avoid automation surprises induced by automatic actions, when the actions are indispensable in ensuring system safety in emergencies.

The following example illustrates how important it is to choose an appropriate LOA to ensure comfort and safety of semi-autonomous human–machine systems.

Table 12.3 Scales of levels of automation (expanded version)

1.	The computer offers no assistance; the human must do it all
2.	The computer offers a complete set of action alternatives, and
3.	narrows the selection down to a few, or
4.	suggests one, and
5.	executes that suggestion if the human approves, or
6.	allows the human a restricted time to veto before automatic execution, or
6.5	executes automatically after telling the human what it is going to do, or
7.	executes automatically, and then necessarily informs the human
8.	informs the human after execution only if he/she asks
9.	informs the human after execution if it, the computer, decides to
10.	The computer decides everything and acts autonomously, ignoring the human

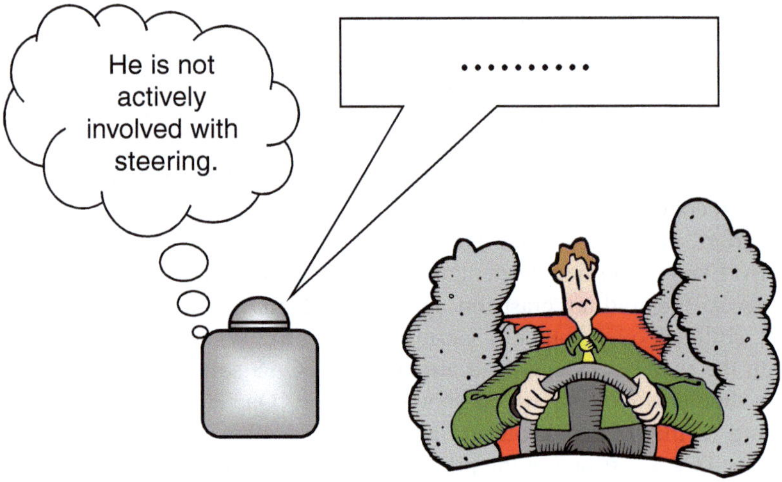

Fig. 12.10 What should the computer say to the minimally involved driver?

Example 10 Suppose a man is driving a car in which the lane keeping assistance (LKA) is operational. LKA is a system that recognizes the lane through image processing technology and provides the driver with assisted steering torque to keep the car in the center of the lane. Suppose the computer determines, by monitoring moment-to-moment steering torque, that the driver has not been actively involved in the steering task for a while. The computer decides it is appropriate to return the steering task to the driver. How should the computer return the steering task to the driver, and what should the computer say to the driver in this situation? (Fig. 12.10).

There are several alternatives for the computer's message (or action) in the above situation. The simplest alternative would be for the computer to mention to the driver, "You seem to be bored." The LOA of this strategy is positioned at level 4. However, the driver may not respond at all, either if he disagrees with the comment, or if he failed to catch the message due to drowsiness.

The second alternative would be for the computer to make a more explicit suggestion, by saying, "Shall I let you drive yourself?" The LOA of this strategy is set at level 5. If the driver does not reply, the computer cannot do anything further, and the lane-keeping task will still be performed by the automation.

The third alternative would be for the computer to give a stronger message, such as, "I will hand over control to you in a few seconds." The LOA of this strategy is positioned at level 6. In this case, the driver is given the right to invoke a veto. If the driver is too slow in responding to the message within the allowed time, the computer puts the LKA into its standby state. Then the driver has to take over control even if he/she does not wish to do so.

The fourth alternative would be for the computer to give the following message after it has deactivated the LKA: "I have just handed over control to you." The LOA of this strategy is set at level 7. In this case, the driver may be upset if he/she was not ready to take over control from the automation.

The most extreme case would be for the computer to hand over control to the driver *silently*. The LOA of this strategy is set at eight or higher. In other words, the computer says nothing to the driver, even though it has already put the LKA into its standby state. Suppose the car approaches a lane boundary some time later. The driver may expect the LKA to steer the wheel appropriately, because he is under the impression that the automation is still in its active mode. The driver would be very surprised to see that the lane boundary continues approaching contrary to expectations.

As the above example illustrates, if the LOA is not chosen appropriately, some undesirable event may occur. In designing human–machine systems, it is important to predict how the design will affect humans and change their behavior [67].

There are three approaches that are useful in selecting an appropriate LOA, each of which is illustrated with an example below.

Selection of an Appropriate LOA via Theoretical Analysis Suppose an engine fails during the takeoff roll of an aircraft. The pilot must decide whether to continue the climb-out (Go) or to abort the takeoff (No-Go). The standard decision rule for an engine failure is stated as follows: (a) reject the takeoff, if the aircraft speed is below V1; and (b) continue the takeoff, if V1 has already been reached. The critical speed V1 is called the *takeoff decision speed* at which the pilot must apply the first retarding means in the case of a No-Go. Inagaki [59] has proven mathematically, based on the following assumptions, that decision authority must be traded between human and automation in a situation-adaptive manner to ensure takeoff safety.

1. An alert is given to the human pilot when a sensor detects an "engine failure." However, the sensor can give a false alert.
2. The pilot's understanding of the given situation may not be correct. Let C denote that an alert is correct, and F that an alert is false. Let "c" denote the pilot's judgment that the alert is correct, and "f" that the alert is false. In addition to the conventional hit ("c"|C), miss ("f"|C), false alarm ("c"|F), and correct rejection ("f"|F), we introduce ("h"|C) and ("h"|F), where "h" denotes "hesitation", that is, the pilot hesitates in deciding whether the alert is correct or false.

3. Two policies are distinguished for cases of "h": (i) trustful policy (TP), in which the given alert is trusted and the engine is assumed failed; and (ii) distrustful policy (DP), in which the given alert is distrusted and the engine is assumed to be working.
4. An incorrect or late decision can cause cost, Z, which varies depending on the situation. Three types of conditional expected loss are distinguished. (i) An inappropriate liftoff is made based on an incorrect Go decision, where an emergency landing is required after reducing the weight of the aircraft to its maximum landing weight by dumping fuel. (ii) An unnecessary abort of the takeoff is made owing to an incorrect No-Go decision. (iii) An overrun accident is caused by an inappropriate RTO (rejected takeoff) action in excess of V1.

The conditional expected loss, E[Z | engine failure alert], was evaluated for each case in which a Go/No-Go decision and its associated action is made by an Automated System (AS), a human with TP, and a human with DP, respectively. The four phases are distinguished based on the time point at which the engine failure alert is issued.

Phase 1. An engine failure alert is set off at a speed way below V1. Then $L_{DP} \leq L_{TP} \leq L_{AS}$, which means that the human pilot must be in authority even if there is the possibility of delay or an error in his/her decision.

Phase 2. An engine failure alert is issued before, but close to V1. An RTO can be initiated before V1 if the human responds without any hesitation. We have $L_{DP} \leq L_{TP}$. There is no fixed order relation between L_{AS} and L_{TP}, or between L_{AS} and L_{DP}.

Phase 3. An engine failure alert is issued almost at V1, where no human pilot can initiate RTO by V1, but the automated system can. We have $L_{DP} \leq L_{TP}$, but no fixed order relation exists between L_{AS} and L_{TP}, or between L_{AS} and L_{DP}.

Phase 4. An engine failure alert is given almost at V1, where neither a human pilot nor the automated system can initiate RTO by V1. Then we have $L_{AS} \leq L_{DP} \leq L_{TP}$, which implies that the automation should have authority for decision and control [58, 59].

Selection of an Appropriate LOA via Cognitive Experiments Another important result in Inagaki [59] is that for a human pilot to be in authority at all times and for every occasion, design of the human interface needs to be changed so that more direct information, such as "Go" or "Abort" messages, can be given explicitly to the human pilot. With the human interface, we have $L_{AS} = L_{DP} = L_{TP}$ in Phase 4.

A flight simulator for a two-engine aircraft has been implemented, and a cognitive experiment with a factorial design, mapping onto (Control mode) × (Phase) × (Human interface design) was conducted. For the control mode, a manual (M) control mode and a situation-adaptive autonomy (SAA) mode were distinguished. In the M-mode, humans have full authority for decision and control. In the SAA-mode, on the other hand, the computer can choose an appropriate LOA for decision and control, and may take over control to continue the takeoff if it decides that it is not possible for humans to initiate the RTO before V1 is reached.

Experimental results show that even though the human interface, with the ability to give "Go" and "Abort" messages, was effective in allowing a correct decision to be made, some overrun accidents did occur under M-mode. Under SAA-mode, on the other hand, no overrun accidents occurred [60].

Selection of an Appropriate LOA via Computer Simulations Suppose a human is driving with the ACC and LKA operational on the host vehicle. While observing that the automation behaves correctly and appropriately, it is natural for the driver to trust the automation. Sometimes he/she may place excessive trust in the automation. In such cases, the driver may fail to focus his/her attention on the driving environment, and may pay attention inappropriately to some non-driving tasks (such as using a mobile phone, manipulation of the on-board audio system, and so on). Suppose the ACC recognizes that the deceleration rate of the target vehicle is much greater than the maximum deceleration rate with which the ACC can cope using the ordinary automatic brake. Which of the following design alternatives are appropriate?

Scheme 1. An engine failure alert is set off at a speed way below V1. Then $L_{DP} \leq L_{TP} \leq L_{AS}$, which means that the human pilot must be in authority even if there is the possibility of delay or an error in his/her decision.

Scheme 2. An engine failure alert is issued before, but close to V1. An RTO can be initiated before V1 if the human responds without any hesitation. We have $L_{DP} \leq L_{TP}$. There is no fixed order relation between L_{AS} and L_{TP}, or between L_{AS} and L_{DP}.

Scheme 3. An engine failure alert is issued almost at V1, where no human pilot can initiate RTO by V1, but the automated system can. We have $L_{DP} \leq L_{TP}$, but no fixed order relation exists between L_{AS} and L_{TP}, or between L_{AS} and L_{DP}.

Based on discrete-event models for dynamic transition of driver's psychological states and driving environments, Monte Carlo runs were performed to analyze the complacency effect and compare the efficacy of schemes 1–3. It was observed that when the driving is peaceful and the ACC continues to operate successfully in its longitudinal control, the driver is more likely to rely on the ACC, and his/her vigilance deteriorates. If the target vehicle decelerates rapidly in such cases, the driver needs time to recognize what is happening and thus may not be able to cope with the situation in a timely manner, even if an emergency-braking alert has been given. The number of collisions under LOA-4 was significantly higher than that under either LOA-6 or LOA-6.5. A higher LOA is more effective in ensuring car safety under time criticality, especially when the driver has been inattentive [61].

12.11 Concluding Remarks

This chapter discussed the issue of authority and responsibility as well as overtrust in and overreliance on the ADAS. It is not easy to obtain a clear answer for any of these issues. The arguments in this paper suggested that the phrase 'human-centered automation' may be misleading. Sheridan [6] distinguished 10 different meanings of human-centered automation, while Hollnagel and Woods [38] stated that "human-centeredness is an attractive but ill-defined concept" (p. 128). Human-centered automation has been developed to resolve various costs incurred by careless introduction of automation (viz., technology-centered automation). However, the term 'human-centeredness' can conjure an image of a 'humans versus machines' structure that tries to claim that the final authority is given only to the human and requires that the machine holds a subordinate position to the human.

An important viewpoint is that "humans and machines are 'equal' partners", and this seeks human–machine coagency "by shifting the focus from human and machine as two separate units to the joint cognitive system as a single unit" ([38], p. 67). If we seek human–machine cooperation toward common goals under the recognition that the human and machine have their own limitations, it would not be wise to assume strictly that "the human must be in command". Therefore, should not the term 'function-centeredness' [62] replace the phrase 'human-centeredness' in order to express human–machine coagency in the form of *function congruence* [63], where functions are distributed among agents by taking into account "the dynamics of the situation, specifically the fact that capabilities and needs may vary over time and depend on the situation" ([63], p. 44), or in the form of situation-adaptive autonomy where the human and the machine trade authority dynamically depending on the situation [64, 65]?

References

1. Sheridan TB (1992) Telerobotics, automation, and human supervisory control. MIT Press, Cambridge, MA
2. Bainbridge L (1983) Ironies in automation. Automatica 19(3):775–779
3. Rasmussen J, Goodstein LP (1987) Decision support in supervisory control of high-risk industrial systems. Automatica 23(5):663–671
4. Woods D (1989) The effects of automation on human's role: experience from non-aviation industries. In: Norman S, Orlady H (eds) Flight deck automation: promises and realities, NASA CR-10036. NASA-Ames Research Center, Moffett Field, pp 61–85
5. Billings CE (1997) Aviation automation—the search for a human-centered approach. LEA, Mahwah
6. Sheridan TB (2002) Humans and automation: system design and research issues. Human Factors and Ergonomics Society & Wiley, Santa Monica
7. Endsley MR (1995) Towards a theory of situation awareness in dynamic systems. Hum Factors 37(1):32–64
8. Wickens CD (1994) Designing for situation awareness and trust in automation. In: Proceedings of IFAC integrated systems engineering, Baden-Baden, Germany, pp 77–82
9. Sarter NB, Woods DD, Billings CE (1997) Automation surprises. In: Salvendy G (ed) Handbook of human factors and ergonomics, 2nd edn. Wiley, New York, pp 1926–1943
10. Parasuraman R, Molloy R, Singh IL (1993) Performance consequences of automation-induced 'complacency. Int J Aviat Psychol 3(1):1–23
11. Moray N, Inagaki T (2000) Attention and complacency. Theor Issues Ergon Sci 1(4):354–365
12. Ferrell WR, Sheridan TB (1967) Supervisory control of remote manipulation. IEEE Spectr 4 (10):81–88

13. Sarter NB, Woods DD (1995) How in the world did we ever get into that mode? Mode error and awareness in supervisory control. Hum Factors 37(1):5–19
14. Dornheim M (1995) Dramatic incidents highlight mode problems in cockpits. Aviat Week Space Technol 142(5):57–59
15. Rouse WB (1991) Design for success: a human centered approach to designing successful products and systems. Wiley, New York
16. Fitts PM (ed) (1951) Human engineering for an effective air-navigation and traffic-control system. The Ohio State University Research Foundation, Columbus
17. Hancock PA, Scallen SF (1998) Allocating functions in human-machine systems. In: Hoffman RR et al (eds) Viewing psychology as a whole. American Psychological Association, Washington, DC, pp 509–539
18. Price HE (1985) The allocation of function in systems. Hum Factors 27(1):33–45
19. Sharit J (1997) Allocation of functions. In: Salvendy G (ed) Handbook of human factors and ergonomics, 2nd edn. Wiley, New York, pp 301–339
20. Grote G, Ryser C, Wafler T, Windischer A, Weik S (2000) KOMPASS: a method for complementary function allocation in automated work systems. Int J Hum-Comput Stud 52:267–287
21. Rouse WB (1988) Adaptive aiding for human/computer control. Hum Factors 30(4):431–443
22. Parasuraman R, Bhari T, Deaton JE, Morrison JG, Barnes M (1992) Theory and design of adaptive automation in aviation systems, Progress report no NAWCADWAR-92033-60. Naval Air Development Center Aircraft Division, Warminster, PA
23. Scerbo MW (1996) Theoretical perspectives on adaptive automation. In: Parasuraman R, Mouloua M (eds) Automation and human performance. LEA, Mahwah, pp 37–63
24. Moray N, Inagaki T, Itoh M (2000) Adaptive automation, trust, and self-confidence in fault management of time-critical tasks. J Exp Psychol Appl 6(1):44–58
25. Scallen SF, Hancock PA (2001) Implementing adaptive function allocation. Int J Aviat Psychol 11(2):197–221
26. Scerbo MW, Freeman FG, Mikulka PJ, Parasuraman R, Di Nocero F, Prinzel III LJ (2001) The efficacy of psychophysiological measures for implementing adaptive technology. NASA/TP-2001-211018
27. Inagaki T (2003) Adaptive automation: sharing and trading of control. In: Hollnagel E (ed) Handbook of cognitive task design. LEA, Mahwah, pp 147–169
28. Parasuraman R, Sheridan TB, Wickens CD (2000) A model for types and levels of human interaction with automation. IEEE Trans Syst Man Cybern 30(3):286–297
29. FAA (2011) Introduction to TCAS II version 7.1 booklet HQ-111358. Washington, DC
30. Bresley B, Egilsrud J (1997) Enhanced ground proximity warning system. Boeing Airliner, pp 1–13
31. Billings CE (1992) Human-centered aircraft automation: a concept and guidelines, vol 103885, NASA technical memorandum. NASA-Ames Research Center, Moffett Field
32. Cacciabue PC (2004) Guide to applying human factors methods: human error and accident management in safety critical systems. Springer, London
33. Wickens CD, Lee JD, Liu Y, Becker SEG (2004) An introduction to human factors engineering, 2nd edn. Prentics-Hall, Upper Saddle River
34. Orlady HW, Orlady LM (1999) Human factors in multi-crew flight operations. Ashgate, Aldershot
35. Endsley MR, Kiris EO (1995) The out-of-the-loop performance problem and the level of control in automation. Hum Factors 37(2):3181–3194
36. Parasuraman R, Riley V (1997) Humans and automation: use, misuse, disuse, abuse. Hum Factors 39(2):230–253
37. Inagaki T, Stahre J (2004) Human supervision and control in engineering and music: similarities, dissimilarities, and their implications. Proc IEEE 92(4):589–600
38. Hollnagel E, Woods DD (2005) Joint cognitive systems: foundations of cognitive systems engineering. CRC Press, Hoboken

39. Inagaki T (2006) Design of human-machine interactions in light of domain-dependence of human-centered automation. Cognit Technol Work 8(3):161–167
40. Inagaki T, Kunioka T (2002) Possible automation surprises in the low-speed range adaptive cruise control system. In: IASTED international conference on applied modelling and simulation, Cambridge, MA, pp 335–340
41. ITARDA (2003) Anecdotal report on traffic accident investigations and analyses (in Japanese). ITARDA, Tokyo, Japan
42. Scott WB (1999) Automatic GCAS: "you can't fly any lower". Aviat Week Space Technol 150 (5):76–79
43. Kingsley-Jones M, Warnick G (2006) Airbus studies emergency traffic avoidance system to act without pilots. Flight International 22 Mar 2006
44. Kaminski-Morrow D (2009) Airbus A350 could be equipped with automatic emergency descent system. Flight International 15 Aug 2009
45. Inagaki T, Sheridan TB (2012) Authority and responsibility in human-machine systems: probability theoretic validation of machine-initiated trading of authority. Cognit Technol Work 14(1):29–37
46. Inagaki T, Itoh M, Nagai Y (2006) Efficacy and acceptance of driver support under possible mismatches between driver's intent and traffic conditions. In: Proceedings of HFES 50th annual meeting, San Francisco, CA, pp 280–283
47. Inagaki T, Itoh M, Nagai Y (2007a) Driver support functions under resource-limited situations. In: Proceedings of HFES 51st annual meeting, Baltimore, MD, pp 176–180
48. Inagaki T, Itoh M, Nagai Y (2007) Support by warning or by action: which is appropriate under mismatches between driver intent and traffic conditions? IEICE Trans Fundam E90-A (11):264–272
49. Inagaki T (2011) To what extent may assistance systems correct and prevent 'erroneous' behaviour of the driver? In: Cacciabue PC et al (eds) Human modelling in assisted transportation. Springer, Milan, pp 33–41
50. Lee JD, Moray N (1992) Trust, control strategies and allocation of function in human-machine systems. Ergonomics 35(10):1243–1270
51. Mosier K, Skitka LJ, Heers S, Burdick M (1998) Automation bias: decision making and performance in high-tech cockpits. Int J Aviat Psychol 8:47–63
52. Meyer J (2001) Effects of warning validity and proximity on responses to warnings. Hum Factors 43(4):563–572
53. Sheridan TB, Parasuraman R (2005) Human-automation interaction. In: Nickerson RS (ed) Reviews of human factors and ergonomics, vol 1. Human Factors and Ergonomics Society, Santa Monica, pp 89–129
54. Inagaki T (2010) Traffic systems as joint cognitive systems: issues to be solved for realizing human-technology coagency. Cognit Technol Work 12(2):153–162
55. Ladkin PB (2002) ACAS and the south German midair. Technical note RVS-Occ-02-02. http://www.rvs.uni-bielefeld.de/publications/Reports/
56. Learmount D (2002) Questions hang over collision. Flight International, 8
57. Inagaki T, Moray N, Itoh M (1998) Trust self-confidence and authority in human-machine systems. In: Proceedings of IFAC man-machine systems, Kyoto, Japan, pp 431–436
58. Inagaki T (1999) Situation-adaptive autonomy: trading control of authority in human-machine systems. In: Scerbo MW, Mouloua M (eds) Automation technology and human performance: current research and trends. Lawrence Erlbaum Associates, Mahwah, pp 154–159
59. Inagaki T (2000a) Situation-adaptive autonomy for time-critical takeoff decisions. Int J Model Simul 20(2):175–180
60. Inagaki T, Takae Y, Moray N (1999) Automation and human interface for takeoff safety. In: Proceedings of tenth international symposium on aviation psychology, Columbus, OH, pp 402–407
61. Inagaki T, Furukawa H (2004) Computer simulation for the design of authority in the adaptive cruise control systems under possibility of driver's over-trust in automation. In: Proceedings of IEEE SMC conference, The Hague, The Netherlands, pp 3932–3937

62. Hollnagel E (2006) A function-centered approach to joint driver-vehicle system design. Cognit Technol Work 8:169–173
63. Hollnagel E (1999) From function allocation to function congruence. In: Dekker SWA, Hollnagel E (eds) Coping with computers in the cockpit. Ashgate, Brookfield, pp 29–53
64. Inagaki T (1993) Situation-adaptive degree of automation for system safety. In: Proceedings of 2nd IEEE international workshop on robot and human communication, Tokyo, Japan, pp 231–236
65. Inagaki T (2000b) Situation-adaptive autonomy: dynamic trading of authority between human and automation. In: Proceedings of HFES 44th annual meeting, San Diego, CA, pp 3.13–3.16
66. Jordan N (1963) Allocation of functions between man and machines in automated systems. J Applied Psychology 47(3):161–165
67. Hollnagel E (2003) Prolegomenon to cognitive task design. In: Hollnagel E (ed) Handbook of cognitive task design. LEA, Mahwah, pp 3–15

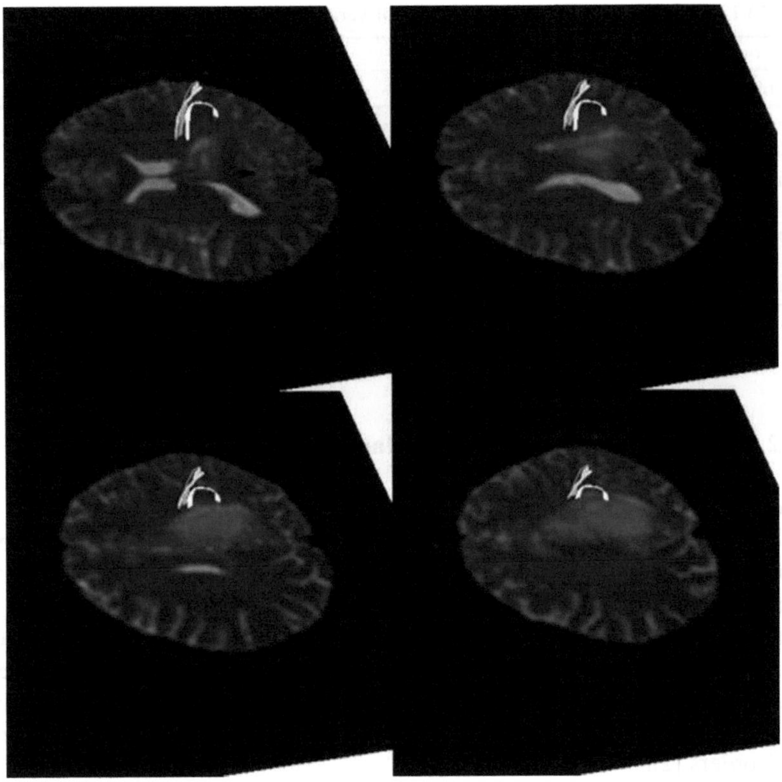

Fig. 13.2 Diffusion tensor image shows two bundles of motor nerves which are displaced laterally by tumor. The lateral bundle is from the motor area of hand, another is from foot area

and software is called 'GAMA – Generalized Automatic Multi-focal Analyzer of water diffusion.' GAMA (Figs. 13.3 and 13.4) works on Volume-One software [6] as a plug-in now.

13.3.3 Grey Matter

Grey matter is primarily made of the body of neurons. The grey matter on the brain surface is called the "cortex." The cortex of the cerebrum is called "cerebral cortex" and is known to be associated with various functions depending on the area stimulated. This is called "functional cortical mapping."

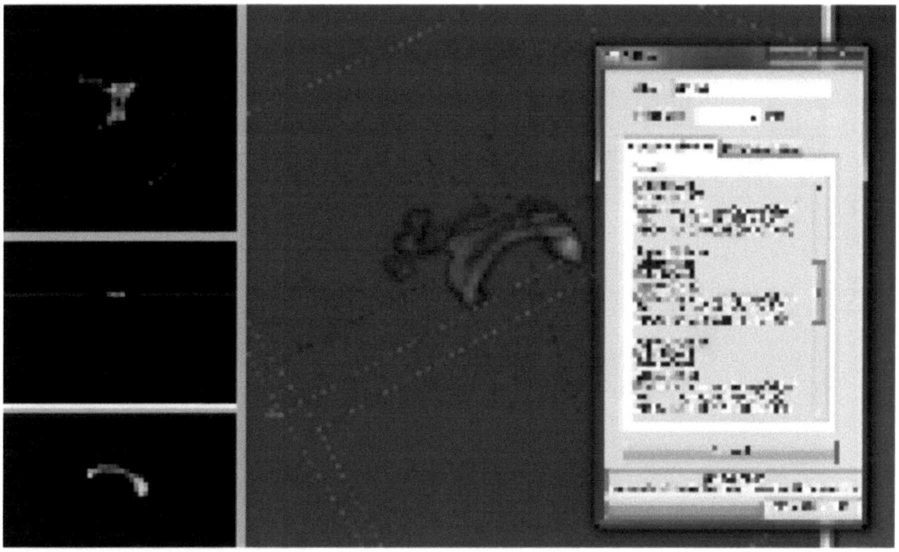

Fig. 13.3 The 3D image and measuring results of corpus callosum on GAMA

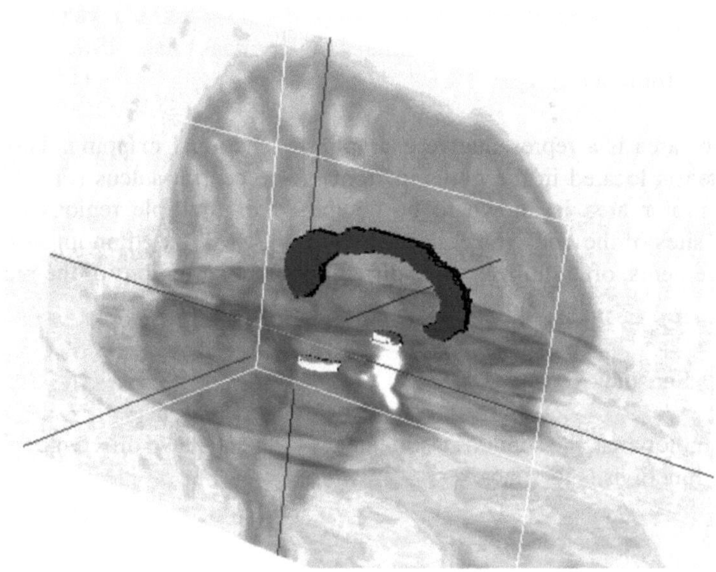

Fig. 13.4 GAMA automatically detects corpus callosum and cerebral peduncles, and reorieent them for measurement from series of diffusion tensor images

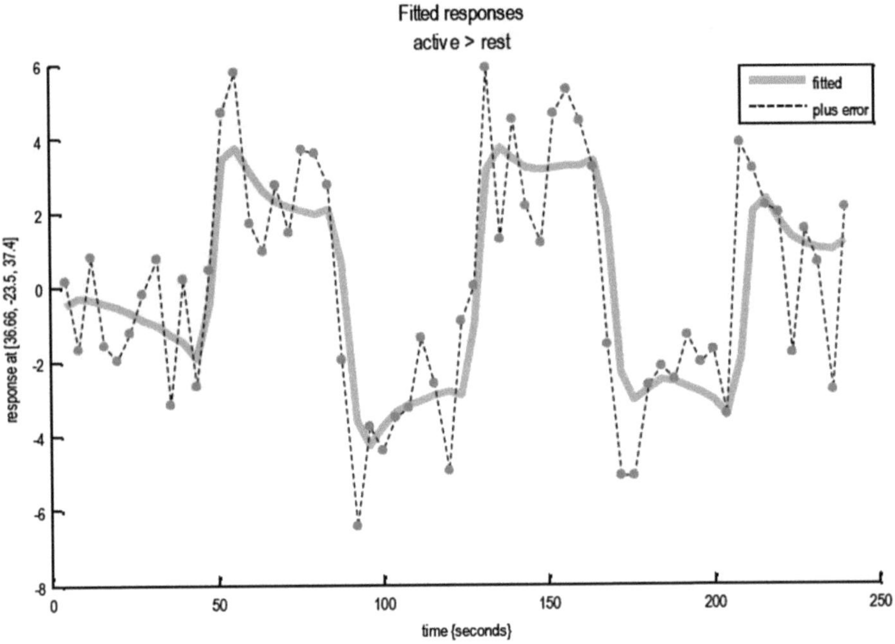

Fig. 13.7 Time-intensity curve on primary motor area during the repetition task of finger tap

a landmark is likely to make functional mapping difficult. In such cases, fMRI is useful in estimating functional mapping of the brain and contributes to improving the accuracy of a surgical plan, shortening of the operation time and so on (Figs. 13.8 and 13.9).

Similar to the white matter described in the section on visualization of the white matter, grey matter is not homogeneous in structure. A change in a structure can lead to a change in tissue water diffusion as mentioned above. We have been studying a method to estimate intracranial pressure, with the compression-caused structural variation serving as an indicator. This approach may perhaps contribute to diagnose diseases involving intracranial pressure such as hydrocephalus and subdural hematoma [8, 9].

13.3.4 Other Nervous System Functions

There are too many nervous system functions to describe here. Some interesting functions are picked up.

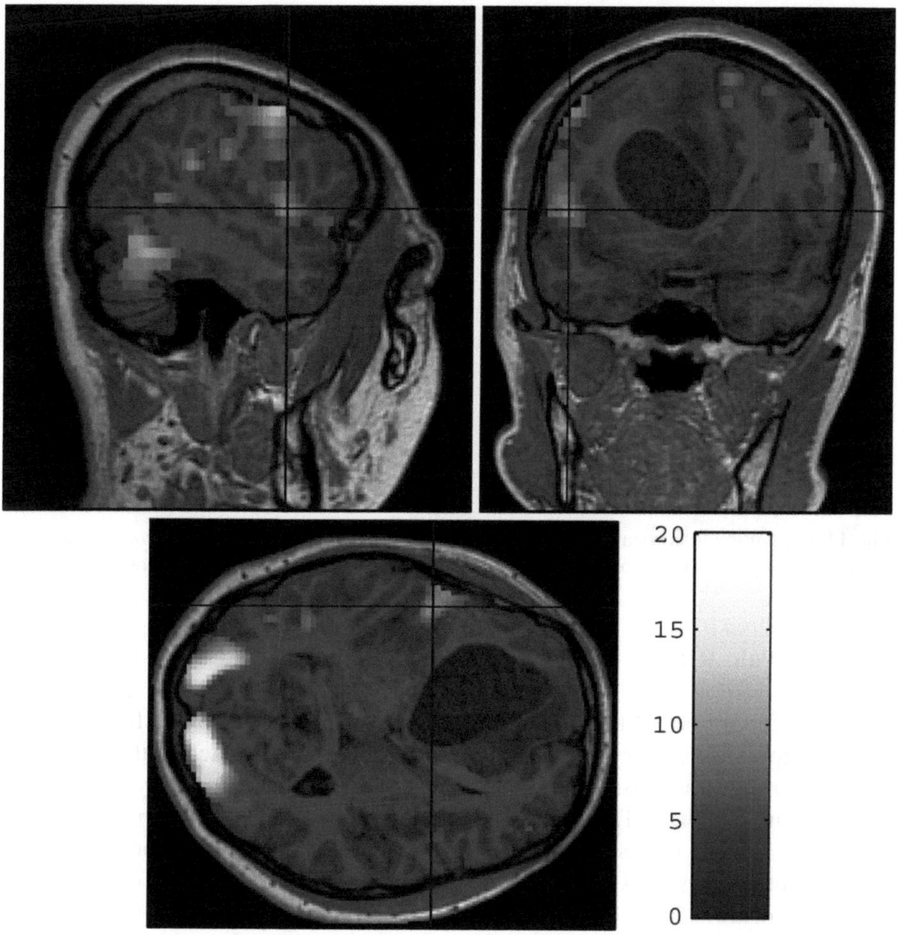

Fig. 13.8 Moterspeech area (Broca's area) and visual cortices are activated in the functional MRI. We can see the distance between tumor and eloquent area

13.3.4.1 Lateral Inhabitation

When signals are transmitted from one neuron to another, the cell occasionally receives input of the suppression system from a neighboring neuron. This is called "lateral inhabitation" and is considered to represent contrast enhancement during information transmission. With this system, the neuron receiving positive input from another neuron that has received intense input, releases intense output, while the surrounding neurons release less potent output due to suppression. In this way, the stimulated site is emphasized during the transmission of signals, resulting in signal amplification. An example of this mechanism is seen in neural ganglions where this mechanism contributes to enhance the contrast of visual input [10].

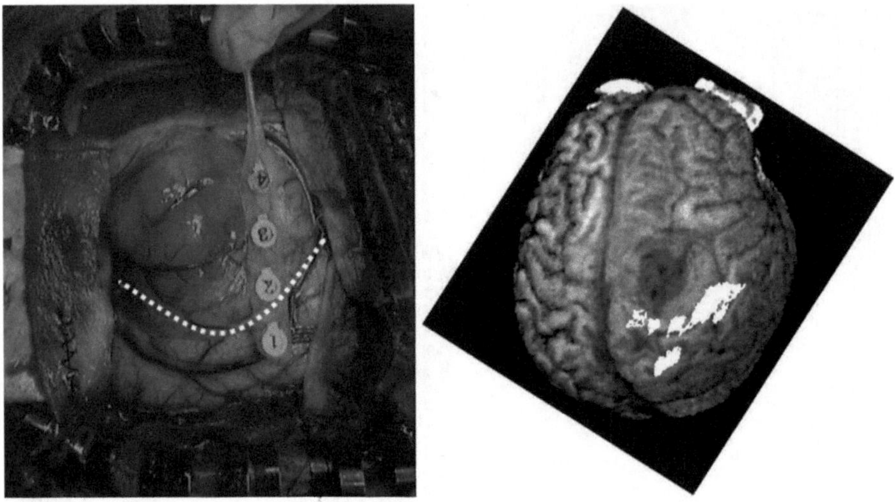

Fig. 13.9 Tumor and cortical electorodes for cortical mapping of motor area. *Broken line* shows central sulcus just posterior of motor area. It is similar to fMRI acquired pre-operatively

13.3.4.2 Pain Relief

At the posterior horn of the spinal cord, the pain sense input from C fibers and the sensory input from Aα or Aβ fibers involve another input mediated by the intercalate neuron during transmission of the information to the secondary neurons in the afferent pathway. This intercalated neuron mediates the information in an excitatory manner in case of tactile sense and in a suppressive manner in that of pain sense; besides, this neuron transmits the signal in a suppressive manner to secondary neurons in the afferent pathway. For this reason, the input of pain sense is transmitted in a suppressive manner if the pain sense is accompanied by tactile sense (e.g., rubbing) as compared to the case where only the pain sense is transmitted.

Furthermore, the presence of a nervous system involved in the transmission of pain sense in a suppressive manner has been confirmed in the spinal cord, distal to the brain. Also a morphine-like substance called "endogenous opioid" that is known to suppress pain has been detected within the brain.

Pain is a sense the most important and most dreadful. The clarification of pain would lead the voyage of discovery of brain [11].

13.4 Neuroelectrical Measurements

Here, methods available to measure neuroelectrical activity are outlined based on the preceding descriptions of neurophysiology and anatomy.

13.4.1 *Single Unit Recording*

This electrical activity can be recorded by micro-electrodes inserted into nerve cells. This method is called "single unit recording" because it yields records from each individual cell.

13.4.2 *Electroencephalography (EEG)*

EEG is a record of changes in brain potential based on the above-mentioned nerve cell activity. EEG can be divided into scalp EEG (taking records from the scalp), electrocorticogram (taking records with electrodes directly placed on the brain surface after craniotomy) and deep EEG (taking records with electrodes inserted into deep brain tissue such as the hippocampus). The records taken with the macro-electrodes used for these EEG techniques differ from the above-mentioned records from single nerve cells taken with microelectrodes (single unit recording) but they represent changes in the electrical field and potential arising from the combined electrical activities of multiple nerve cells (local field potential). That is, the latter records reflect both the changes in the local areas around the electrodes and those in areas distant from the electrodes. They may also reflect the activity/change of elements other than that of nerve tissue (e.g., glia).

Changes in electrical potentials in the brain can be divided into changes in direct current potential, slow potential changes and changes in alternating current potential. Generally, EEG measures alternating current components and classifies the waves into δ wave (−4 Hz), θ wave (4–8 Hz), α wave (8–13 Hz), β wave (13–20 Hz) and γ wave (20 Hz-). If these electrical activities are subjected to A/D conversion, yielding digital data, it will be possible to incorporate various analyses into BMI for clinical use. At present, the motor output type BMI is often used in combination with β range desynchronization and γ range synchronization, but even the slower waves and direct current potentials can contain clinically significant information.

13.4.2.1 Scalp EEG

Scalp EEG is usually used for diagnosis in clinical cases. This technique of EEG uses about 20 electrodes arranged according to the internationally standardized method. Attempts have also been made to use a larger number of electrodes for more detailed analysis or research purposes. When healthy individuals remain still with the eyes closed, quite rhythmic α activity accompanied by gradual increase/decrease in amplitude is visible predominantly in the occipital region. The origin of such rhythmic wave has been estimated to be located in the thalamus-cerebral cortex circuit, although its origin has not been definitely identified. If the

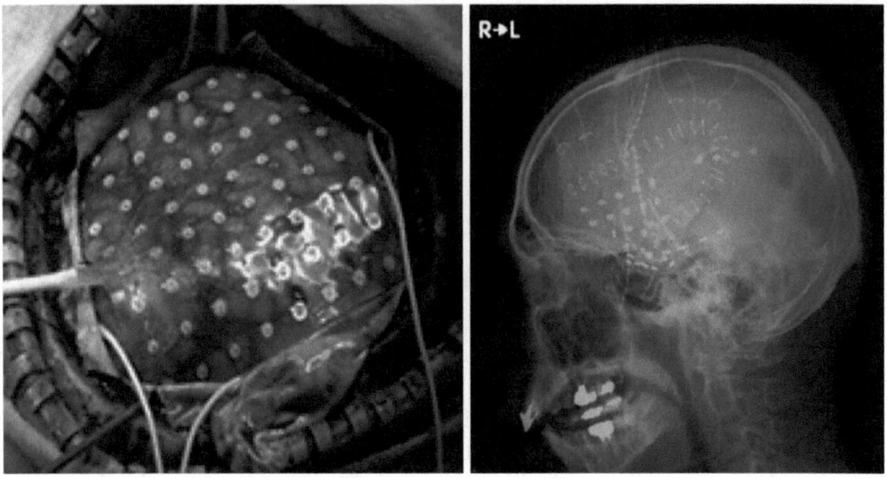

Fig. 13.10 Cortical mapping using multiple electrodes

individuals open the eyes or make mental activity, α activity is suppressed, and β activity or more rapid activity becomes predominant. This is accompanied by disappearance of the synchronized activity seen during α activity (desynchronization). In the frontal lobe, similar desynchronization is noted associated with motion of the extremities. The range activity seen at rest is called μ activity. It is known that during motion, the activities of μ and β ranges are suppressed. During sleep, slow waves of θ and δ ranges increase, probably reflecting decrease in cerebral cortex activity and increase in deep brain waves. Characteristic patterns corresponding to the depth and phase of sleep are visible.

If loaded with stimuli of certain frequencies (light, sound, etc.), brain activity is driven by the given frequency (photo-driving, steady-state response). For this reason, brain activity may also be viewed as a group of non-linear vibrators. Based on this view, attempts have been made to control nervous activity using stochastic resonance, etc.

13.4.2.2 Electrocorticogram (ECoG)

Although scalp EEG is noninvasive, there is some distance between the scalp and brain tissue. Besides, bone and skin are interposed between the scalp electrodes and brain tissue. For these reasons, scalp EEG records attenuated potentials from wide electrical fields. If the electrodes are placed directly on brain surface, changes in narrower fields can be recorded. Clinically, brain surface electrodes (subdural electrodes) or deep electrodes are kept inserted to identify the focus of abnormal epileptic activity before surgical treatment of epilepsy (Fig. 13.10). It is also possible to stimulate the brain surface from outside via these electrodes, as utilized in functional mapping that will be described later. ECoG also has similar advantages when it is used for BMI, enabling observation of synchronization identical to active brain areas (primarily the γ range) in addition to desynchronization associated with brain activity. Because the γ range has high frequency and low amplitude, sufficient observation is often impossible with scalp EEG.

13.4.2.3 Magnetoencephalography (MEG)

Magnetoencephalography measures changes in magnetism with a high sensitivity sensor (SQUIDS element) as an indicator of brain activity, instead of measuring electrical potentials. This technique can yield more information than scalp EEG because it involves less attenuation and is also capable of catching changes in the horizontal direction and so on. Because this technique requires a large-sized device, it is not used directly for BMI at present, but it is expected to contribute greatly to advancing brain function research.

13.5 Brain-Machine-Interfaces (BMI)

In this section, several clinical applications of BMI will be introduced.

13.5.1 EEG and BMI

As described above, brain nerve activity recordings can be divided into unit recording and field potential recording. From the standpoint of decoding multiple unit records, multiple electrodes of fro type have been developed. The use of this type of electrode allows acquisition of detailed records, but it involves shortcomings such as cell destruction by electrode insertion, inability to maintain the electrodes inserted for long periods of time, inability to take extensive records and so on. Subdural electrodes are invasive but do not injure the nerve cell itself and can yield more information than scalp EEG. There is also the idea that more global information can be obtained from field potentials. Thus, research and development in this field are now being advanced from standpoints tailored to the objectives.

13.5.2 Evoked Potential

This technique records EEG corresponding to various sensory stimuli (or electrical stimuli to sensory nerves). Although the records obtained with this technique are very small changes in potential, averaging of summated potentials with a stimulus serving as the trigger enables identification of the evoked potential appearing certain time after application of the stimulus. Clinically, this technique is primarily used to check for disorders in transmission through each sensory pathway from the periphery to the center. The evoked potentials measured with this technique include somatosensory evoked potentials, acoustic evoked potentials, visual evoked potentials, and so on. Because summation takes some time, information cannot be obtained on a real-time basis with this technique.

13.5.2.1 Event Related Potential (ERP)

This pertains to changes in potentials arising from cognitive/mental activity loading such as prediction, attention and so on. This kind of potential has a longer latency than the sensory evoked potentials mentioned above. They occasionally assume the form of slow potential change. A positive wave of about 300 ms (P300) is a representative pattern. With BMI, it is possible to discern only the stimulus to which the individual pays attention among the multiple stimuli presented. This technique has been clinically applied to selection of letters, direction (forward, backward, right, left), and so on.

13.5.2.2 Electrical Stimulation of Brain and Brain Function Mapping

If the brain surface is electrically stimulated, it is possible to excite or suppress nervous function. In this way, it is possible to estimate the brain function played by the stimulated site. This is called "brain function mapping." Clinically, this technique is used to determine the extent of planned brain resection and intraoperative monitoring. Brain function mapping is carried out either using chronic subdural electrodes or during surgery. Mapping of the speech area of the brain requires the patient's response and is therefore carried out with chronic subdural electrodes or during surgery while keeping the patient awake.

If the motor area is stimulated, the corresponding motion (e.g., hand motion in response to stimulation of the hand motor area) is induced; that is, a positive sign is noted. Regarding speech function, stimulation of motor speech center (Broca's area) results in a negative sign (ceased speech).

13.5.3 Functional Neurosurgery and Neuromodulation

Functional neurosurgery is intended to adjust and control the nervous function of patients with functional diseases (e.g., motor disorder, intractable pain, epilepsy and so on) using surgical methods. Historically, certain therapeutic efficacy has been obtained by partial resection/destruction of nervous tissue. Recently, electrical stimulation has begun to replace such past methods. According to the most recent technique, electrodes and other devices for stimulation are implanted surgically for

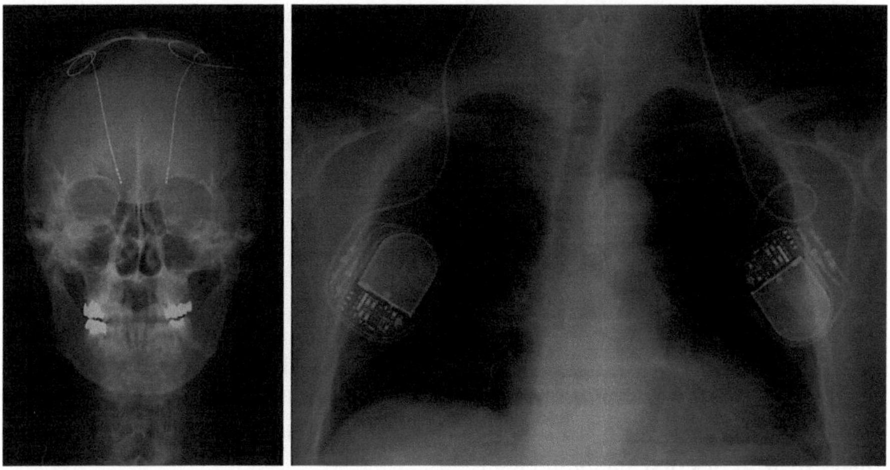

Fig. 13.11 DBS electrodes and generators

use in electrical stimulation. As compared to surgical resection/destruction, this technique is advantageous in reversibility (stimulation can be discontinued) and adjustability (the conditions and extent of stimulation can be adjusted).

Although this technique is being used in clinical practice, the mechanism for the action of electrical stimulation involves many open questions and this technique has been advanced mainly in an empirical manner. Electrical stimulation is sometimes applied to the same site under varying conditions (e.g., varying frequencies) to achieve different clinical efficacy.

In recent years, attempts have also been made to treat spasm and pain through serial infusion of drugs into the spinal canal from an implanted device. These treatment attempts are collectively called "neuromodulation." This kind of method may also be called BMI of the direct manipulation type.

13.5.3.1 Deep Brain Stimulation (DBS)

Electrodes are inserted into deep areas of the brain (e.g., into the thalamus and basal ganglia) to stimulate these areas. To enable electrode insertion into the right place, a special technique called "stereotactic brain operation" is applied (Fig. 13.11). The site corresponding to the diseases or symptoms is selected for stimulation. The electrical stimulus generator is usually implanted subcutaneously into the precordia, and the conditions for stimulation can be adjusted and changed from above the skin using a specific programmer [12].

Representative diseases (brain sites to be stimulated) indicated for DBS are Parkinson's disease (hypothalamic nucleus, thalamus, and pallidum), dystonia (pallidum), and intractable pain (thalamus). Now DBS for treatment of epilepsy is under clinical trial in Europe and USA. With this technique, the appearance of attack waves is perceived by the sensor to begin stimulation (an on-demand type stimulator).

In addition, attempts have also been made recently to apply DBS to treatment of cluster headache (hypothalamus), obesity (hypothalamus) and some psychiatric diseases such as depression and obsessive/compulsive disorder. In Japan, however, surgical treatment of psychiatric diseases is currently prohibited.

13.5.3.2 Motor Cortex Stimulation

This is aimed at treating intractable pain (neuropathic pain). It has not been fully explained as yet why stimulation of the motor area alleviates this kind of pain. In recent years studies on the effects of motor area stimulation on paralyzed motor function have been carried out. Stimulation is either made from outside the dura mater or with inserted subdural electrodes.

13.5.3.3 Spinal Cord Stimulation

This is used to treat intractable pain. It is more correct to say that this technique alleviates the pain through superimposing another stimulus at the painful site, rather than causing disappearance of pain. The technique of spinal cord stimulation has been developed on the basis of the gate control theory for pain, i.e., based on the idea that the pain suppression system is activated by stimulation of the dorsal column. However, it has recently been shown that the efficacy of spinal cord stimulation cannot be fully explained by this theory alone.

Spinal cord stimulation is used not only for pain relief but also for treatment of consciousness disturbance. More recently, it was reported that this technique was effective against dysbasia associated with Parkinson's disease and that it induced walking in patients with motor paralysis secondary to spinal cord injury. Because this technique involves epidural insertion of electrodes, it enables less invasive treatment.

13.5.3.4 Vagal Nerve Stimulation

The vagus nerve is stimulated in an ascending manner at the left neck. This is used for treatment of intractable epilepsy. In the USA and some other countries, this technique has been approved to treat depression.

13.5.3.5 Transcranial Direct Current Stimulation (tDCS)

Attempts have been to attach electrodes onto the scalp and apply direct current. This technique has been reported to activate the nervous activity below the anode.

For treatment, this technique is used as a means of suppression or excitation. Improvement in function of paralyzed extremities has been reported.

13.5.3.6 Transcranial Magnetic Stimulation (TMS)

Lately, a technique that involves stimulation of the cerebral cortex with pulsed magnetism of 1 Tesla class (via the skull) instead of electrical stimulation has become widely used. Now, this technique is clinically utilized to measure the velocity of nerve conduction to the periphery (through stimulation of the motor area) and to evaluate excitation of the cerebral cortex. Studies regarding control of nervous activity with this technique, by which suppressive stimulation and excitatory stimulation can be applied as needed, are now under way. The effects of this technique on depression, Parkinson's disease, motor paralysis, intractable pain, etc. are now under evaluation.

13.5.3.7 Other Neuromodulation

In addition to the techniques listed above, many other techniques of neuromodulation are now under research and development, including FES (functional electrical stimulation) aimed at stimulating motion by direct stimulation of muscles, and so on.

13.6 Perspectives from the Standpoint of Engineering

There is much room for improvement of the current devices (such as electrodes and stimulators) in terms of size reduction of the generator, improvement of stimulation conditions, automated adjustment of stimulation conditions, and so on. For example, it is desirable to develop a safer and more reliable technique for inserting the device at an optimum position of the living body in close cooperation with researchers in the field of engineering.

In recent years, research on neuromodulation has been conducted through light stimulation, rather than electrical stimulation with electrodes. Electrical stimulation with electrodes is poor in selectivity, since it stimulates every tissue and cell in the vicinity of the electrodes. To resolve this problem, research on a technique for selective nerve stimulation with light is under way; according to such technique, rhodopsin protein, showing frequency-specific reaction with a particular ion channel, is implanted by genetic engineering and light is applied to this protein. If this technique is fully advanced, it will enable achievement of selective effects through application of light of an appropriate wavelength after insertion of an optical fiber instead of deep electrodes.

With the current method of electrical stimulation for treatment, the nerves are forced to become suppressed or excited by electrical stimulation, and the symptoms tend to relapse after discontinuation of stimulation. However, in patients with some diseases, relapse of symptoms does not occur after discontinuation of stimulation, suggesting that flexibility of some nature remains in such cases. Consequently, a desirable direction of research from now on may be the development of techniques of neuromodulation that provide "support" to the healing potential inherent in the living body, guiding it to achieve "healing" eventually.

References

1. Basser PJ (1995) Inferring microstructural features and the physiological state of tissues from diffusion-weighted images. NMR Biomed 8(7–8):333–344
2. Osuka S et al (2010) Mild encephalitis/encephalopathy with a reversible splenial lesion: evaluation by diffusion tensor imaging. Two case reports. Neurol Med Chir (Tokyo) 50(12):1118–1122
3. Ashburner J, Friston KJ (1999) Nonlinear spatial normalization using basis functions. Hum Brain Mapp 7(4):254–266
4. Smith SM et al (2006) Tract-based spatial statistics: voxelwise analysis of multi-subject diffusion data. Neuroimage 31(4):1487–1505
5. Mori S, Oishi K, Faria AV (2009) White matter atlases based on diffusion tensor imaging. Curr Opin Neurol 22(4):362–369
6. Masutani Y et al (2003) MR diffusion tensor imaging: recent advance and new techniques for diffusion tensor visualization. Eur J Radiol 46(1):53–66
7. Ogawa S et al (1990) Oxygenation-sensitive contrast in magnetic resonance image of rodent brain at high magnetic fields. Magn Reson Med 14(1):68–78
8. Osuka S et al (2010) Diffusion tensor imaging in patients with adult chronic idiopathic hydrocephalus. Neurosurgery 67(5):E1474
9. Osuka S et al (2010) Evaluation of ventriculomegaly using diffusion tensor imaging: correlations with chronic hydrocephalus and atrophy. J Neurosurg 112(4):832–839
10. Aizawa T, Katayama S (1956) Lateral summation and inhibition in the human retina. Tohoku J Exp Med 64(3–4):349–360
11. Melzack R (2008) The future of pain. Nat Rev Drug Discov 7(8):629
12. Alesch F et al (1995) Stimulation of the ventral intermediate thalamic nucleus in tremor dominated Parkinson's disease and essential tremor. Acta Neurochir (Wien) 136(1–2):75–81

Part IV
Management Technology for Next-Generation Systems

Chapter 14
Roboethical Arguments and Applied Ethics: Being a Good Citizen

Takeshi Kimura

Abstract This chapter is designed to draw students' attention to roboethical arguments as a part of Science, Technology, and Society (STS). They need to be aware of the political implications of various kinds of robot technology. Their good intentions in developing their technology do not automatically mean that it will turn out to be beneficial as it was designed to be. A young student in robot technology needs to learn to be a good citizen and to develop accountability.

Keywords Roboethics • Politics and robot technology • Accountability • Responsibility • Good citizen

14.1 Introduction

This chapter intends to encourage young graduate students in Robotics Engineering to broaden their perspectives and to pay more attention to social, cultural, and ethical issues as part of STS (Science, Technology, and Society). Most robotics engineers are very conscientious in their work and are eager to contribute to the betterment of human society. In the secluded space of the laboratory, where young engineers are allowed to focus on discussing, formulating, and developing their ideas, they do not feel the social pressures that exist beyond the walls of the laboratory. Rather, they feel they are being supported by a society that encourages them to test their ideas. Yet in designing and producing next-generation robotics technology, good intentions do not guarantee that the products will be automatically accepted as ethically sound by society unless these engineers consider carefully the ethical, cultural, and psychological implications for society of the robot technology. Needless to say, what would be regarded as ethically sound depends on

---

T. Kimura (✉)
Faculty of Humanities and Social Sciences, University of Tsukuba, Tsukuba, Japan
e-mail: takeshi-kimura.fw@u.tsukuba.ac.jp

Y. Sankai et al. (eds.), *Cybernics: Fusion of human, machine and information systems*, DOI 10.1007/978-4-431-54159-2_14, © Springer Japan 2014

the culture and history of a particular society, though there are certain areas of robotic technology that would be universally acceptable.

In this chapter, I will draw young students' attention to several socially and culturally related issues. In a social setting, robotic engineers face social restrictions, restraints, and pressure. It is the engineers' social responsibility to respond to these. Engineers need to be aware of roboethical issues if they wish to design and construct next-generation robotics and become experts in their field of research. Young robotic students have been mostly educated and trained in science, engineering, and technology. After such studies, some students go on to work in industry while others continue to study and undertake research in an academic setting. To be successful in their respective areas of future work, both kinds of students need to learn to understand the perspectives of manufacturers, users, and policymakers and respond to these accordingly.

14.2 Roboethics and Progressing Robot Technology

When Gianmarco Veruggio coined the term "roboethics" in 2002, he made a list of areas within robotic technology that call for roboethical concerns: humanoids, artificial bodies, industrial robotics, adaptive robot servants, distributed robotic systems, outdoor robotics, surgical robotics, biomechatronics, health care and quality of life, military robotics, educational robot kits, robot toys, entertainment robotics, and robotic art. Since then, roboethical arguments have gradually gained currency among intellectuals. In 2006, Veruggio wrote as follows:

> Like Nuclear Physics, Chemistry or Bioengineering, in a few years, Robotics could also be placed under scrutiny from an ethical standpoint by the public and Public Institutions (Governments, Ethics Committees, Supranational Institutions). Feeling the responsibilities involved in their practices, an increasing number of roboticists from all over the world, in cross-cultural collaboration with scholars of Humanities, have started deep discussions aimed to lay down the Roboethics, the ethics that should inspire the design, manufacturing and use of robots [1].

Around the same time, Peter M. Asaro argued that there are at least three issues with regard to roboethics: the ethical system that is built into robots; the ethics of robotic engineers who design and use robots; and the ethics of how ordinary individuals respond to robots. According to Asaro, the best approach is to consider all three issues simultaneously. Then, he emphasized that "what we should want from a robot ethics is primarily something that will prevent robots, and other autonomous technologies, from doing harm, and only secondarily something that resolves the ambiguous moral status of robot agents, human moral dilemmas, or moral theories [2]." What interests Asaro is mainly the issue of safety. Asaro was arguing on a theoretical basis, with little reference to actual developments in robot technology, but there has in fact been considerable progress in this area.

In 2007, Japan's Ministry of Economy, Trade and Industry compiled the Guideline for Securing Safety for the Next Generation Robot Technology, whose publication signaled that robot technologies had reached the stage where they would soon be introduced into the public sphere. And as we know, in the city of Tsukuba, with the participation of AIST, the New Energy and Industrial Technology Development Organization's Project for Practical Applications of Service Robot began in 2009, whose primary goal is to "establish safety verification technology [3]." In 2010, the Robot Safety Center opened and is now carrying out a 5-year-project. So now the question emerges, who and which institution is responsible for securing safety in designing and manufacturing robots? Graduate students in robotic engineering will need to face this question sometime in the future since one of the main goals of engineering research is to contribute to society through technological innovation; this means that their own robotic technology will be introduced into society.

In the academic sphere, robotics scholars have become aware of the ethical implications with regard to robot technology; they have observed the rapid development of roboethical concerns. In 2007, Chiba University in Japan announced its Robot Ethics Charter. In 2009, a collection of essays entitled *Ethics and Robotics*, edited by Rafael Capurro and Michael Nagenborg, was published in Germany [4]. In 2011, *Robotics & Automation* magazine published a special edition—"Robo Ethics: Defining Responsibility to Protect Humankind [5]." In Japan, the term roboethics is also gaining academic currency. A philosophy scholar, Kanji Ishihara of the University of Tokyo, and a robotic engineer, Atsuo Takanishi of Waseda University, are working together on the issue of roboethics. These developments mean that the ethical examination of these next-generation robot technology will soon be part of real life.

Once in a class room, I asked a group of non-engineering students whether or not in the light of coming Japan's aging society, they would like to have an autonomous robot take care of their elderly parents in the future if such robot technology became available. Interestingly enough, most of them said no. Only one or two responded that only if such a robot could be sufficiently safe would it be worthwhile considering. Their replies made me aware that there are some significant differences between robot engineers (and industry and government) and ordinary people in terms of expectations. On the other hand, the popularity of such robots as ASIMO and HRP-4 Mimu indicates that ordinary individuals really enjoy watching and observing such advanced robot technology almost as entertainment. Robot toys such as AIBO and Pleo have been popular among both children and grown-ups. Yet most students do not realize that advanced robotics technology is already used in these and many other products. The DaVinci robotic surgical system is being employed in many hospitals around the world.

These social developments are new both to ordinary people and to robotics scholars. However, as experts in the field, robotics scholars are required to address the implications of introducing and incorporating robot technology into daily life. Young graduate students are still young enough to be flexible in their thinking and are able to develop an ethical sense related to their own engineering research.

14.3 Political Dimensions to Technology

For a scholar in the humanities, one impressive feature about researchers in robotics engineering is that regardless of whether or not they are able to achieve their research goals, those engineers are very conscious about the fact that they wish to make a positive contribution to society through technology. Their attitude should be admired, yet the whole matter is rather complex. Historically, technology has always played major roles in changing human society in many different ways, and human society has gained a lots from technological developments and innovations.

At the same time, by placing technology in a social context, it can be said that technology has a political dimension or that technology embodies social relations. Langdon Winner argues that technology or artifacts may have political dimensions in two ways: technological arrangements as a form of order; and inherently political technology [6]. With the first of these ways, employing a certain technology can enhance the power and authority of a particular group of people. The political consequences of the employed technology indicate that this transcends the simple categories of what was or was not the intention behind developing the technology. The second of the two ways is to employ a type of technology that is inherently political. The atomic bomb is an example of this, and it assumes an authoritarian and centralized political system. On the other hand, solar energy is more democratic; it assumes a decentralized social and political system. With the first of Winner's two ways, it could be said that there is a sort of technological determinism whereby technology can determine the political shape of a society. For example, auto engines using fossil fuels have changed how people produce, work, transport, and even reside. Television has changed how people spend their leisure time at home. It has completely changed global society. Now the next-generation robotic technology is advancing into society, and it can be expected to contribute to social change. But there are questions as to how it will change society. In what form will it make a contribution to society? Will it bring about a positive change? What kind of positive changes will robot technology bring into social life? Military robots certainly belong to Winner's second category of inherently political technology, which assumes a strong, centralized political authority. Most Japanese robotics researchers refuse to be involved in any enterprise that contributes to the military employment of robot technology. Yet at the same time, as socially responsible individuals, young robotics engineers need to arrive at their own opinions in this regard.

It is clear that modern technologies have created problems for society and exerted some negative impacts: certain kinds of technology have inflicted harm on people's lives. Many critics have traced the cause of this kind of negative impact and the harm inflicted upon human societies by modern technology back to a modern philosophical view of the relationship between mind and matter. This view is a sort of materialistic view of a creature, as exemplified by Descartes. There is a well-known drawing of a goose whose inner structure is made up of machinery that embodies this notion of a material and physical body devoid of any life-giving essence. This viewpoint embraces a strong dualistic division between the material structure and mental dimension. The body is a mechanical entity without any mental capacity. Thus, “robot” is used to refer to a human who lacks mental activity but functions like a machine. There is of course a strong negative connotation in the usage of this term, and young robotics engineers need to know that some negative implications are evoked by the term “robot.”

A question arises concerning the relationship between this inherent view of robotics and materialism. As long as robot technology is employed as a means of production in a factory, this question does not tend to surface. However, the next-generation robotics will aim at incorporating robot technology into human life and society. In one area, it will aim at creating a fusion of the human body with robot technology. In another area, it will aim at a fusion of the human mind with robot technology. Brain-Machine Interface (BMI) technology is already being developed. Needless to say, technology using BMI will be very beneficial for some physically and socially challenged individuals. I admit that there is a strongly positive dimension to the possibilities with BMI. Yet at the same time, it is necessary to ask whether introducing robot technology into society might promote the dualistic view of mind and matter noted above. Are robotics engineers promoting the dualistic materialism of human beings and human society? Are robotics engineers helping dualistic materialism prevail in society by introducing the next-generation robot technology? Since a robot will be a part of society, there is also an issue about the relationship of robotics to that society. Young robotics students need to ask whether their robot technology might contribute to further materialization and technologicalization of a society. They need to know that some people are opposed to such materialization and technologicalization, and they need to know that as engineers their work will not always be welcomed. Asking these questions about dualistic materialism will make robotics students become aware of the social significance of their profession. They will be designing new robot technology in a laboratory, but they will not be separate from society. They are carrying out their work in a society, and they have to learn to respond in a responsible manner to criticisms of their work.

It is very necessary then for young robotics students to share publicly their views regarding future society if they intend to contribute to the betterment of society using their new robot technology. In doing so, they need to be aware that society does not operate in the same way as a laboratory. In the laboratory, students and professors together form a group of engineers, sharing basic interests and concerns, exchanging their ideas and views, and discussing how they might pursue their dreams. It is a kind of social club, in which young robotics students acquire professional skills and knowledge but also develop a sort of social and professional personality that allows them to be initiated into a professional circle. This circle is shared by professors, advisers, close collaborators and friends, who are the ones who will make a value judgment. After a short period spent observing the progress of robot technology in Japan, I as an outsider to the field have to say that I have seen some very innovative robot technologies, which have won admiration and praise from the fellow professionals of the engineers however, I was unable to see any valuable social importance of these technologies in terms of a permanent contribution to society. It may seem odd, but a highly praised robot technology could lack any enduring social values that makes it survive beyond the life span of its inventor. Once the robotics engineer retires from an institutional position, I wonder if his or her robot technology will fall into oblivion—become just a piece of history, not a social reality. Therefore, it is necessary for young robotics students to consider if what they are trying to create will survive beyond their time of professional practice. In other words, does robot technology have any social usefulness in a practical sense? It is one thing that young robotics engineers are interested in designing and constructing new technology, but it is another thing whether their prospective technology will really be socially useful and acceptable. Many young robotics engineers working in next-generation robotics need to learn to articulate their view of the practical relationship between society and their technology.

From the above discussion, it is now clear that graduate students in robotic engineering need to develop communicative skills. The graduate program in engineering, whose function and structure is similar to that of other graduate programs in natural sciences, social sciences, and humanities, is a path that many young students take to become professionals. Yet the very same path imposes a limitation on young students in terms of their personality traits, communication ability, and knowledge. On many occasions, it is found that young students who study in a certain area of research eventually face difficulties in communicating and discussing other intellectual topics and issues beyond their specialist fields. Many would call this compartmentalization.

If young students in robotic engineering are to learn to communicate their views and ideas to people outside an academic setting, they need to develop skills in talking to such people and answering their concerns, which may be rudimentary and lacking in sophistication, but the safety concerns of those individuals have to be addressed. In addition, robotics engineers need practice in dealing with the strict regulations imposed by the government, which sees and treats robotic technology in a social context and as part of the social environment. Engineering students are not so familiar with these two areas of social interactions. However, the next-generation robotics technology that they intend to develop will be directly related to the lives of ordinary individuals as well as to various legal aspects, whose articulation and ratification is the government's responsibility. Robotics students need to learn to talk and negotiate with these two different sectors if they wish their technology to become eventually accepted by and incorporated into society.

14.4 What a Text of Engineering Ethics Teaches

Young graduate students in robot technology also need to know what and how young graduate students in other areas of research are thinking in terms of the relationship between robot technology and society. A better intellectual relationship with other young students in humanities and the social sciences will help robotics engineers develop their communication skills. Thus, they should be encouraged to engage in good social occasions that involve intellectual conversations with students from other disciplines.

It may be useful for young students in robotics technology to know what a graduate student in ethics thinks about technological ethics. If a young graduate student in ethics were to examine a textbook on engineering ethics from an ethical perspective, he would notice that it is full of concrete examples of problematic cases caused by technology [7]. Becoming suspicious about the intent of engineering ethics, he would argue that engineering ethics is more oriented toward educating students in engineering than about considering ethical principles, even though any ethical judgment of each concrete case of an engineering problem assumes some general ethical principles. The ethics student would list three types of ethical knowledge from the perspective of inquiring into the relationship between general ethical principles and a particular judgment: deductivism, principlism, and particularism. He would find some problems with deductivism. Deductivism begins with a general ethical principle and then proceeds to apply it to a concrete case to make a judgment. It implies that a general ethical principle can be systematized. But the ethics student would be quite suspicious about the possibility of a general ethical principle being independently systematized from concrete cases because it would implies that the general ethical principle does not have any context. A scholar like J. Dancy denies any roles of a general ethical principle, whatever it may be. The ethics student refers to this as particularism. He himself tries to avoid both deductivisim and particularism, but he supports principlism. Principlism admits the impossibility of the systematization of ethical principles, yet it claims the applicability of general principles. Referring to Tom L. Beauchamp, Dancy lists six criteria with which an ethical principle can maximize the totality of ethical judgments: logical coherence, support by arguments, intuitive understanding, compatibility with rational confidence other than a moral base, comprehensiveness, and simplicity.

It would be useful for a young robotics student to hear this kind of argument by the ethics student so as to understand how the other is thinking and discussing in terms of applied ethics just as it would be useful for the ethics student to learn what graduate students in engineering are studying under the name of technology ethics. However, for engineers, the most important matter is of course dealing with technological problems and solving them safely in a practical setting. Therefore, it is reasonable enough for them to learn about many concrete cases of technological accidents and problems. Yet it is also important for robotics students to know that by narrowly focusing on concrete cases, they also miss the chance to broaden their thinking and understand the perspectives of ordinary individuals and students working in other research areas. Of course, it is very important that these engineers are able to solve practical technological problems and not just be able to talk about them with humanities students. But at the same time, it would be useful for robotics students to acquire some basic principles and ideas in ethics (though there is no particularly definitive ethical code that they would be recommended to refer to).

Within a secluded academic setting, young robotics engineers do not feel any social restrictions and social pressures. Rather, they enjoy having the privilege of being able to think and conduct their experiments freely. However, a question is to what extent young robotics engineers are expected to pay attention to these social, cultural, and ethical concerns. While they devote their time and energy to designing and constructing the projects of their respective laboratories, they are allowed to focus just on what they are doing there. Yet it is precisely at this time when they are given the freedom to think that they need to start to familiarize themselves with these social, cultural, and ethical concerns before going out into society, knowing that during high school and undergraduate studies they were more concerned with taking courses in the natural sciences and engineering, not so much in studying the humanities and social sciences. Also, young robotics engineers need to know that throughout their long careers, they will work on a variety of themes, each of which will have different social, cultural, and ethical connotations, to which they will be expected to react with responsibility. They will need to learn to become responsible robotics engineers, that is, to become not only good researchers but also good citizens.

14.5 Good Citizens, Accountability and Responsibility

Becoming a good engineer is not at odds with becoming a good citizen. To become good citizens, robotics engineers need to learn to be aware of accountability. Whether or not they will actually be required to account for their inventions or their actions to the society beyond their laboratory walls is an issue, but they always have to consider their accountability in their designing and manufacturing efforts. The reason is that academic research is supported mainly by society. When I once attended an academic meeting in robot technology, it struck me as odd that similar technology was being tried, developed, and designed separately at several different universities and research institutes. There are of course so many detailed technological differences even in the design and construction of similar kinds of technology. Let's me add quickly that in an academic meeting in the humanities, there are many presentations on similar topics and on same philosophers. Therefore, in this regard, I am not arguing that robotics researchers should not freely choose their own area of study. I am arguing that robotics researchers need to learn to develop accountability in choosing and designing a specific type of robot technology because their research and work are supported by society. When I discovered that it sometimes costs over 1 million dollars to design a new type of robot technology whose technology is remarkably innovative, but whose practicality is extremely limited and—more critically—has not yet been applied in any practical situation is, I wondered which is more useless, the humanities or basic engineering research. I acknowledge that a long series of successive technological development is necessary so that practical robot technology will actually materialize and that the basis of technological research, out of which a few innovations do emerge, needs to be broad. Nevertheless, considering the high expectation that robot technology could contribute to the well-being of individuals and to the betterment of social conditions, robotic engineers need to present their ideas and plans not only to their respective professional circles but also to society at large. Young graduate students in robotic technology need to learn not only to focus on what they want to do, but also learn to design and develop the sort of robot technology that ordinary people want to see applied in their ordinary lives. In this regard, robotics students need to be more conscious about how general and universal their particular type of robot technology may be. In other words, they need to assess how many people would be able to gain any benefit from using their technology. They need to learn to respond to the wishes and demands of ordinary citizens by designing and creating what those people want the robotic engineers to design and create their robot technology for the sake of providing benefits to society in general.

Furthermore, young graduate students in robot technology need to understand their responsibilities regarding designing and constructing robots and introducing them into society because the presence of a robot in the home or in a social setting may affect human relationships. This is somewhat different from the point argued by Hans Jonas in his seminal work *The Imperative of Responsibility: In Search of an Ethics for the Technological Age* [8]; however, if there is even a slight chance that introducing some kind of robot technology into human society might have an injurious effect on human psychology, that would be against the expectations of most young graduate students in robot technology. My argument is that young robotics students learn to think about the extent to which they feel responsibility in designing and developing their technology. In most cases, robotics students only see what they are designing and creating directly in front of them. They largely feel responsibility for what they are designing and constructing. But they also need to learn to feel responsibility for what they assume would not happen. In other words, they have to learn to imagine what negative impacts their robot technology may introduce or to give consideration to the worst-case scenario that their robot technology could engender.

Related to the above issue, young graduate students in robotic technology need to develop a critical perspective with regard to robot technology itself. For example, they need to be able to answer possible questions concerning the military employment of robot technology [9]. Technological advancement is remarkable. Yet, advances in robot technology often result in the ability to kill human beings, even though they may be enemies. In Japan, most robotics scholars assume that robot technology is employed only for the sake of promoting social well-being and represents a peaceful use of technology. However, around the globe, the military employment of robot technology is very common. Young graduate students in robotics engineering need to develop their own perspectives on this issue.

14.6 Conclusion

Advances in robot technology stir excitement and expectation. Crowds of people gathering to watch a humanoid robot such as ASIMO and Mimu run, dance, sing, and do other performances has become a familiar scene in Japan. Robot technology clearly fascinates people. Yet most ordinary people are not aware of the ethical and cultural implications of incorporating and introducing the next generation of robot technology into human society. It is the responsibility of robotics engineers to explain what is at stake in bringing about robot-human interactions.

Graduate students in robotic engineering are still young and flexible enough to learn to communicate their ideas and views about the near future, when various kinds of robot technology will become more incorporated into human society. These students need to be aware of many social, ethical, and even political implications of introducing certain types of robot into an aging society such as Japan. It is also their professional responsibility to understand many ethical and political implications of their own robot technology. It is expected that young robotics researchers through their technology will make a contribution toward the betterment of society in the future.

References

1. Gianmarco V, Operto F (2006) Roboethics: a bottom-up interdisciplinary discourse in the field of applied ethics in robotics. Int Rev Inf Ethics 6:3
2. Asaro PM (2006) What should we want from a robot ethics? Int Rev Info Ethics 6(12):10–16
3. Robot Safety Center (ed) Robot safety center brochure. http://robotsafety.jp/multimedia/RSC_Brochure(101227).pdf
4. Capurro R, Nagenborg M (eds) (2009) Ethics and robotics. Akademische Verlagsgesellschaft, Heidelberg
5. IEEE (2011) Robo ethics: defining responsibility to protect humankind. Robotics & Automation Magazine 18(1). http://ieeexplore.ieee.org/stamp/stamp.jsp?tp=&arnumber=5751964
6. Winner L (1980) Do artifacts have politics? Daedalus 109(1):121–136
7. Kanasugi T (2004) Some remarks on the methodology of engineering ethics education: the significance of principles and case studies. Kagaku Kagakushi Ronso 6:23–44
8. Jonas H (1985) The imperative of responsibility: in search of an ethics for the technological age. The University of Chicago Press, Chicago/London
9. Kimura T (2011) Amerika ni okeru roboto gijutsu no gunji riyo ni kansuru robo eshikkusu teki ichi kosatsu. Tsukuba Daigaku Chiiki Kenkyu 32:1–16

Chapter 15
Safety and Ethical Issues in the Development of Human Assistive Robots

Koji Hasebe, Hiroaki Kawamoto, Kiyotaka Kamibayashi, and Akira Matsushita

Abstract Recent advances in robot technology have led to the practical use of various human assistive robots. With the increase in such robots, there comes a demand to establish a social system that ensures the safety of the users and protects trial subjects. In this chapter we give an overview of the safety and ethical issues in the development of human assistive robots. We first describe the recent standardization activities for the safety of human assistive robots. We next discuss an ethical issue in the development of robots and introduce our proposed stepwise development process for protection of trial subjects.

Keywords Human assistive robots • Safety • Standardization • Clinical trial • Ethical review • Guideline

15.1 Introduction

The development of the robotics technology in recent years has brought numerous inventions for human-assistive robots, such as electric powered wheelchairs, myoelectric prosthesis, and wearable robots. In particular, there are high expectations of

K. Hasebe (✉)
Department of Computer Science, University of Tsukuba, 1-1-1 Tennodai, Tsukuba 305-8573, Japan
e-mail: hasebe@cs.tsukuba.ac.jp

H. Kawamoto • A. Matsushita
Center for Cybernics Research, University of Tsukuba, 1-1-1 Tennodai, Tsukuba 305-8573, Japan
e-mail: kawamoto@golem.kz.tsukuba.ac.jp

K. Kamibayashi
Faculty of Health and Sports Sciences, Doshisha University, 1-3 Tatara Miyakodani, Kyotanabe-shi, Kyoto-fu 610-0394, Japan
e-mail: kkamibay@mail.doshisha.ac.jp

Y. Sankai et al. (eds.), *Cybernics: Fusion of human, machine and information systems*, DOI 10.1007/978-4-431-54159-2_15, © Springer Japan 2014

the human-assistive robots for the support of nursing care and other welfare, as they provide a direct means to improve the quality of life for the elderly and physically disabled and alleviate the workload of the caretakers.

What needs to be considered first in making such human assistive technologies more widespread are the reduction in price and the improvement of usability. To achieve these goals, it is important to overcome both the technical challenges, specifically, the improvement of physical and physiological assistance technologies and communication network technologies that link devices at distant locations, as well as to make these up-to-date technologies safe and reliable, so that users can utilize them without anxiety. Human assistive technology is a field that has seen dramatic development in recent years. Together with the rapid increase in product commercialization, these technologies have already been used in various situations. There are, however, suggestions that technological advances are given priority over the establishment of a social infrastructure for the safe usage and that their preparation has not matched the speed of development. Unlike industrial robots, human assistive robots are expected to be used by and in the presence of large groups of people, or in the absence of specialists. Introducing legislation that makes it mandatory for companies to ensure safety, and clarifying where the responsibility lies in the case of an accident is therefore necessary for the technology to be fully adopted. In addition, standardization is also required in order to allow customers to objectively evaluate the safety of the purchased device. For industrial robots, there already exist standard safety requirements. However, as discussed in the following section, safety requirements for service robots that are intended for humans are still at the stage of forming a standard. Related to this standardization, legislation that assigns negligence liability for device safety between manufacturers and users should also be introduced. Most recent human-assistive devices also possess data transmission function. Data security is thus also an important issue for the safe and reliable usage of devices. In the case of human-assistive devices, the important challenge is not only the confidentiality of personal information, which has recently become a social problem, such as information leakages from PCs, but also the security of control programs against hacking in order to prevent malfunctions.

In addition to securing safety of the users, one must have specific consideration for the safety of the environment in which the devices are being developed in the field of human-assistive technology. Analogous to pharmaceutical products and medical devices, an increasing number of clinical trials (i.e., human trials) are now being done in the field of development for human-assistive devices. Unlike the field of drug development, where safety protocols for subjects and ethical guidelines are established, there is still a lack of understanding about ethical guidelines in the field of engineering, which includes human-assistive technology.

Based on the above discussed problems, this chapter mainly consists of two sections. In the first half (Sects. 15.2), Sect. 15.2.1 describes the background for standardization, followed by discussions on the current situation, challenges and trends regarding standardization on security in Sect. 15.2.2. Problems regarding data security are reported in Sect. 15.2.3. Section 15.2.4 discusses legislative issues, such as the Product Liability Act. In the latter half (Sect. 15.3), problems concerning ethical guidelines during development are discussed. The ethical review process for phased robot development proposed by the authors is also presented.

15.2 Current Situation and Challenges Regarding the Standardization of Safety for Human-Assistive Robots

15.2.1 Background

Traditionally, the control of machine tools has been done by humans or by simple relays. Based on a large amount of experience from accidents regarding machine safety, a so-called fault tolerance or fault avoidance techniques, such as dual circuit system, which increases redundancy, have been established. Concurrently, methods of identifying the hazard sources such as FTA (Fault Tree Analysis) [1], HAZOP (Hazard and Operability Study) [2], or FMEA (Failure Modes and Effect Analysis) were also established. Based on such techniques and methods, the International Organization for Standardization (ISO) and the International Electrotechnical Commission (IEC) have conjointly formulated the ISO/IEC Guide 51 [3], the guideline for safety aspects as the international standard for machine safety, which was then refined as ISO 12100 [4] and established as the standard. Following such movement, the safety of industrial robots is also being standardized as ISO 10218 [5] mentioned earlier.

As a result of rapid development of engineering and information processing technology, modern robots are now being controlled by complex algorithms programmed on microcomputers and thus, their safety can no longer be ensured by only controlling the physical stability of the machinery (such as damaged or defect components). In addition to physical safety aspects, methods ensuring safety for control software must be thoroughly considered. For human-assistive devices introduced thus far, the distance between the human and the machine are extremely close. A minor bug in the control software could lead to a serious accident and methods to ensure their safety is thus strongly needed. In the case of robots, simply shutting down the system is often insufficient to remove the risk caused by malfunction or failure of the machine.

Under such circumstances, standards and guidelines that mention safety of software as one method to ensure safety of the devices are being published by various industries. Among them, the IEC 61508 (Functional Safety of Electrical/Electronic/Programmable Electronic Safety-related Systems) [6], which summarizes the functional safety requirements for a safety-related system that uses a computer is drawing increasing attention. In this standard, the notion of "functional safety" is defined as "safety that is ensured by controlling the hazard source using safety-related system". That is, the safety provided by mechanism that ensures safety (called “safety-related system”) even when the system is in a dangerous condition (for example an air-bag system for cars during crush). The IEC 61508 is a collection of best-practices when building a safety-critical system and provides a general standard for a computer-based safety-related system. The number of industries such as medical devices, railways, and industrial machines have published their standard based on the IEC 61508. For automobile industry, the standard was formulated in 2011 as the ISO 26262 [7]. Having these as background, this standard is also drawing attention from the field of robotics.

There will be a number of difficulties if the field-specific standard for robots was formulated by simply refining the IEC 61508. The first problem arises from the wide variety of forms in robots. Unlike aircraft or automobiles, where field-specific standards are already set, robots vary greatly in their form, nature, and usage depending on their purposes and thus it seems difficult to form a unifying standard that is applicable to the safety of all kinds of robots. Second, IEC 61508 is a standard that is originally intended for large-scale systems such as chemical plants, and thus it is difficult to directly expand its content to robots. In fact, IEC 61508 is a huge standard comprised of eight parts (Part 0–7) that encompass the entire life-cycle of a system, starting from the safety analysis, design, development, installation of devices, repair, and dismantling. Formation of field-specific standard based on such a large-scale standard would involve a huge amount of discussion and interpretation of individual standards. Lastly, the problem of ensuring software safety still remains. Design and development of software are defined as parts of the life-cycle of the whole system in IEC 61508, and their requirements are listed in Part 3 of the standard. For example, the V-model is recommended for the software development process and methods/techniques expected to be used at each stage of development, for instance, specification formation, architecture design, module design, coding, and tests, are defined according to the degree of safety requirement and the Safety Integrity Level (SIL) of each stage. However, the details of how these methods/techniques should be implemented are not specified in the standard, and thus the degree of implementation is often a subject of debate across the industry where there is still no clear agreement. In the field of robotics, it is often the case that developers independently develop control software according to the device. Formulation of methods/techniques for ensuring safety in one standard framework would thus involve large amount of work. For the above-mentioned reasons, a field-specific standard based on the IEC 61508 has not been formulated, despite intense attention from the field of robotics.

15.2.2 Trends in Standardization in Recent Years

As illustrated in the previous section, standardization of safety regarding human-assistive technology is far from complete. There are, however, noteworthy developments. A few representative examples, mainly from Japan, are introduced in the following section.

In 2008, the Japanese Ministry of Economy, Trade and Industry formulated and published a safety guideline for next-generation robots. This is aimed at robots that share the operating range and existence range with humans (so called "next-generation robots" in the guideline) and has indicated the basic thought on the future safety on such robots. As mentioned before, the form of service robots including human-assistive devices spans a wide range. This guideline does not aim to categorize the variety of robots, but extracts the common features of all robots. It also presents the basic principle for reducing risk resulting from manufacturers, supervisors, sellers and users of the robot.

The New Energy and Industrial Technology Development Organization (NEDO) have announced the "Project for Practical Applications of Service Robot", a 5-year project starting from 2009, as a part of "Project for Open Innovation Promotion by Utilizing Basic Robotic Technology" promoted by the Ministry of Economy, Trade and Industry and "the Pioneering Project for Accelerating Social Returns" promoted by the Cabinet Office. This project is intended to establish evaluation methods and standards for ensuring safety in service robots, which is expected to provide one solution to the labor shortfall due to the declining birthrate and ageing population. By proposing the established standard as an international standard for safety, the project aims to expand domestically produced robots to international markets in the future. Four types of robots will be developed in this project. They are: mobile operation robots that mainly rely on human maneuver (wheelchair-to-bed transfer system using detach-and-attachable type bed); mobile operation robots with mainly autonomous control (security robots); wearable robots (for elderly people and those with physical disabilities in the lower limbs); and vehicle robots. Research will be carried into developing risk standards, assessment methods, risk reduction methods, and safety validation methods for each type of robot. These safety standards are expected to require both static and dynamic safety tests for every 16 test items regarding mechanical, electrical and functional safety. Furthermore, there are plans to propose the developed methods and protocols for test and evaluation as international standards. This project also considers the possibility of forming a centralized "robot safety base" inside the Tsukuba area in Ibaraki Prefecture.

As mentioned earlier, the only international safety standard for robots that exist thus far is the ISO 12018 formulated by the ISO and thus has often been referred to when discussing safety assurance of robots. ISO 10218 in actuality is a standard for industrial robots and is not necessarily adequate for human-assistive devices and service robots. For example, the standard includes placing a safety fence between human and the robot as one of the requirements. In the recent years, there has been an effort at the ISO/TC184/SC2 [8] (Subcommittee for the Technical Committee 184) to formulate new international safety standards for service robots (called the "robots in personal care" in the committee).

Lastly, we would like to point out other important issues outside the formulation of standards. For the standards to be prevailed, a consensus must be formed across industries and people that are related to the field. Moreover, it is also important that the certification system is appropriately formed and that the standards for approval and evaluation are clear. It is often pointed out in the discussion about the slow adoption rate of the IEC 61508 in Japan, that there is no institute that could certify the IEC 61508 in Japan and one must apply through a limited certification organization in order to receive certification. Due to this limited availability of organization, there is often the problem that the certification standard for software is unclear, hampering the spread of certification. Considering the above discussed issues, the development of certification organizations is as necessary as the formulation of the standards for the recognition of safety standards for human-assistive technology.

15.2.3 Problems Concerning Information Security for Human-Assistive Robots and their Standardization

As discussed in previous sections, human-assistive devices have developed to perform complex behavior according to the diverse environments and needs of the users, controlled by programs that run on embedded microcomputers. In addition, with the advance of information transmission technology, a growing number of devices now transfer personal information. For example, some heart pacemakers implanted in patient bodies now have functions to record and transmit their physiological information, so that doctors can access them. Moreover, recent research on artificial hearts has come up with a system that can transfer information such as pulse to doctors at a remote location. Such a function is expected to develop further, and data transmission technology is also essential for commercialization of watch-over technology and next-generation living environments.

On the other hand, as seen in the leaks of personal information via personal computers that have become a social problem in recent years, the problem of information security must be thoroughly considered. Roughly speaking, current information security technology utilizes encoding techniques such as RSA or DES and protocol suites that include encryption such as IPSec. These technological elements are developed to a high standard, but the techniques to combine these methods to ensure information security is yet to be improved.

The issue of information security is particularly important in human-assistive devices not only from the personal information point of view but also from protecting the control software from malicious hacker attacks. Further development in information security is thus essential in order to improve convenience in human-assistive devices. Several efforts are being made to establish such technologies as the research into security verification method using the formal method to which industries recently pay attention. This is a method for describing program specifications using mathematical language and mathematically proving their safety. Research into this method and introduction to industries started in the 1970s, but they are still not in full use. Further advances in this field, which would allow them to be utilized by human-assistive technology, are expected.

Standardization is important not only from the technical aspect, but also from the security aspect discussed in the previous section. The existing standards on data security are, for example, ISO/IEC 15408 (common criteria) [9] for IT-devices and IEC 62304 [10] for information security on control software for medical devices. However, there is clearly a need of mentioning information security discussed thus far in the safety standard for robots that is currently being formulated, as it integrates human-assistive technology and information transfer technology.

15.2.4 Legal Issues Regarding Human-Assistive Robot

Thus far, we have mainly discussed standardization for safety assurance as the essential social basis for human-assistive technology and its problems. There are, however, other problems of social basis that needs to be concerned.

Human-assistive devices are designed for situations in living environments such as nursing care and households. Cases where users are injured are expected to happen. Civil Code defines "negligence" as tort cases, but there are also laws such as the Product Liability Act, which assigns liability for damages caused by product defects. With the Product Liability Act, the manufacturers could be held responsible for damage caused by accidents with the product if the victim can prove that the accident was caused by a defect of the product. Devices developed by physiological, motion, and life-support technologies are also subject to the Product Liability Act. For next-generation robots and next-generation living-environments, high-level intelligent control and adaptive control systems that could, to a certain extent, perform autonomous judgment and decision making are required when necessary. This introduces a new risk of causing damage due to a misjudgment of the software in addition to the mechanical defect. As discussed before, it is impossible to manufacture a device that guarantees "absolute safety" and thus the risk of damage caused by mechanical systems must be considered.

In such cases where responsibility and authority are defined by certain regulation, both the manufacturer and the user must share the understanding of possible risk. That could cause to expand the use of new human-assistive devices. The role of legislation is to increase the predictability of such risk. On the other hand, great difficulties are expected for cases and events that do not fit with the new legislation.

One way of enforcing rules as a social norm is to use legal binding force. In other words, to stipulate it as a national law, whose implementation is guaranteed by the court. However, legal stipulation is a double-edged sword as there is a risk of misconception that "only what is defined by the law is allowed." In addition, its enactment and revision take a long time.

This is where guidelines published by the industries play an important role. There is no legal binding force to guidelines, but in the real economic society, companies feel a certain sense of binding and obey the guideline. Clear protocol and evidence are needed for compulsory execution of laws, whereas guidelines do not involve forcible exercises. The guidelines are "voluntarily" met without having the need of clear evidences. To make one follow rules, we must consider what is to be legally defined and what is to be left for the voluntary framework according to the circumstances, and make sure the rules are not biased towards any interested parties.

Further to such legal issues, social insurance for medical benefit and administrative policy enforcement as public services are also important. From the point of infrastructure for social basis the demand for introducing devices that support, enhance and augment human function is high. In the same way as a public utility whose main function is nursing care and welfare, human-assistive devices may contribute to the improvement of public welfare and form a new social production base. However, in order to be widely accepted by society, it is vital to have co-operation from companies such as medical device manufacturers who would take the responsibilities for production, distribution and clinical trials. Efforts to reduce the financial load for the users must also be made. For example, for embedded devices such as heart pacemakers, patients and the family often consider whether the product could be subsidized to be most important and not the technical advantage.

15.3 Ethical Problems Regarding the Development of Human-Assistive Robot

15.3.1 Background

The previous section discussed the social and legislative problems regarding the safety of devices following recent years of technological development in robotics. Ethical problems also remain, in particular, what is often suggested by the developers is the ethical question raised during clinical trials under the developing situation described hereafter.

Clinical trials are vital for developing human-assistive robots. Increasing number of ethical reviews are thus being done for clinical trials in the field of engineering. However, it is only recent that ethical reviews are carried out for the field outside of medicine and thus, number of engineers are finding it difficult to form the experimental protocol or to have the understanding of the ethical review per se. These difficulties are not simply due to engineers' lack of experience for clinical trials. For example, as Yamauchi et al. [11] suggested, this could be largely due to a few fundamental differences in the nature of the research and development methods of the medical and engineering fields.

One characteristic of the development process of human-assistive robots is that clinical trials are carried out from the early stage of development and the device is developed through number of try-and-error process. Moreover, this development process does not define a clear architecture at the beginning, nor does it get accomplished by refining the configuration. Instead, it is done by repeating the short cycle of experiments verifying technical solutions for the requirements specification and adaptation to the newly found improvements/changes. In other words, experiments carried out in the process of robot development are strongly exploratory. On the other hand, research and development in medicine (especially in the field of drug development, which is a typical example) has the characteristic that the nature of their clinical trials gradually shifts from exploratory to verification, and the specifications for developed products such as new drugs are systematically defined. The principle of such gradational and gradual phased development process is the protection of human subjects and scientific experimental design, and the process is being summarized as various guidelines used today.

The gap between the characteristics of the development process in the field of robotics and that of medicine is the main reason why engineers are finding it difficult to understand the ethical review standards. Consequently, directly applying the guidelines formulated for drug development to the clinical trials of robot development would be considerably difficult. The difference in procedures is also an element that is hampering the mutual understanding of the engineers and the ethical committee.

15.3.2 Attempts to Formulate the Guideline for Clinical Trials

In order to solve the above-mentioned problems, we are currently preparing to formulate guidelines for clinical trials targeted at developers of human-assistive robots. As a first step, we have proposed a protocol for clinical trials in development of human-assistive robots that incorporates the idea of stepwise procedure established in the medical field [12, 13]. The basic idea of the proposed protocol is to segment the series of clinical trials into multiple phases and to suggest a stepwise method for experiments. With this segmentation, we aim to clarify the requirements for individual experiments in robot development from both the ethical and scientific points of view. In addition, this guideline is also expected to aid the ethical committee in understanding the purpose of the experiments carried out by the engineers and to be the "common language" for the ethical review process. In this section we introduce the phases for clinical trials and discuss the issues on formulating them into the guideline.

15.3.3 Outline of the Clinical Trial Processes in Drug Developments

What is accepted as the standard guideline for clinical trials in drug development is the 1998 Agreement by the International Conference on Harmonization (ICH). Guidelines from individual countries are also based on this Agreement. The guideline requires clinical trials to be done in a stepwise manner. The purpose for such a stepwise procedure is to first limit the possible side-effects to a small number of subjects and gradually widen the clinical trial to patients after giving full consideration to the subjects' safety. At the same time, by gradually sliding the purpose of the trial from the exploratory stage to objective verification for the effect it allows one to design and analyze clinical trials. These ideas are based on the Nuremberg Code [14], the Belmont Report [15], the Declaration of Helsinki [16], and the Code of Federal Regulations Title 45 [17]. Specifically, the series of clinical trials carried out during the drug development are separated into the following four phases.

Phase I: Based on results from the non-clinical study, test drugs are administered to human subjects for the first time. The main purpose of this phase is to confirm the safety of the tested drug on humans. Subjects in this phase are, in principle, healthy male volunteers.

Phase II: Trials on patients are first done in this phase. The safety and effectiveness of the test drug are evaluated. Exploratory trials to set the aim for the future clinical trials are carried out. The subjects will be patients with the target disease. Trials are first done on adult male subjects with light symptoms and gradually expanded to a larger number of patients. In addition, double-blind comparative studies are required to the extent possible in the latter stage of this phase in verifying the effectiveness of the tested drug.

Phase III: This phase confirms the therapeutic efficacy of drugs to the intended indication(s). Both comparative clinical trial and open clinical trial are carried out on large number of subjects from the patient group with intended indication (s). Based on the data obtained from this phase, a new drug application is finally being done.

Phase IV: Follow-up trials done after the manufacturing approval is granted to the drug and made commercially available (Post Marketing Surveillance Trials). The objective of this phase is to control if the drugs are adequately used and prevent side-effects by monitoring the data from large number of patients.

15.3.4 Clinical Trial Process for Human-Assistive Robot Development

15.3.4.1 Aim and Approach

The clinical trial process for human-assistive robot development introduced here is defined by incorporating the characteristics of the development process in engineering (especially in the field of robotics) into the stepwise clinical trials as seen in drug development process. We thus categorized the series of clinical trials into different phases depending on their purpose and the subjects that are involved, analogous to the "general guideline for clinical trials."

The purpose of stating such processes for clinical trials is to allow engineers to see at which stage within the whole process of the experiment they are about to perform is positioned. As mentioned earlier, exploratory experiments and changes in designs are done throughout the development, from the early stage of designing to the later stages of development. What is often criticized by the ethical committee as the "uncertainty about the endpoint" in clinical trials done in the engineering field stems from such characteristics of the development in engineering. In that sense, the proposed process could aid engineers to design and analyze scientific clinical trials and to clarify the endpoints according to each step, while gradually shifting from the exploratory pilot stage to the validation stage at which the usefulness of the developed device is verified, especially for the experiments at the validation stage. In addition, as seen in the previous sections, it is important to fully understand each stage of the trials from the point of view of the safety of the subjects. Laying down such ideas into the protocol would aid the engineers in understanding the problems in experimental protocol that were often suggested by the ethical committee. On the other hand, to find technical solutions at the early stage of development, researchers often become subjects of their own experiment. Strictly limiting such activity from the ethical point of view has a danger of strongly hampering the speed of development. We therefore named such clinical trials at the very early stage as Phase 0 and regard the safety of subjects (i.e., the researchers themselves) as the issue in work safety rather than the subject of ethical review, as suggested by Yamauchi et al. [11].

15.3.4.2 Outline of Phases

Having the key factors mentioned in the previous section, the proposed process is described according to the time-line. Table 15.1 shows the main objective, subject of clinical trial, possibility to change the design, and the necessity of the ethical review for each phase. The devices considered hereafter are mostly assistive devices for patients with diseases such as the rehabilitation assistant robots and power-assist devices. It does not contain the development of devices for healthy people or a specific disease.

Phase 0: Pilot exploratory experiments are done, and basic design that satisfies the requirement specification is made in this phase. The design is made through a rapid cycle of verification by simple clinical trials (i.e., trying out the prototype device) and modification based on the improved results. The objective of this phase is to build the first prototype, which will be used in clinical trials in the following phases. As discussed earlier, the subjects in this phase are the researchers themselves (or the member of collaboration group from the same lab unit). Ethical reviews for individual trials carried out in this phase are thus unnecessary. The safety of a series of experiments is specified instead. In other words, the safety of the prototype is confirmed by the hazard analysis that is done prior to the trial. In addition, further safety measures, such as prohibition of

Table 15.1 Outline of each phase

	Main objective	Subjects of clinical trial	Change in design	Ethical review
Phase 0	Formation of the first prototype	Developer	Allowed	Not needed
Phase I	Verification of the safety and performance of the device	Healthy subjects	Allowed	Needed
Phase II	Data acquisition for further verifying experiments	Patients with target disease	Allowed	Needed
Phase III	Efficacy and safety validation of the device and formulation of the final design	Patients with target disease (with larger subject group than Phase II)	Not allowed	Needed
Phase IV	Post-marketing surveillance trial	Customer/consumer	Not allowed	Not needed

carrying out the trial alone, or installation of an emergency shutdown system, are encouraged during the trial. The trial environment is also taken into consideration from a safety perspective. These items are expected to be confirmed using a checklist at the beginning of each trial.

Phase I: Based on the trial results from Phase 0, trials on humans other than researchers are carried out first in this phase. A limited amount of device improvements through trial-and-error are allowed, but the main objective of this phase is to confirm safety of the device when used. In principle, subjects are healthy adult volunteers. The main purpose of the trials carried out in this phase is to assess and confirm the comprehensive safety of the human-assistive robots. Considering the characteristics of such robots, this is done from the following three points of view.

(a) The hazards intrinsic to the device
(b) The hazards due to users, such as improper use of the device
(c) The hazards caused by contact between the device and the user

Furthermore, based on expected usage of the device, the trials for, e.g., motion angle, velocity, torque are tested from a fully safe range and gradually increased to the limit where their safety is secured. Hazards identified in these trials are reflected in the design and the process is repeated until its safety reaches a final acceptable level.

The transition from Phase 0 to Phase I implies that the development has left the try-and-error stage and entered the stage where objective experiments involving third-person as subjects are carried out. As described earlier, the uncertainty of endpoint that is often criticized by the ethical committee stems from the ambiguous border between the exploratory stage at Phase 0 and the verification stage from Phase I. It is important for the engineers to be aware of such stepwise implementation of the experiments and to formulate hypotheses and define endpoints required at each phase objective.

Phase II: Trials with patients (or expected primary user of the device) are carried out first at this phase. In the first half of Phase II, various clinical trials are carried out assuming realistic usage of the device. For a rehabilitation assistant robot, for example, one could test the training sequences and operating times using the most recent prototypes. Effectiveness of prototype usage for various target disease groups could also be investigated at this phase. Specifically, trial subjects are patients with minor and stable symptoms at the earlier stage of this phase, and their number is gradually increased, including patients with more serious symptoms. Similarly to Phase I, changes in design can be made if the trials reveal possible improvements. However, the margin of design change is limited to that where the safety of device can be clearly guaranteed from hazard analysis and experimental results. The verification of the design formulated thus far starts from the latter half of Phase II. Prototypes used in the verification trials are therefore limited to those with designs formulated until the earlier half of Phase II. Trial subjects are also limited to patient groups where positive effects from device usage have been confirmed during the earlier stages. The number of subjects, on the other hand, will be increased from the earlier half of Phase II to the scale where statistical analysis on efficacy and reproducibility could be carried out. Changes in design during the experiment will not be allowed from the latter half of Phase II.

Phase III and Phase IV: Validation trials are carried out in Phase III to decide the final design and specification of the device for commercialization. In order to make the validation more concrete, the trials will be on a large-scale with a large subject group and will be carried out in multiple facilities. In the following Phase IV, information regarding the safety of the manufactured robots and defect cases under appropriate usage will be collected. Investigation on safety based on the reports from the users and additional trials, if necessary, will be carried out by the manufacturers.

15.3.5 Problems in Formulating the Guideline

In order to develop the process reviewed in previous section into a full guideline for clinical trials, it must be refined by considering the detailed development process. In this section, we introduce our discussion on safety analysis methods as an example of guideline formulation.

As introduced in the previous section, from the point of subject safety, all hazard sources of the prototype must be analyzed prior to the clinical trial and full safety measures must be taken. Hazard analysis methods that are widely known and used are, for example, FMEA, HAZOP, and FTA. These methods has the advantage that they complement each other, but carrying out a detail analysis using any of these methods is very expensive, both time and work-wise. Initial stages of development, for example, Phase 0, involves a large amount of experiments using simple prototypes. It is thus unrealistic to carry out the full hazard analysis using these methods above for all the experiments. We thus propose a method in which the experimenter carries out a simple analysis by considering a pre-defined list of possible injuries which occur in clinical trials of robot development as the top incidents in the FTA (we will use ICD-10 [18] endorsed by the WHO as one of the reference).

Specifically, we first create a list of possible injuries such as "bone fracture" and "incised wound" in the guideline. Developers will select the relevant items from the list considering the experimental paradigm and the form and characteristics of the prototype used in the trial. Furthermore, the developer would name the possible causes of the selected items based on the FTA (e.g., "cutting burr from the prototype" for "incised wounds"). Through this process, hazard sources that need to be controlled are identified. This is the detailed proposal for the "safety analysis using checklist" done in Phase 0.

For the safety analysis for the overall development process, we are considering a method that associates the process of design refinement and the progress of clinical trial phases. In other words, a relatively simple safety analysis will be carried out at the early phase of development. Using the results from the safety analysis carried out in the preceding phases, the analysis will be refined as this phase progresses. Details of this regulation that encompass the entire development process are currently being specified by checking the consistency with the Guide 51, i.e., the standards for the basic concept of safety design, and IEC 61508, i.e., standards on functional safety.

Further issues remain other than the safety analysis mentioned before, such as re-examination protocols for ethical reviews following inevitable design changes, and detailed definition of each phase. These are currently being discussed by considering more concrete development processes.

15.4 Conclusions

This chapter presents an overview of issues in achieving widespread applications of human-assistive robots from the points of view of social infrastructure and ethics. First, the current situation and challenges concerning the standardization of the safety aspects of robots are described. Guidelines are currently being formulated, but method to bridge the gap between the safety measures stemming from the difference in human-assistive robots and other devices remains open.

Ethical problems related to the development of human-assistive robots and the clinical trial process proposed by the authors are introduced in the latter half. Proposed approach is based on the stepwise clinical trials adopted in drug development as the standard process, and segments the series of clinical trials carried out during the development of a human-assistive robot into multiple phases. By defining these phases, we aim to assist engineers in positioning their series of experiments onto different stages and to comprehend the appropriate hypothesis and endpoints when formulating an individual experiment protocol. This trial process will be refined in further detail. Our final goal is to formulate the guideline for clinical trials during the development of human-assistive robots.

References

1. IEC (2006) IEC 61025 Ed. 2.0–Fault tree analysis (FTA)
2. IEC (2001) IEC 61822 Ed. 1.0–Hazard and operability studies (HAZOP studies)–application guide
3. ISO/IEC (1999) ISO/IEC Guide 51: safety aspects–guidelines for their inclusion in standards
4. ISO (2010) ISO 12100: 2010–Safety of machinery–general principles for design–risk assessment and risk reduction
5. ISO (2011) ISO 10218-1 and 2: robots and robotic devices–safety requirements for industrial robots–Part 1: Robots, Part 2: Robot systems and integration
6. IEC (1998–2000) IEC 61508: functional safety of electrical/electronic/programmable electronic safety related systems
7. ISO (2011) ISO 26262: 2011 (Part 1–8)–Road vehicle
8. ISO TC 184/SC 2 (2011) ISO/CD 13482–Robots and robotic devices–safety requirements
9. ISO/IEC (2012) ISO/IEC 15408: evaluation criteria for IT security (ver. 3.1, rev. 4)
10. IEC (2006) IEC 62304: medical device software–software life cycle processes
11. Yamauchi S (2009) Studies in science and engineering and ethical review–report on ethical studies in clinical trials for welfare devices (in Japanese). Jpn Soc Wellbeing Sci Assistive Technol
12. Hasebe K, Kawamoto H, Matsushita A, Kamibayashi K, Sankai Y (2010) Towards a guideline for clinical trials in the development of human assistive robots. In: IEEE international conference on robotics and biomimetics (ROBIO 2010), Tianjin, China, pp 751–756
13. Hasebe K, Kawamoto H, Matsushita A, Kamibayashi K, Sankai Y (2011) Stepwise process of clinical trials in safety-conscious development of human assistive robots. In: IEEE international conference on robotics and biomimetics (ROBIO 2011), Phuket, Thailand, pp 50–55
14. Mitscherlich A, Mielke F (1949) The Nuremberg Code, doctors of infamy: the story of the Nazi medical crimes. Schuman, New York, pp xxiii–xxv (Reprinted from Trials of war criminals before the Nuremberg Military Tribunals under Control Council Law, vol 2, no 10. U.S. Government Printing Office, Washington, DC, pp 181–182)
15. The National Commission for the Protection of Human Subjects of Biomedical and Behavioral Research (1979) The Belmont Report-ethical principles and guidelines for the protection of human subjects of research, Washington, DC
16. World Medical Assembly (1996) Declaration of Helsinki. (As printed in JAMA. 277(11):925–926 (1997) or at www.wma.net for 2008 version)
17. Federal Government of the United States (2005) Code of federal regulations, Title 45-Public Welfare, Department of Health and Human Services, Part 46: Protection of Human Subjects
18. WHO (2007) International statistical classification of diseases and related health problems 10th revision (ICD-10)

Chapter 16
Standards and Statutes: 'Soft' Law and 'Hard' Law

Masao Yanaga

Abstract Standards have been widely applied successfully in various areas, especially with regard with information technology. After a brief look at the process for setting standards, we will review the intellectual property and competition law issues as they regard these standards. There is also an overview of the important role of standards in establishing damages. Finally, the reasons why standards as a sort of 'soft law' are often preferred to statutes are discussed.

Keywords Standards • Hard law • Soft law • Intellectual property • Competition policy • Civil liability

16.1 What is a Standard?

A standard can be defined as any set of technical specifications that either provide or are intended to provide a common design for a product or process.

Setting the anticompetitive effect of standardization aside, standardization significantly increases consumer benefits in many markets. This is particularly the case with so-called *network markets*[1] where the value of a product to a particular consumer is a function of how many other consumers use the same (or a compatible) product (e.g. telephone network, computer operating system) since standards control interoperability in a network market.

Even in *non-network markets,* standard setting might have beneficial effects. In this sort of market, standards often govern the quality or safety of a product.

---

[1] In this type of market, we can observe a phenomenon known as "tipping", in which a dominant technology or player defines the standard for an industry, resulting in "winner-take-all" economies of scale and scope.

M. Yanaga (✉)
Department of Business Sciences, University of Tsukuba, Bunkyo-ku, Japan
e-mail: yanaga.masao.ff@u.tsukuba.ac.jp

Y. Sankai et al. (eds.), *Cybernics: Fusion of human, machine and information systems*, DOI 10.1007/978-4-431-54159-2_16, © Springer Japan 2014

Table 16.1 Coordinative standards and regulative standards ([2], p. 246)

	Coordinative standards	Regulative standards
Aim	Interoperability, compatibility	Prevention of negative externalities
Mode of generation	Negotiation of agreement among 'interested' actors/ emergence in markets	Hierarchical political governance
Normative character	Convention, voluntary	Legal rule, mandatory
Area of validity	Industries, markets (techno-economic units)	States (political units)
Economic effects	Reduction of transaction costs/positive externalities	Internalization of negative externalities

In addition, standards can facilitate competitive markets for replacement parts or service, for example, in durable-goods industries. Moreover, medical doctors and many other professionals must meet minimum licensing standards set in order to protect and advance both the private interests of patients (clients, consumers) and the interests of society at large.

There might be another classification of standards: mandatory (regulative) standards and voluntary (coordinative) standards. "Regulative standards – often in the form of maximum or minimum requirements and limits – aim at preventing negative externalities through internalization, i.e. imposing the externalities on those who have induced them". "Coordinative standards, such as protocol and interface specifications, on the other hand, frequently aim at promoting interoperability and compatibility of technology in order to reduce transaction costs and to generate positive externalities" [1] (Table 16.1).

16.2 Standard-Setting Organizations

A standard may arise from the *operation of the market* (*de facto* standards). "Market" or "*de facto*" standards are common in "network industries" where consumers benefit by adopting products or processes adopted by others. In this case, there exists no standard setting organization.

On the other hand, there are a lot of codified standards. Technical specifications for standards are typically formally adopted by a standard-setting organization, either private or governmental/public.

16.2.1 International Organization for Standardization (ISO)

The ISO (International Organization for Standardization) is the world's largest developer and publisher of International Standards. The ISO is a network of the national standards institutes of countries, one member per country, which is a *non-governmental organization* that forms a bridge between the public and private sectors. Many of its member institutes are part of the governmental structure of their countries, or are mandated by their governments while other members have their roots exclusively in the private sector, having been set up by national partnerships of industry associations.

16.2.2 Japanese Industrial Standards Committee (JISC)

Japanese Industrial Standards (JIS), which are set by the competent Ministries (i.e. the Ministry of Economy, Trade and Industry; the Ministry of Education, Culture, Sports, Science and Technology; the Ministry of Environment; the Ministry of Internal Affairs and Communications; the Ministry of Agriculture, Forestry and Fisheries; the Ministry of Land, Infrastructure and Transport; and the Ministry of Health, Labor and Welfare), are national standards (Article 11, Industrial Standardization Act), in the same manner as the ANS (American National Standards) of the ANSI in the US or the BS (British Standards) of the BSI in the UK.

The Japanese Industrial Standards Committee (JISC) is a consultative body for the competent ministries. It consists of many national committees and plays a central role in standardization activities in Japan The JISC is the official Japanese representative to both the International Electrotechnical Commission (IEC) and the ISO.

The JIS are established or revised on the basis of a consensus among producers, consumers, regulators and related parties. The JIS, which cover industrial and mineral products, have been influenced by the standards established by various industrial associations for their specific needs, or the standards established by many companies called for by the company standards (e.g. operation manuals, products specifications etc.). In other words, the need for common practices in companies belonging to the same industrial sector leads to the establishment of industrial association standards, and the same need in terms of wider applications has promoted the establishment of JIS.

16.3 Standard Setting Process

16.3.1 Input Legitimacy and Output Legitimacy/Substance and Process

In most cases, specifications and standards are developed by and for the interested parties themselves as a consensus-driven activity. Accordingly, the legitimacy of the standards or specifications rests heavily on the wide participation/involvement of stakeholders. In addition, in networked society, for example, it is difficult to ignore technology standards—whether they are the informal *de facto* ones or the more formal *de jure* ones emanating from formal standards-setting organizations. One consequence of this pivotal role of standards is that the perceived legitimacy of the standardization process as well as the substance of the standards themselves requires care and attention.

Werle and Iversen [1] have pointed out a tendency to think of the legitimacy-deficit in terms of '*input legitimacy*' criteria, while they have observed at the same time a tendency for standards-setting organizations to orient efforts towards achieving '*output legitimacy*', by developing standards which are regarded by diverse groups of legitimizing stakeholders as 'good standards'. The *input legitimacy* focuses on the 'production' of a standard (i.e. the standardization process) while the *output legitimacy* addresses the 'product' (i.e. the standards themselves). According to Werle and Iversen [1], high input legitimacy is characterized by a *due process*, that is, ensuring stakeholder representations, hopefully maintained by a highly-respected standards-setting organization. They define output legitimacy, on the other hand, as being a situation in which "all 'interests' are considered (but not directly represented) in the standardization process; external tracking and monitoring of standardization by stakeholder and advocacy groups; and decision-making in an open inclusive discourse (arguing) to the benefit of all standards addressees", in addition to its perception as a 'good standard' by interested parties.

16.3.2 An Example: Japanese Industrial Standards (JIS)

To establish a JIS standard, the Japanese Industrial Standards Committee (JISC) must duly follow the procedure stipulated by the competent ministerial ordinance, deliberate on the proposed industrial standard, and report the results to the competent minister(s) (Fig. 16.1). In addition, when the competent minister officially acknowledges that the proposed industrial standard which JISC reported to have to be established complies with opinions of all persons who have a vested interest in it, would not unfairly discriminate against persons who are under the same type of conditions, and is otherwise suitable, it must be established as an industrial standard under Article 13 of the Industrial Standardization Act. Furthermore, according to the official procedure provided by the ordinances of the competent ministry, the proposed industrial standard must be deliberated on by JISC (including working groups if applicable) which shall be composed of committee members and special members, who determine whether or not the standard complies with opinions of committee members, users, consumers, and all others who have a vested interest in it. In this case, it is also stipulated that when there are minority opinions in the decision, and when committee members or special members so request it, then the opinions must be described in reports of the standard (Enforcement Regulation for Industrial Standardization Act, Article 2 *quater*).

Opportunities are guaranteed for reporting opinions, etc., to persons with a vested interest. First, when there is a plan to create a JIS draft, public notice must

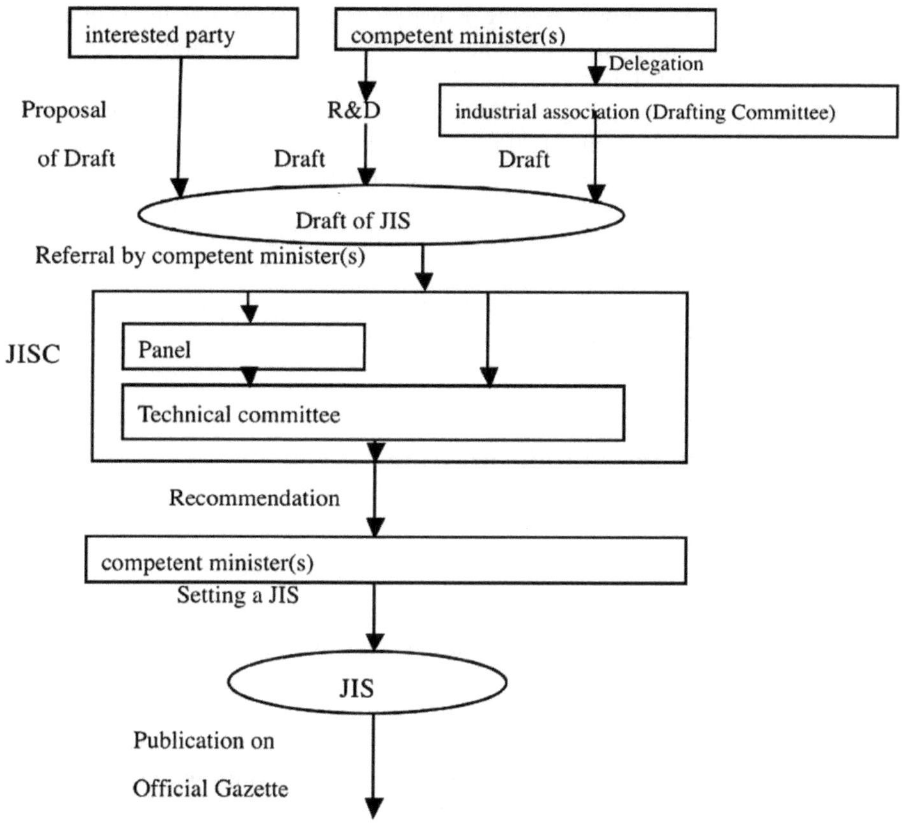

Fig. 16.1 Flow of setting JIS

be given at least 3 weeks prior to the event, and if there are persons with a vested interest in the proposed JIS (such as manufacturers, sellers, and consumers of products, that are covered by the JIS proposal in question, as well as persons, companies. etc., possessing rights such as patents for technologies related to the proposed JIS), they may, regardless of their nationality, present their opinions (usually in written form) to the committee that is drafting the proposed JIS.

In addition, the JIS action plan is publicly released at least once every 6 months. If there are any parties with a vested interested in proposals for setting or revising a JIS standard, regardless of their nationality they may express their opinions at subcommittees and expert committees of the JISC that are deliberating on the JIS proposal in question.

Furthermore, before establishing or revising a JIS standard, there must public announcements for providing opportunities for submitting opinions based on Article 4, Section 1 of the WTO/TBT Agreement, as well as for gathering information about patents, etc. related to the JIS patent policy. There is a 60-day period for soliciting opinions.

In addition to the above, finding a need for industrial standardization, the competent minister may hold public hearings to solicit the opinions of persons or parties having a vested interest. Therefore, the JISC, or persons/parties with a vested interest in industrial standards, can request the Minister to hold a public hearing to reflect the opinions of all persons with a vested interest, or to determine whether or not the application of said standard would unjustly affect persons who are subject to similar conditions. Upon such a request, the Minister will examine the facts clearly presented at the public hearing, and if it is determined that the industrial standard must be revised, then the standard shall be discussed at the JISC, and the revision must be properly deliberated upon, as per Article 18 of the Industrial Standardization Act.

16.4 Antitrust and Standardization

16.4.1 Antitrust Issues

While standardization may increase some benefits to consumers, it might be undesirable to the extent that standardization of a single product reduces consumer choice. In addition, standard-setting organizations (SSOs) may be able to impede competition, effectively acting as a cartel with the power to reduce output by excluding certain kinds of products. This is partly because an SSO sometimes wields economic power because it consists of the largest companies in the industry, and partly because some SSOs may wield direct legal control over a market, either directly (e.g. in cases where the legislatures delegate to professional associations the power to control entry into the profession) or indirectly (in cases where an SSO adopts standards that are incorporated into or referred to in statutes enacted by legislatures).

Accordingly, we find two main types of antitrust issues in the context of standards setting: procedural issues, which address the method by which the standard was set, and substantive issues, which concern the content of the standard adopted.

16.4.2 Japanese Antimonopoly Act and Standardization

The Japanese Antimonopoly Act (AMA) stipulates that no company or individual may engage in private monopolization or unreasonable restraint of trade (Article 3). ‘Private monopolization’ is defined as “business activities, by which any individual, organization or company, or any combination thereof, excludes or controls the business activities of other individual or companies, thereby causing, contrary to the public interest, a substantial restraint of competition in any particular field of trade" (Article 2, paragraph 5). In addition, it is forbidden to enter into an international agreement or an international contract that contains matters that may be considered unreasonable restraint of trade or unfair trade practices (Article 6). Moreover, no trade association may engage in activities that (1) substantially restrain competition in any particular field of trade, (2) enter into an international agreement or an international contract as described in Article 6, (3) limit the present or future number of participants in any particular field of business, (4) unjustly restrict the functions or activities of the constituent members (i.e., members of the trade association), and (5) induce or coerce individuals or businesses to engage in unfair trade practices (Article 8).

The Japanese Fair Trade Commission created and published *Guidelines on Standardization and Patent Pool Arrangements.* According to the *Guidelines*, while standardization of specifications by competitors is not assumed to be illegal *per se* under the AMA, it might result in violation of the AMA in cases where the standardization activity restricts competition in related markets or threatens to impede fair competition with restrictions as follows:

1. Restricting prices of new products with specifications: Competitors in the activity jointly fix prices, quota outputs, limit marketing activities etc. of their new products with specifications (unreasonable restraint of trade, etc.).
2. Restricting development of alternative specifications: Competitors in the activity mutually restrict, without due cause, the development alternative specifications or adopt alternative specifications to produce and distribute products with them (unreasonable restraint of trade, dealing on restrictive terms etc.).
3. Unreasonably extending the scope of specifications: Competitors in the activity jointly extend the scope of specifications when doing so is not necessary to ensure compatibility among their products, but only to mutually restrict competition in developing new products (unreasonable restraint of trade, etc.).
4. Unreasonably excluding technical proposals from competitors: Competitors deliberately, without due cause, prevent technical proposals by a specific competitor from being adopted in the development or improvement of the technologies for specifications (private monopolization, discriminatory treatment in a concerted activity, etc.).
5. Excluding competitors from the activities: Competitors deliberately exclude specific competitors from the activity in cases where the competitors are largely not involved in developing and distributing the products with the specifications and do not participate in the activity, and are at risk of being excluded from the market (private monopolization, etc.).

In addition, the *Guidelines* point out that refusing to grant a license might be considered a breach of rules in the AMA if a patent holder has taken part in the standardization activities and is endeavoring to have their patented technologies adopted by the specifications while the patent holder is free to refuse to grant a license under the AMA as long as the patent holder is not involved in the activities. Once specifications are standardized, and if it becomes difficult for companies to develop and produce the products with the specifications, then the activities of patent holders are deemed to constitute private monopolization when they substantially restrict competition in related markets. Alternatively, they may constitute unfair trade practices when they threaten to impede fair competition. This will also apply to cases where a patent holder has not been formally involved in developing the specifications by, for example, colluding with a participant in the activity. If several companies involved in the standard-setting activity jointly conduct such an act, the act is regarded as unreasonable restraint of trade in cases where competition is substantially inhibited and as unfair trade practice (concerted refusal to deal) in cases where competition is not substantially inhibited. Both of these cases are deemed to be a violation of the AMA.

16.5 Intellectual Properties (IP) and Standardization

16.5.1 Intellectual Properties (IP)

Intellectual properties are creations of the mind, such as musical, literary and artistic works, discoveries and inventions, names, symbols and designs, for which a set of exclusive rights are usually recognized and provided by law (in most cases, statutes). Common types of intellectual property rights include copyrights, trademarks, patents, industrial design rights and trade secrets.[2]

16.5.2 Lock-In/Hold-Up Problems and SSOs

16.5.2.1 Lock-In/Hold-Up Problems

After a standard has been adopted and becomes established, there are occasionally cases in which someone claims an intellectual property right (whether patent or copyright) over the existing standard. However, an asymmetry exists between the low *ex ante* cost of choosing an alternative proposed standard and the higher *ex post* cost of abandoning an existing standard in favor of a new standard.

16.5.2.2 Intellectual Property Rights and Standard-Setting Organizations (SSOs)

Many SSOs have policies that address the interplay between the standards they adopt and the IP rights of participants (Table 16.2). The prospect for *ex post*

[2] For details of the situation in Japan, see e.g. Asahi Koma Law Offices, Intellectual Property Rights in Japan, http://www.ictregulationtoolkit.org/en/document.1481.pdf

Table 16.2 Patent policy adopted by selected SSOs

<table>
<tr><th rowspan="2"></th><th rowspan="2">Duty to search</th><th rowspan="2">Disclose/ Declare</th><th colspan="4">License</th><th rowspan="2">Decline to grant a license after standardization</th></tr>
<tr><th>Waiver</th><th>Royalty-free</th><th>RAND</th><th>Reciprocity allowed</th></tr>
<tr><td>ISO/IEC</td><td rowspan="2">Good faith and on a best effort</td><td rowspan="6">○</td><td></td><td rowspan="2">○</td><td rowspan="2">○</td><td rowspan="2">○</td><td rowspan="3">Review the standards</td></tr>
<tr><td>ITU-T/ ITU-R</td><td></td></tr>
<tr><td>ANSI</td><td></td><td></td><td>○</td><td>○</td><td></td></tr>
<tr><td>IEEE</td><td>Reasonable and good faith</td><td>○</td><td>○</td><td>○</td><td></td><td>Regardless of the declination, all standards are subject to periodic review</td></tr>
<tr><td>JISC</td><td></td><td></td><td>○</td><td>○</td><td>○</td><td rowspan="2">Review the standards</td></tr>
<tr><td>W3C</td><td>Receive a disclosure request/ have actual knowledge</td><td></td><td>○</td><td></td><td>○</td></tr>
</table>

"hold-up" is one of the key rationales for requiring patent holders to disclose their patents *ex ante* and to specify *ex ante* the royalty rates that they intend to seek for the use of their patents.

Specifically, many SSOs have policies that prevent the SSO from adopting standards on which some individual or party has (or claims to have) a patent[3] and that call for the SSO to withdraw previously approved standards if it is subsequently discovered that there is a patent that reads on the standard. Many SSOs, however, explicitly disclaim any effort to interpret the patent (or IP) or to determine whether or not a patent reads on a proposed standard.

Secondly, the rules of an SSO usually impose obligations on the SSO participants to search, disclose and license the IP (mainly, patent(s)) that they have. Among these rules, search and disclosure rules obviously impose burdens on the SSO participants. Search rules might be troublesome because of limited knowledge that participants' representatives to the SSO may have on the patent portfolios of the participants. This implies that the scope of the obligation (if any) to search for potentially relevant patents is extremely important. It is not easy to find an appropriate level of disclosure because overdisclosure can be as problematic as underdisclosure. A "core dump" type of disclosure is not very helpful.

Thirdly, participating IP holders whose IPs (usually, patents) have been identified as being relevant to the proposed standard are requested in the SSO's policy to agree to license whichever IPs are "necessary" to make products that comply with the standard to anyone seeking a license. Participating IP holders must commonly agree to license their patents either royalty-free or on RAND (reasonable and non-discriminatory) terms.

[3] Most SSOs, however, make exceptions as long as the patent holder declares that they are willing to license their patent.

16.5.2.3 ISO/IEC (International Electrotechnical Commission)/ ITU (International Telecommunication Union)

Any party participating in the work of ITU, ISO or IEC should, from the outset, inform the Director of ITU-TSB, the Director of ITU-BR, or the offices of the CEO of ISO or IEC, about any known patent or pending patent application, either their own or of another organization. In addition, the patent holder is requested to declare that they are willing to negotiate licenses with other parties on a nondiscriminatory basis on reasonable terms and conditions free of charge or on a non-discriminatory basis with reasonable terms and conditions. Moreover, in cases where the patent holder is not willing to comply with the above provisions, the Recommendation/ Deliverable shall not include provisions that depend on the patent.

16.5.2.4 JIS

When a competent ministry proposes establishing JIS in accordance with Article 11 of the Industrial Standardization Act and requests an entity (contractor) to undertake the drafting of a specific JIS, the contractor shall conduct a patent search for the technology relevant to the draft JIS. If the contractor finds that the draft JIS contains patented technology, they shall then coordinate as necessary with all patent rights holders so that all such rights holders may be able to submit a declaration concerning the treatment of patent rights and licensing in connection with draft Japanese Industrial Standards.[4] However, it is not necessary to extend the patent search beyond such patent rights as are known to the developers of the draft JIS. The same requirement applies in cases where an interested party (applicant) proposes to establish JIS in accordance with Article 12 of the Industrial Standardization Act.

Moreover, the department in charge of the draft JIS must, in conjunction with the announcement of the public comment period, collect information on the existence and names of patent rights holders, etc., related to the draft JIS. In cases where patent rights related to the draft JIS under deliberation are found to include rights of patent holders who have not yet submitted a declaration, the department in charge of the draft JIS shall request those patent holders to submit a declaration. If such a declaration is not submitted, or the patent rights holders have declared that they are unwilling to grant licenses to the patent rights free of charge or on RAND terms, then the department in charge of the draft JIS shall work with contractors and/or applicants to make the necessary amendments to the draft JIS. The JISC may not issue a report until the procedures stipulated above have been satisfactorily completed.

[4] This does not apply in cases where the draft JIS is identical to ISO/IEC standards or where the draft JIS requires minor editorial changes, but remains identical in technical content.

Furthermore, in cases where a JIS-containing technology covered by patent rights is to be established, the JIS shall include a statement in the Foreword about the relevant patent rights and the conditions for granting licenses.

Above all, in cases where those who have submitted a declaration on the use of patent rights under RAND do not, in fact, grant a license under those conditions, which could hinder the good use of the JIS related to the patent rights, then the department in charge of the JIS shall endeavor to ensure appropriate use by making the necessary request to the patent holder(s). Unless appropriate actions are taken, the competent department has to investigate the potential impact on the public interest of revising or repealing the JIS. Based on the results of a study, the competent department must amend the JIS so that it does not include technology covered by the patent rights in question, or withdraw the JIS.

The same rules apply in cases where it is found after the publication of a JIS that the JIS involves patent holders other than those who submitted a declaration on the license to use the patent.

On the other hand, those who would like to be granted a license to implement the patent and meet certain requirements may apply for arbitration for implementing patent inventions, etc., under the Patent Act.

16.6 Civil Liability and Standards

16.6.1 Incomplete Performance

Obligors are liable for the failure to meet the purpose and meaning of their obligations (Civil Code, Article 415). A delivery of defective goods falls within this category. Regulations, quality standards, etc., play an important role in determining whether or not any act of an obligor is consistent with the purpose of the obligation, especially in case of the obligation to deliver goods, when determining whether or not the goods have the required quality.

16.6.2 Seller's Liability for Hidden Defects

If the object of a sale has any hidden defects, the buyer may claim damages. In addition, the buyer is entitled to rescind the contract, provided that he is unable to achieve the purpose of the contract with such a defect (Civil Code, Article 570). In this context, the defect is considered latent in cases where such a defect is what an ordinary buyer is unable to find with ordinary care. This seller's liability is strict liability and the seller is liable unless he proves that the buyer knew or should have known the defect with due care.

In sales contracts, the product will be deemed as defective unless the pre-set implicit or explicit rules, product standards, etc. are complied with.

16.6.3 Product Liability

Manufacturers, etc., are liable for damages when another's life, body or property is injured by a defect in the delivered product which they manufactured, processed, imported, licensed to put their name on, etc. (Product Liability Act, Article 3). In this context, 'defect' is defined as "lack of safety which the product should ordinarily provide, taking into account the nature of the product, the ordinarily foreseeable manner of use of the product, the time when the manufacturer, etc., delivered the product, and other circumstances concerning the product" (Article 2, Paragraph 2).

In addition, a "defect" can be found in cases where the product lacks safety either because there are problems with the design itself (design defect), or because the product was not manufactured according to the design, specifications, etc. (defect in production); and where there are risks involved because the defect cannot be removed from the product, and appropriate information has not been provided about such risks (lack of direction or information) in, for example, the user's manual. When inadequate quality control, inspections, etc., lead to non-compliance with safety standards set by national or public organizations, or corporate/industry voluntary standards, a product has a defect due to inadequate safety. If, as a result of a design that does not meet such safety standards, the product does not meet the safety standards that consumers (users) normally expect, then it has a design defect.

16.6.4 Negligence

A person who intentionally or negligently violates another's rights shall be liable for the losses caused by the act. This provision is abstract enough for the courts to give sufficient discretion in their interpretation. It is said that four elements of tort can be derived from this provision: fault, unlawfulness, victim's loss and causal relationship between the tortious act and the loss (Civil Code, Article 709). It is the widely accepted that negligence is a breach of duty rather than a state of mind. In other words, one is considered negligent if one fails to take appropriate measures to prevent a loss that was foreseen or should have been foreseen. A breach of duty to foresee and prevent a loss constitutes negligence. In this respect, the required standard of care is that of the reasonable person, taking into account the profession of the defendant and the knowledge, competence and experience required for a similar class of people as the defendant. If one has satisfied the standards of the ordinary members of his/her profession, then that person is not deemed as negligent.

When determining whether or not a liability in torts arises, the failure to follow social norms within certain social groups constitutes a violation of duty of care, and there are quite a few cases where negligence has been acknowledged due to the lack of following such norms. However, the reverse case is not always true. In other words, merely following the example set by experts, the industry, etc. can sometimes be interpreted as not doing everything possible to fulfill one's duty of care.

For example, on 16 February 1961, the Japanese Supreme Court ruled that a doctor who had given blood transfusions in accordance with the norms that had existed among his peers, had violated his duty of care (Supreme Court Reports on Civil Matters (*Saiko saibansho minji hanrei shu*), volume 15, no. 2, page 244). That is, a court approves a social norm that maximizes a social group's profit, but if the social norm is disjunct from the public interests, it may give the social group in question incentive to create a model that effectively externalizes losses (e.g. the substandard duty of care in medical practice existing among some doctors).

For example, ordinary customs, ways of thinking, etc., in *Hoshino*'s "partial society" (a society comprised of persons having certain skills, professions, status, etc.) may be mutually suitable for the members of that society, and settling conflicts among those members in the light of the customs and ways of thinking may be appropriate or natural ([3], pp. 568–569). However, that is not the case for one party in an incident or conflict that becomes a problem, where he/she is a third party or ordinary person who does not belong to the partial society. That is, the matter should be settled by the common understanding of the wider society including the two parties. According to *Hoshino*, the customs, ways of thinking, etc. of the partial society should not be the standard for resolving conflicts, although they might be taken into consideration as a mitigating factor ([3], pp. 568–569).

16.7 Soft Law and Hard Law

16.7.1 Soft Law

Hard law is binding legal instruments and laws (typically, statutes and ordinances formulated by a government) in contrast with soft law. *Soft law* is a set of rules that people find binding in the real economy and society though they are not the mandatory rules formulated by the State and, accordingly, are not necessarily enforced by the State. Soft law is rules of conduct which in principle have no legally binding force but which nevertheless may have practical effects. Soft law may be formulated or created either domestically or internationally not only by private bodies, businesses and the market, but also by public bodies and the government.

Traditionally, soft law is common in international (public) law where there are no sovereign governing bodies. Soft law is expressed in, for example, conference declarations, UN resolutions and declarations, and the nonbinding guidelines of international organizations. However, legally non-binding standards such as soft law have been widely applied to technical, professional and international matters (Table 16.3).

16.7.2 Rationales for Soft Law Instruments

A variety of rationales have been given for utilizing soft law instruments over hard law ones.[5]

1. Lower "contracting" costs. Creating an agreement usually entails negotiation or "contracting", i.e., learning about the issue, bargaining, and so forth. When the issue is complex or contentious, soft law might be more appropriate because non-binding norms lower the stakes for the parties involved in the negotiations. Soft law might help agreements to be reached quickly and avoid ratification or other cumbersome domestic procedures.
2. Lower sovereignty costs: While binding agreements might deprive the States involved of the authority to make decisions in the area and lead to the diminution of the States' sovereignty, soft law instruments can promote cooperation among the States while preserving sovereignty.
3. Coping with diversity and flexibility: Soft law allows States to adapt their commitments to their particular situations. It can accommodate diverse legal systems, and can cope better with uncertainty and fast-changing environments.
4. Wide participation: Soft law instruments often allow a variety of interested parties to participate in the process of making. Increased openness allows for more active participation of non-state actors, promotes transparency, enhances agenda setting, and facilitates the diffusion of knowledge.
5. Incrementalism: Soft law may represent a first step on the path to legally binding agreements or hard law. Soft law can also be used as a precursor to hard-law instruments. Soft-law instruments can establish norms and customs as well.

16.7.2.1 Accounting Standards, etc.

Even in cases where non-governmental bodies (i.e. private parties) develop or formulate standards, the legal system sometimes makes such rules a prerequisite. The standard-setting body develops norms while expecting or anticipating that the government will enforce the norms that they themselves set. A typical example of such models is accounting standards. In the relation with financial reports required under the Financial Instruments and Exchange Act, Article 1, Paragraph 1 of the Financial Statements Regulation stipulates that the technical terms, formats, and methods of preparing financial statements that "are not provided in these regulations shall follow the standards of business accounting that are generally accepted as fair and proper". Paragraph 3 stipulates that "accounting standards, developed by

[5] For example, *Ruggie* pointed out that States may turn to soft law for several reasons: to chart possible future directions for, and fill gaps in, the international legal order when they are not yet able or willing to take firmer measures; in cases where they conclude that legally binding mechanisms are not the best tool to address a particular issue; or in some instances, to avoid having more binding measures gain political momentum [5].

Table 16.3 Soft law and hard law (Adapted from Fujita [4])

	Enforced by the state	Not enforced by the state
Formulated by the state	Hard law	Provisions in several statutes (e.g. labor legislation) that appeal to the parties involved to respect good practice and provide no sanctions
Formulated by non-state actors	Accounting standards *Lex mercatoria*	Social norm/business ethics/corporate social responsibility

an organization engaged in the survey, research and development of business accounting standards and meets all of the conditions" prescribed in Paragraph 3, "developed and promulgated under due process, and found that they are likely to be accepted as fair and proper and designated by the Commissioner of the Financial Services Agency" "shall be deemed as business accounting standards that are generally accepted as fair and proper". In addition, Article 431 of the Companies Act states that "accounting in joint stock companies shall follow the business accounting practices that are generally accepted as fair and proper".

The Accounting Standards Board of Japan promulgates various accounting rules, and the Board expects that the rules they are setting will be ultimately enforced as "business accounting standards that are generally accepted as fair and proper" or "business accounting practices that are generally accepted as fair and proper". Of course, this does not mean that there is a guarantee that whatever the Accounting Standards Board may formulate will automatically be accepted and enforced by the State. The government does not simply give private parties *carte blanche* for formulating rules and automatically implement and enforce the rules; however, the legal system does encourage private parties to formulate norms, and the private parties make a concerted effort to respond to such encouragement.

In addition, in regard to auditing standards, the fundamental "Auditing Standards", etc., are formulated by the Business Accounting Deliberation Council, a consultative body for the Financial Services Agency (FSA), while more concrete and detailed norms are formulated as committee reports (practical guides) by the Japanese Institute of Certified Public Accountants in order to converge with the International Auditing Standards on a timely basis.

16.7.2.2 *Lex mercatoria*

Without making enforcement by the State a precondition, the norms, order, etc., that have been voluntarily formed by non-governmental bodies have *ex-post* significance in courts and other venues where the State is involved with settling disputes. For example, there are controversies over whether business practices and trade practices are incorporated in agreements between the contracting parties and whether the courts should determine that some business practices, etc. bind the parties as customary law. Often, the role of *lex mercatoria* becomes a topic of discussion and debate.

Lex mercatoria is a "set of special legal rules, which is non-governmental private law, for international transactions that are not based on traditional sources of law". In Japan, the applicable law for international transactions is determined by the Act on General Rules for the Application of Laws (rules of private international law), but even when Japanese law is applicable, at least part of *lex mercatoria* is also applied, through interpretation of the intentions of the parties concerned, and/or through interpretation and recognition/approval of international business customs (laws). In other words, judicial precedent, through deliberation from the perspectives of reasonableness and fairness, acknowledges *lex mercatoria* as a business custom.

For example, one court[6] ruled that in Japan, the basing of letters of credit on the Uniform Customs and Practice for Documentary Credits (UCP) is "recognized as a business practice. In addition, the settling of commercial bill accounts based on letters of credit, so long as branches of the issuing bank, etc., are not established around the world, will inevitably have to utilize the services of another bank, and if we accept that, then banks, etc. should not make a half-hearted attempt at letters of credit transactions. In order to facilitate letters of credit transactions, it is reasonable to have the risks involved with using another bank's services borne not by the issuing bank, but by the applicant of the letter of credit. The provision of Article 12 (a) of the UCP should be construed as fair and reasonable... The legal relationship based on the contract in the present case should be judged by the UCP".

16.7.2.3 Provisions in Several Statutes

In recent labor legislation, there has been an increasing number of cases involving the obligation to make efforts, in which parties involved in most of the cases have used wording such as "must make an effort" or "should make an effort" about the user, who is the addressee of such regulations. Noncompliance with the requirements to make efforts is not deemed as a violation of the law and does not result in making some acts void so long as the parties involved voluntarily and willfully fulfill their obligations in principle.

In Japan, for example, the Equal Employment Opportunity Act that was promulgated in 1985, stipulates only that "an effort must be made" for equal opportunity to be given for the recruitment, employment, deployment, promotion of employees, and equality in treatment . Furthermore, not undertaking fulfillment

[6] Tokyo District Court, Judgement on May 29, 1987 (*Kin-yu Homu Jijou*, No. 1186, p. 84).

of effort is evaluated neither as a judicial violation, nor as something that may result in liability for damages. As with many other regulations for effort, these regulations for fulfillment of effort are derived through a gradual escalation of sanctions and granting of economic incentives.

In other words, the specifics of fulfillment of effort are indicated with guidelines, etc., with concerned parties encouraged to follow them, and government authorities providing advice, instruction, recommendations, and so on, and economic incentives are provided through such means as monetary benefits. Furthermore, in the relation with fulfillment of effort in Japan, there are examples of public disclosure of the names of companies that do not follow advice, etc. In addition, that are also quite a few economic incentives in place in the form of benefits, etc., that should help promote the enforcement of policies in question.

16.7.3 International Standards as Soft Law

In addition to those discussed in Sect. 16.7.2, in international transactions, etc., similar to the UCP, international organizations and/or private groups establish regulations and prescribe their conformity in the agreement, or international organizations and/or private groups formulate standard agreement formats or standard covenants, and use those formats to promote the standardization of models. Furthermore, there are many international organizations and/or private groups that establish model acts and guidelines and expect relevant parties to voluntary follow them. At the same time, there are quite a few of such organizations and groups that create standards such as ISO 9000s (Quality Management) and international accounting standards and expect relevant parties to voluntarily follow those.

This is partly because of the problem of national sovereignty. It is not easy to set rules that could be enforced internationally. Furthermore, it appears that behind the scenes, it takes a long time to formulate and sign agreements. At the same time, in Japan, there are many cases where models are established in the form of standards, rather than statutes. In the same way, it is considered appropriate to set specialized standards in accordance with advancements in scientific knowledge and technology.

16.8 Legal Status of Standards

In Japan, a number of statutes contain technical regulations providing binding legislative rules for the protection of human life, health, and the environment, for example, and for electronic appliances under the Electrical Appliance and Material Safety Act. These technical regulations should respect JIS where appropriate, under the Industrial Standardization Law. In fact, thousands of JIS items are quoted by the technical regulations in Japan.

However, this does not mean that all standards are incorporated into law or can be referred to explicitly. Regardless, as can be seen in Sect. 16.6, standards, through interpretations of laws or contracts, can influence the success or failure of civil liability. Not only that, but as seen in Sect. 16.7.2, accounting standards, for example, with general provisions included in Companies Act or the Financial Instruments and Exchange Act as a medium, can be understood as being legally binding on parties who make financial statements, and failure to follow accounting standards can sometimes lead to misrepresentation. Furthermore, not only can misrepresentation result in liability, it can also lead to official disciplinary action and be grounds for criminal charges.

Therefore, without incorporation into law and/or explicit reference in the law, there may be issues from the perspective of the legality principle, such as legal binding in standards that are not formulated under democratic control can be approved, and in the law, there may be constitutional issues involved with making dynamic reference[7] to such standards, or problems from the standpoint of legality principles.

This is because the Constitution of Japan stipulates that "the Diet shall be the highest organ of the state power, and shall be the sole law-making organ of the State" (Article 41) and the Constitution does not have any provision for delegating legislative functions to any private bodies. In addition, the legality principle presupposes that only the Diet, which has democratic legitimacy, shall provide for penalties in the form of statutes, with a few limited exceptions.

[7] Reference is not made to the standards at a certain point in time. Rather, when standards are changed, the statutory requirements (regardless of whatever procedures may be involved) are automatically changed in accordance with the revised standards. This is sometimes called incorporation by reference, which is in contrast with static reference.

References

1. Werle R, Iversen EJ (2006) Promoting legitimacy in technical standardization. Sci Technol Innov Stud 2(1):19–39
2. Werle R (2002) Standards in the international telecommunications regime. In: Guerrieri P, Scharrer H-E (eds) Trade, investment and competition policies in the global economy: the case of the international telecommunications regime. Nomos, Baden-Baden, pp 243–282
3. Hoshino E (1965) Yuketsu ni yoru baidoku kansen ni tsuite no ishi no kashitsu sekinin (Doctor's negligence in blood transfusion that caused syphilitic infection). Hogaku Kyokai Zasshi 81 (5):565–572 (in Japanese)
4. Fujita T (2006) Kihan no shiteki keisei to kokka ni yoru enforcement: shokanshu/torihiki kanko wo sozai to shite (Private Ordering and Enforcement by the State: taking business customs and trade practices as examples), COESOFTLAW-2006-2. http://www.j.u-tokyo.ac.jp/coelaw/COESOFTLAW-2006-2.pdf, (in Japanese)
5. Ruggie J (2007) Report of the special representative of the Secretary-General on the issue of Human Rights and Transnational Corporations and other business enterprises, A/HRC/4/35, Office of the High Commissioner on Human Rights, Geneva
6. Anton JJ, Yao DA (1995) Standard-setting consortia, antitrust, and high-technology industries. Antitrust Law J 64(1):247–265
7. Gersen JE, Posner EA (2008) Soft law. Public law and legal theory working paper, no 213. University of Chicago, Chicago
8. Lemley MA (1996) Antitrust and the internet standardization problem. Conn Law Rev 28(4):1041–1094
9. Ly FD (1997) Uniform commercial law and international self-regulation. Dir Com Int 11(3):519–547

Index

Y. Sankai et al. (eds.), *Cybernics: Fusion of human, machine and information systems*, DOI 10.1007/978-4-431-54159-2, © Springer Japan 2014

MIX
Papier aus verantwortungsvollen Quellen
Paper from responsible sources
FSC® C105338

If you have any concerns about our products,
you can contact us on
ProductSafety@springernature.com

In case Publisher is established outside the EU,
the EU authorized representative is:
Springer Nature Customer Service Center GmbH
Europaplatz 3, 69115 Heidelberg, Germany

Printed by Libri Plureos GmbH
in Hamburg, Germany